PROGRESS IN CLINICAL AND BIOLOGICAL RESEARCH

1983 TITLES

Vol 115: **Prevention of Hereditary Large Bowel Cancer,** John R.F. Ingall, Anthony J. Mastromarino, *Editors*

Vol 116: **New Concepts in Thyroid Disease,** Roberto J. Soto, Gerardo Sartorio, Ismael de Forteza, *Editors*

Vol 117: **Reproductive Toxicology,** Donald R. Mattison, *Editor*

Vol 118: **Growth and Trophic Factors,** J. Regino Perez-Polo, Jean de Vellis, Bernard Haber, *Editors*

Vol 119: **Oncogenes and Retroviruses: Evaluation of Basic Findings and Clinical Potential,** Timothy E. O'Connor, Frank J. Rauscher, Jr., *Editors*

Vol 120: **Advances in Cancer Control: Research and Development,** Paul F. Engstrom, Paul N. Anderson, Lee E. Mortenson, *Editors*

Vol 121: **Progress in Cancer Control III: A Regional Approach,** Curtis Mettlin, Gerald P. Murphy, *Editors*

Vol 122: **Advances in Blood Substitute Research,** Robert B. Bolin, Robert P. Geyer, George Nemo, *Editors*

Vol 123: **California Serogroup Viruses,** Charles H. Calisher, Wayne H. Thompson, *Editors*

Vol 124: **Epilepsy: An Update on Research and Therapy,** Giuseppe Nisticò, Raoul Di Perri, H. Meinardi, *Editors*

Vol 125: **Sulfur Amino Acids: Biochemical and Clinical Aspects,** Kinya Kuriyama, Ryan J. Huxtable, and Heitaroh Iwata, *Editors*

Vol 126: **Membrane Biophysics II: Physical Methods in the Study of Epithelia,** Mumtaz A. Dinno, Arthur B, Callahan, Thomas C. Rozzell, *Editors*

Vol 127: **Orphan Drugs and Orphan Diseases: Clinical Realities and Public Policy,** George J. Brewer, *Editor*

Vol 128: **Research Ethics,** Kåre Berg, Knut Erik Tranøy, *Editors*

Vol 129: **Zinc Deficiency in Human Subjects,** Ananda S. Prasad, Ayhan O. Çavdar, George J. Brewer, Peter J. Aggett, *Editors*

Vol 130: **Progress in Cancer Control IV: Research in the Cancer Center,** Curtis Mettlin and Gerald P. Murphy, *Editors*

Vol 131: **Ethopharmacology: Primate Models of Neuropsychiatric Disorders,** Klaus A. Miczek, *Editor*

Vol 132: **13th International Cancer Congress,** Edwin A. Mirand, William B. Hutchinson, and Enrico Mihich, *Editors.* Published in 5 Volumes: Part A: **Current Perspectives in Cancer.** Part B: **Biology of Cancer (1).** Part C: **Biology of Cancer (2).** Part D: **Research and Treatment.** Part E: **Cancer Management**

Vol 133: **Non-HLA Antigens in Health, Aging, and Malignancy,** Elias Cohen and Dharam P. Singal, *Editors*

See pages following the index for previous titles in this series.

PROGRESS IN CANCER CONTROL IV
Research in the Cancer Center

PROGRESS IN CANCER CONTROL IV
Research in the Cancer Center

**Proceedings of the Progress in Cancer Control Meeting
Held in Bethesda, Maryland
January 21 and 22, 1983**

Editors

Curtis Mettlin

Director
Cancer Control and Epidemiology
Roswell Park Memorial Institute
Buffalo, New York

Gerald P. Murphy

Director
Roswell Park Memorial Institute
Buffalo, New York

ALAN R. LISS, INC., NEW YORK

Address all Inquiries to the Publisher
Alan R. Liss, Inc., 150 Fifth Avenue, New York, NY 10011

Copyright © 1983 Alan R. Liss, Inc.

Printed in the United States of America.

Library of Congress Cataloging in Publication Data

Progress in Cancer Control Meeting (1983 : Bethesda, Md.)
    Cancer control research in the cancer center.

    (Progress in clinical and biological research ; v. 130)
    Bibliography: p.
    Includes index.
    1. Cancer—Congresses. 2. Cancer—Prevention—Congresses. I. Mettlin, Curtis. II. Murphy, Gerald
Patrick. III. Series. [DNLM: 1. Neoplasms—Prevention
and control—Congresses. 2. Research—Congresses.
W1 PR668E v.130 / QZ 200 P9652p 1983]
RC261.A2P76   1983   616.99′4   83–48142
ISBN 0–8451–0130–7

Contents

Contributors . . . . **xi**

Preface
Curtis Mettlin and Gerald P. Murphy . . . . **xvii**

Welcome
Gerald P. Murphy . . . . **xix**

Viewpoints on Cancer Control
Tim Lee Carter **1**

International Resources for Cancer Control
R. Lee Clark **3**

Cancer Control Research Programs of the National Cancer Institute
Jerome W. Yates, Peter Greenwald, and Carlos E. Caban **19**

Cancer Prevention and Control by the American Cancer Society
Alfred Goldson and Diane J. Fink **29**

Cancer Control Research in American College of Surgeons Approved Programs
Charles R. Smart **37**

Occupational Cancer and Cancer Institutes
Anders Englund **47**

Lifestyles and Cancer Prevention
Guy R. Newell **55**

Linking Resources: Cancer Centers and Health Departments
Dwight T. Janerich, Kathleen Carlton, Edward Fitzgerald, and
Philip C. Nasca **67**

I. Patient and Public Education About Cancer

Meeting the Educational Needs of Adolescents With Cancer
Barbara D. Blumberg **85**

Project Choice: Evaluating a School-Age Cancer Prevention and Risk-Reduction Curriculum
David Docter, Terry Janicki, and Connie Hansen **91**

Pharmacists' Role in Smoking Prevention and Cessation
Nancy McCormick-Pickett, Sharon Natanblut, Pamela W. Gelfand,
and A. Gerald Franz **99**

Cancer Prevention/Detection Behavior by the Public: Lessons From Three Surveys
Gary D. Murfin and David A. Wagstaff 103

Community-Based Cancer Education for the Elderly
Edna Kane-Williams and Jack E. White 113

Cancer and the Elderly: A Cancer Control Challenge
Barbara Rimer, Wendy L. Jones, Christine Wilson, David Bennett, and
Paul F. Engstrom 123

Skin Cancer/Melanoma Knowledge and Behavior in Hawaii: Changes During a Community-Based Cancer Control Program
P. H. King, G.D. Murfin, K.L. Yanagisako, D.A. Wagstaff, G.L. Putnam,
F.L. Hajas, and S.C. Berger 135

Population-Based Assessment of the Characteristics of Potential Users of a Cancer Information Service (CIS)
Sharon R. Haymaker, Laura L. Morlock, David D. Celentano, Donna
S. Cox, and T. Phillip Waalkes 145

Applying Marketing Techniques to Promotion of the Cancer Information Service
Russell C. Sciandra and Judith A. Stein 153

A Methodology for Cancer Control Utilizing Cancer Information Service Data
Dorothy Eckert 161

Communications Strategies, Cancer Information and Black Populations: An Analysis of Longitudinal Data
Les Butler, Gary King, and Jack E. White 171

Consumer Education Modifies Cancer Phobia – Behavioral Changes Create a New Health Problem
Charlene T. Luciani and Jack S. Gruber 183

Newspaper Coverage of Laetrile Clinical Trials Results
Robert W. Denniston, Rose Mary Romano, and Holly Keck 193

II. Cancer Etiology, Prevention, and Detection

Characteristics of Women With Cervical Intraepithelial Dysplasia
Robert Michielutte, Robert A. Diseker, Wayne T. Corbett, and
W. Joseph May 203

The Acquired Immune Deficiency Syndrome
Peter W.A. Mansell, Guy R. Newell, and Evan M. Hersh 217

Cancer Control: X-Ray Induced C3HBA Tumor Regression and Prevention of Its Regrowth by β-Carotene or Vitamin A
Eli Seifter, Jacques Padawer, Giuseppi Rettura, Paul Goodwin, and
Stanley M. Levenson 237

A Method for Estimating the Potential Effects of Primary and Secondary Prevention Activities in High Risk Populations
John P. Enterline and Ellen B. Gold 249

Ohio's Mortality-Based System for Identification of Cancer
Intervention Program Sites
William S. Donaldson 261

Some Issues Concerning Community Based Chronic Disease
Control Programs
Emil Berkanovic, Barry Gerber, Helene Brown, and Lester Breslow 271

Community Cancer Control of Los Angeles (CCC/LA): Breast
Examination Training (BET) Centers
Claudia Lee 283

Breast Self-Examination Post Mastectomy: Empirical Findings
and Their Implications
Prakash L. Grover, Zili Amsel, Andrew M. Balshem, Barbara Kulpa,
and Paul F. Engstrom 293

A Precise Method of Manual Breast Self-Examination
H.S. Pennypacker, Mark Kane Goldstein, and Gerald H. Stein 305

Determining the Quality of Breast Self-Examination and Its
Relationship to Other BSE Measures
Joyce Mamon and Jane Zapka 313

The Relationship Between Breast Self-Examination Frequency,
Technique, and Breast Lump Detection
Annlouise Assaf, K. Michael Cummings, and Debra Walsh 323

Validation of Breast Self-Examination Practice Related to
Frequency and Competency of BSE
David D. Celentano 331

Multisite Cancer Screening of Women in a Rural Population
Ned D. Rodes, Charles W. Blackwell, and Dinah K. Pearson 341

Risk Factors and Physician Delay in the Diagnosis of Breast
Cancer
Mary Lou Finley and Anita Francis 351

Family Physicians' Beliefs About Cancer Screening Tests
K. Michael Cummings, Curtis Mettlin, Louis Lazar, and
Kenneth B. Frisof 361

III. Treatment, Rehabilitation, and Data Management

Criteria Setting and Adherence to Criteria for Managing Cervical,
Breast and Endometrial Cancer Among Community Physicians
Wesley C. Fowler, Jr., Anne C. Freeman, Barbara S. Hulka, Arnold D.
Kaluzny, Shirley P. O'Keefe, and Michael J. Symons 371

Compliance With Chemotherapy: Theoretical Basis and
Intervention Design
Jean L. Richardson, C. Anderson Johnson, Judith Selser, Leonard A.
Evans, Connie Kishbaugh, and Alexandra M. Levine 379

Important Gaps in Patients' Knowledge Prior to Chemotherapy
Wendy L. Jones, Barbara Rimer, Paul F. Engstrom, Michael Levy,
Anthony Paul, Robert Catalano, and Ruth Peter 391

Recent Progress and Results of Modern Radiation Therapy in
Medulloblastoma
H.W. Chin and Y. Maruyama 401

Evaluation of a Coordinated Community Approach to Hospice
Services: An Abstract
M.E. Grobe, D.M. Ilstrup, D.L. Ahmann, J.C. Miller, M. Gillard,
H. Haycock, and D. Jacobsen 411

Clergy as Intermediary—An Approach to Cancer Control
Delores G. Askey, Dorothy Parker, Darralyn Alexander, and
Jack E. White 417

Demonstration of the Effectiveness of the Professional Education
Component of a Comprehensive Cancer Control Project Using
Serial "Patterns of Care" (POC) Studies
William P. Vaughan, Laura L. Morlock, Raymond E. Lenhard, Gregory
P. Rausch, Stanley P. Watkins, Joyce M. Kane, and T. Phillip Waalkes 425

Colorectal Cancer Patient Rehabilitation and Continuing Care
Needs: A Preliminary Assessment of Services Provided by a
Voluntary Cancer Agency
William A. Stengle and Dorothy Eckert 433

Cancer Rehabilitation Issues for Occupational and Physical
Therapists: A Conference Report
Patricia D. Lynch, Sarajane Schaefer, and Dorothy Eckert 443

Quality of Cancer Care Evaluation in Italy
A. Liberati, G. Masera, G. Tognoni, and M.G. Zurlo 455

Data Bases for Patterns of Care Studies in Defined Populations
Lorenz J. Finison, Paul Jacques, Sharon J. Spaight, William Fine,
W. Bradford Patterson, Richard Clapp, Cynthia Burghard, and
Vincent O'Sullivan 465

The University of Texas M.D. Anderson Hospital Patient
Surveillance System
Vincent F. Guinee and Luceli Cuasay 477

Statewide Cancer Management Outlines: An Aid in Patient-
Oriented Cancer Control
T.C. Hall, G. Batten, G.D. Murfin, R.N. Denney, and P.H. King 483

A Program to Encourage Early Detection and Treatment of Breast
Cancer by Giving Information and Emotional Support
Rose Kushner 493

Index 503

Contributors

D.L. Ahmann, Mayo Comprehensive Cancer Center, Mayo Clinic, Rochester, MN 55905 **[411]**

Darralyn Alexander, Howard University Cancer Center, Washington, DC 20060 **[417]**

Zili Amsel, The Fox Chase Cancer Center, Philadelphia, PA 19111 **[293]**

Delores G. Askey, Howard University Cancer Center, Washington, DC 20060 **[417]**

Annlouise Assaf, Cancer Control and Epidemiology, Roswell Park Memorial Institute, Buffalo, NY 14263 **[323]**

Andrew M. Balshem, The Fox Chase Cancer Center, Philadelphia, PA 19111 **[293]**

Grover Batten, Cancer Center of Hawaii, University of Hawaii-Manoa, Honolulu, HI 96813 **[483]**

David Bennett, The Fox Chase Cancer Center, Philaldelphia, PA 19111 **[123]**

S.C. Berger, Cancer Center of Hawaii, University of Hawaii-Manoa, Honolulu, HI 96813 **[135]**

Emil Berkanovic, School of Public Health, University of California, Los Angeles, CA 90024 **[271]**

Charles W. Blackwell, Cancer Research Center, Columbia, MO 65205 **[341]**

Barbara D. Blumberg, Office of Cancer Communications, National Cancer Institute, Bethesda, MD 20205 **[85]**

Lester Breslow, School of Public Health, University of California, Los Angeles, CA 90024 **[271]**

Helene Brown, School of Public Health, University of California, Los Angeles, CA 90024 **[271]**

Cynthia Burghard, Massachusetts Health Data Consortium, Waltham, MA 02154 **[465]**

Les Butler, Howard University Cancer Center, Washington, DC 20060 **[171]**

Carlos E. Caban, Division of Resources, Centers, and Community Activities, National Cancer Institute, Bethesda, MD 20205 **[19]**

Kathleen Carlton, Bureau of Chronic Disease Prevention, New York State Department of Health, Albany, NY 12237 **[67]**

Tim Lee Carter, National Cancer Advisory Board, Tompkinsville, KY 42167 **[1]**

Robert Catalano, The Fox Chase Cancer Center, Philadelphia, PA 19111 **[391]**

David D. Celentano, The Johns Hopkins Oncology Center and The Johns Hopkins School of Hygiene and Public Health, Baltimore, MD 21205 **[145, 331]**

Hong W. Chin, Department of Radiation Medicine, University of Kentucky, Lexington, KY 40536 **[401]**

Richard Clapp, Department of Public Health, Commonwealth of Massachusetts, Boston, MA 02116 **[465]**

The boldface number in brackets indicates the opening page of the contributor's article.

R. Lee Clark, The University of Texas System Cancer Center M.D. Anderson Hospital and Tumor Institute, Houston, TX 77030 **[3]**

Wayne T. Corbett, Bowman-Gray School of Medicine, Winston-Salem, NC 27103 **[203]**

Donna S. Cox, The Johns Hopkins Oncology Center and The Johns Hopkins School of Hygiene and Public Health, Baltimore, MD 21205 **[145]**

Luceli Cuasay, Department of Patient Studies, University of Texas M.D. Anderson Hospital, Houston, TX 77030 **[477]**

K. Michael Cummings, Cancer Control and Epidemiology, Roswell Park Memorial Institute, Buffalo, NY 14263 **[323, 361]**

Ruth N. Denney, Cancer Center of Hawaii, University of Hawaii-Manoa, Honolulu, HI 96813 **[483]**

Robert W. Denniston, Office of Cancer Communications, National Cancer Institute, Bethesda, MD 20205 **[193]**

Robert A. Diseker, Bowman-Gray School of Medicine, Winston-Salem, NC 27103 **[203]**

David Docter, Fred Hutchinson Cancer Research Center, Seattle, WA 98104 **[91]**

William S. Donaldson, Comprehensive Cancer Center, Ohio State University, Columbus, OH 43210 **[261]**

Dorothy Eckert, Evaluation Department, Division of Epidemiology, Michigan Cancer Foundation, Detroit, MI 48201 **[161, 433, 443]**

Anders Englund, International Union Against Cancer, Geneva, Switzerland **[47]**

Paul F. Engstrom, The Fox Chase Cancer Center, Philadelphia, PA 19111 **[123, 293, 391]**

John P. Enterline, The Johns Hopkins University Oncology Center and Department of Epidemiology, Baltimore, MD 21205 **[249]**

Leonard A. Evans, Division of Hematology, Department of Medicine, University of Southern California, Los Angeles, CA 90031 **[379]**

William Fine, Division of Cancer Control, Dana-Farber Cancer Institute, Boston, MA 02115 **[465]**

Lorenz J. Finison, Division of Cancer Control, Dana-Farber Cancer Institute, Boston, MA 02115 **[465]**

Diane J. Fink, American Cancer Society, New York, NY 10017 **[29]**

Mary Lou Finley, Social Epidemiology Program, Fred Hutchinson Cancer Research Center, Seattle, WA 98104 **[351]**

Edward Fitzgerald, Bureau of Chronic Disease Prevention, New York State Department of Health, Albany, NY 12237 **[67]**

Wesley C. Fowler, Jr., Department of Obstetrics-Gynecology and the Cancer Research Center, University of North Carolina, Chapel Hill, NC 27514 **[371]**

Anita Francis, Social Epidemiology Program, Fred Hutchinson Cancer Research Center, Seattle, WA 98104 **[351]**

A. Gerald Franz, Office of Cancer Communications, National Cancer Institute, Bethesda, MD 20205 **[99]**

Anne C. Freeman, The Cancer Research Center, University of North Carolina, Chapel Hill, NC 27514 **[371]**

Kenneth B. Frisof, Wayne State University, Detroit, MI 48202 **[361]**

Pamela W. Gelfand, Office of Cancer Communications, National Cancer Institute, Bethesda, MD 20205 **[99]**

Barry Gerber, School of Public Health, University of California, Los Angeles, CA 90024 **[271]**

Margaret Gillard, Mayo Comprehensive Cancer Center, Mayo Clinic, Rochester, MN 55905 **[411]**

Ellen B. Gold, Department of Epidemiology, The Johns Hopkins University, Baltimore, MD 21205 **[249]**

Alfred Goldson, Howard University Cancer Center, Washington, DC 20060 **[29]**

Mark Kane Goldstein, Center for Ambulatory Studies, University of Florida and Corporation for Public Medicine, VA Medical Center, Gainesville, FL 32602 **[305]**

Paul Goodwin, Department of Radiology, Albert Einstein College of Medicine, Yeshiva University, New York, NY 10461 **[237]**

Peter Greenwald, Division of Resources, Centers, and Community Activities, National Cancer Institute, Bethesda, MD 20205 **[19]**

Mary Ellen Grobe, Mayo Comprehensive Cancer Center, Mayo Clinic, Rochester, MN 55905 **[411]**

Prakash L. Grover, The Fox Chase Cancer Center, Philadelphia, PA 19111 **[293]**

Jack S. Gruber, School of Medicine, Wright State University, Dayton, OH 45401 **[183]**

Vincent F. Guinee, Department of Patient Studies, University of Texas M.D. Anderson Hospital, Houston, TX 77030 **[477]**

F.L. Hajas, Cancer Center of Hawaii, University of Hawaii-Manoa, Honolulu, HI 96813 **[135]**

Thomas C. Hall, Cancer Society of Hawaii, University of Hawaii-Manoa, Honolulu, HI 96813 **[483]**

Connie Hansen, Fred Hutchinson Cancer Research Center, Seattle, WA 98104 **[91]**

H. Haycock, Mayo Comprehensive Cancer Center, Mayo Clinic, Rochester, MN 55905 **[411]**

Sharon R. Haymaker, The Johns Hopkins Oncology Center and The Johns Hopkins School of Hygiene and Public Health, Baltimore, MD 21205 **[145]**

Evan M. Hersh, Departments of Cancer Prevention and Clinical Immunology, University of Texas M.D. Anderson Hospital and Tumor Institute, Houston, TX 77030 **[217]**

Barbara S. Hulka, Department of Epidemiology and the Cancer Research Center, University of North Carolina, Chapel Hill, NC 27514 **[371]**

Duane M. Ilstrup, Mayo Comprehensive Cancer Center, Mayo Clinic, Rochester, MN 55905 **[411]**

Deborah Jacobsen, Mayo Comprehensive Cancer Center, Mayo Clinic, Rochester, MN 55905 **[411]**

Paul Jacques, USDA Nutrition Research Center on Aging at Tufts University, Boston, MA 02111 **[465]**

Dwight T. Janerich, Division of Community Health and Epidemiology, New York State Department of Health, Albany, NY 12237 **[67]**

Terry Janicki, Fred Hutchinson Cancer Research Center, Seattle, WA 98104 **[91]**

C. Anderson Johnson, Division of Hematology, Department of Medicine, University of Southern California, Los Angeles, CA 90031 **[379]**

Wendy L. Jones, The Fox Chase Cancer Center, Philadelphia, PA 19111 **[123, 391]**

Arnold D. Kaluzny, Department of Health Policy and Administration and the Cancer Research Center, University of North Carolina, Chapel Hill, NC 27514 **[371]**

Joyce M. Kane, The Johns Hopkins Oncology Center and School of Hygiene and Public Health, Baltimore, MD 21205 **[425]**

Edna Kane-Williams, Howard University Cancer Center, Washington, DC 20060 **[113]**

Holly Keck, Office of Cancer Communications, National Cancer Institute, Bethesda, MD 20205 [193]

Gary King, Howard University Cancer Center, Washington, DC 20060 [171]

P.H. King, Cancer Center of Hawaii, University of Hawaii-Manoa, Honolulu, HI 96813 [135, 483]

Connie Kishbaugh, Division of Hematology, Department of Medicine, University of Southern California, Los Angeles, CA 90031 [379]

Barbara Kulpa, The Fox Chase Cancer Center, Philadelphia, PA 19111 and Department of Epidemiology and the Cancer Research Center, University of North Carolina, Chapel Hill, NC 27514 [293]

Rose Kushner, Breast Cancer Advisory Center, Rockville, MD 20850 [493]

Louis Lazar, Millard Fillmore Hospital, Buffalo, NY 14209 [361]

Claudia Lee, Cancer Control, Memorial Hospital Medical Center, Long Beach, CA 90801-1428 [283]

Raymond E. Lenhard, The Johns Hopkins Oncology Center and School of Hygiene and Public Health, Baltimore, MD 21205 [425]

Stanley M. Levenson, Department of Surgery, Albert Einstein College of Medicine, Yeshiva University, New York, NY 10461 [237]

Alexandra M. Levine, Division of Hematology, Department of Medicine, University of Southern California, Los Angeles, CA 90031 [379]

Michael Levy, The Fox Chase Cancer Center, Philadelphia, PA 19111 [391]

Alessandro Liberati, Laboratory of Clinical Pharmacology, Mario Negri Institute, 20157 Milano, Italy [455]

Charlene T. Luciani, School of Medicine, Wright State University, Dayton, OH 45401 [183]

Patricia D. Lynch, Comprehensive Cancer Center of Metropolitan Detroit, Detroit, MI 48201 [443]

Nancy McCormick-Pickett, Office of Cancer Communications, National Cancer Institute, Bethesda, MD 20205 [99]

Joyce Mamon, School of Hygiene and Public Health, Johns Hopkins University, Baltimore, MD 21205 [313]

Peter W.A. Mansell, Departments of Cancer Prevention and Clinical Immunology, University of Texas M.D. Anderson Hospital and Tumor Institute, Houston, TX 77030 [217]

Yosh Maruyama, Department of Radiation Medicine, University of Kentucky, Lexington, KY 40536 [401]

Giuseppe Masera, Cattedra di Puericultura, Università di Milano, 20157 Milano, Italy [455]

W. Joseph May, Bowman-Gray School of Medicine, Winston-Salem, NC 27103 [203]

Curtis Mettlin, Roswell Park Memorial Institute, Buffalo, NY 14263 [xvii, 361]

Robert Michielutte, Bowman-Gray School of Medicine, Winston-Salem, NC 27103 [203]

Jane C. Miller, Mayo Comprehensive Cancer Center, Mayo Clinic, Rochester, MN 55905 [411]

Laura L. Morlock, The Johns Hopkins Oncology Center and The Johns Hopkins School of Hygiene and Public Health, Baltimore, MD 21205 [145, 425]

Gary D. Murfin, Cancer Center of Hawaii, University of Hawaii-Manoa, Honolulu, HI 96813 [103, 135, 483]

Gerald P. Murphy, Roswell Park Memorial Institute, Buffalo, NY 14263 [xvii, xix]

Philip C. Nasca, Bureau of Chronic Disease Prevention, New York State Department of Health, Albany, NY 12237 [67]

Sharon Natanblut, Office of Cancer Communications, National Cancer Institute, Bethesda, MD 20205 [99]

Guy R. Newell, Department of Cancer Prevention, University of Texas M.D. Anderson Hospital and Tumor Institute, Houston, TX [55, 217]

Shirley P. O'Keefe, The Cancer Research Center, University of North Carolina, Chapel Hill, NC 27514 [371]

Vincent O'Sullivan, Cancer Registry Program, Brockton Hospital, Brockton, MA 02402 [465]

Jacques Padawer, Department of Anatomy, Albert Einstein College of Medicine, Yeshiva University, New York, NY 10461 [237]

Dorothy Parker, Howard University Cancer Center, Washington, DC 20060 [417]

W. Bradford Patterson, Division of Cancer Control, Dana-Farber Cancer Institute, Boston, MA 02115 [465]

Anthony Paul, The Fox Chase Cancer Center, Philadelphia, PA 19111 [391]

Dinah K. Pearson, Cancer Research Center, Columbia, MO 65205 [341]

H.S. Pennypacker, Center for Ambulatory Studies, University of Florida and Corporation for Public Medicine, VA Medical Center, Gainesville, FL 32602 [305]

Ruth Peter, The Fox Chase Cancer Center, Philadelphia, PA 19111 [391]

Georgia L. Putnam, Cancer Center of Hawaii, University of Hawaii-Manoa, Honolulu, HI 96813 [135]

Gregory P. Rausch, The Johns Hopkins Oncology Center and The Johns Hopkins School of Hygiene and Public Health, Baltimore, MD 21205 [425]

Giuseppi Rettura, Department of Surgery, Albert Einstein College of Medicine, Yeshiva University, New York, NY 10461 [237]

Jean L. Richardson, Division of Hematology, Department of Medicine, University of Southern California, Los Angeles, CA 90031 [379]

Barbara Rimer, The Fox Chase Cancer Center, Philadelphia, PA 19111 [123, 391]

Ned D. Rodes, Cancer Research Center, Columbia, MO 65205 [341]

Rose Mary Romano, Office of Cancer Communications, National Cancer Institute, Bethesda, MD 20205 [193]

Sarajane Schaefer, Comprehensive Cancer Center of Metropolitan Detroit, Detroit, MI 48201 [443]

Russell C. Sciandra, Cancer Information Service, Roswell Park Memorial Institute, Buffalo, NY 14263 [153]

Eli Seifter, Departments of Surgery and Biochemistry, Albert Einstein College of Medicine, Yeshiva University, New York, NY 10461 [237]

Judith Selser, Division of Hematology, Department of Medicine, University of Southern California, Los Angeles, CA 90031 [379]

Charles R. Smart, Commission on Cancer, American College of Surgeons, Chicago, IL 60610 and Latter Day Saints Hospital, Salt Lake City, UT 84143 [37]

Sharon J. Spaight, Division of Cancer Control, Dana-Farber Cancer Institute, Boston, MA 02115 [465]

Gerald H. Stein, Center for Ambulatory Studies, University of Florida and Corporation for Public Medicine, VA Medical Center, Gainesville, FL 32602 [305]

Judith A. Stein, Division of Resources, Centers, and Community Activities, National Cancer Institute, Bethesda, MD 20205 [153]

William A. Stengle, Planning and Program Development, Michigan Cancer Foundation, Detroit, MI 48201 [433]

Michael J. Symons, Department of Biostatistics and Cancer Research Center, University of North Carolina, Chapel Hill, NC 27514 [371]

Gianni Tognoni, Laboratory of
Clinical Pharmacology, Mario Negri
Institute, 20157 Milano, Italy **[455]**

William P. Vaughan, The Johns
Hopkins Oncology Center and The
Johns Hopkins School of Hygiene and
Public Health, Baltimore, MD 21205
[425]

T. Phillip Waalkes, The Johns
Hopkins Oncology Center and The
Johns Hopkins School of Hygiene and
Public Health, Baltimore, MD 21205
[145, 425]

David A. Wagstaff, Cancer Center of
Hawaii, University of Hawaii-Manoa,
Honolulu, HI 96813 **[103, 135]**

Debra Walsh, Computer Center,
Roswell Park Memorial Institute,
Buffalo, NY 14263 **[323]**

Stanley P. Watkins, The Johns
Hopkins Oncology Center and The
Johns Hopkins School of Hygiene
and Public Health, Baltimore, MD
21205 **[425]**

Jack E. White, Howard University
Cancer Center, Washington, DC
20060 **[113, 171, 417]**

Christine Wilson, The Fox Chase
Cancer Center, Philadelphia, PA
19111 **[123]**

William P. Vaughan, The Johns
Hopkins Oncology Center and The
Johns Hopkins School of Hygiene and
Public Health, Baltimore,
MD 21205 **[425]**

Karen L. Yanagisako, Cancer Center
of Hawaii, University of Hawaii-
Manoa, Honolulu, HI 96813 **[135]**

Jerome W. Yates, Division of
Resources, Centers, and Community
Activities, National Cancer Institute,
Bethesda, MD 20205 **[19]**

Jane Zapka, Division of Public
Health, University of Massachusetts,
Amherst, MA 01003 **[313]**

Maria G. Zurlo, Cattedra di
Puericultura, Università di Milano,
20157 Milano, Italy **[455]**

Preface

At the founding of the majority of cancer centers in the United States, these centers of medical excellence focused on research in basic science and clinical oncology. Few of them had significant programs in cancer control research. In the past such research was often relegated to settings which had only marginal involvement in the cancer problem and had little access to cancer patients and defined populations, essential to cancer control research. The growth of national and international cancer programs has changed this situation dramatically. In recent decades cancer control research has become an integral aspect of the research, treatment, and education missions of cancer centers in the United States and abroad. Consequently, these centers have developed special expertise in the form of research resources and highly trained cancer control investigators capable of contributing rigorous research on interventions in the community to reduce cancer morbidity and mortality.

This volume reflects the progress which has been achieved in cancer control research in the cancer center. It reports the proceedings of a conference held in Bethesda, Maryland, January 21 and 22, 1983. These proceedings constitute the fourth volume on Progress in Cancer Control we have reported. Earlier volumes focused on issues in cancer screening and communications and on regional approaches to cancer control. Future volumes may concentrate on yet other areas of the growing and increasingly specialized science of cancer control. Cancer control research in cancer centers is a dynamic and diverse national resource. These reports only represent part of this activity and one point in time. We expect this research to continue and, we hope, to be stimulated by the sharing of methodologies, hypotheses, and findings reported here.

The first section of this volume includes reports from invited speakers who presented their perspectives on broader issues of cancer control research. In subsequent sections, the reports of investigators from different centers on their special research endeavors are presented in the order they appeared on the conference program.

The editors are grateful to the conference participants and to the several sponsoring organizations for their involvement.

Curtis Mettlin
Gerald P. Murphy

Welcome

It is a great pleasure to acknowledge the sponsorship of this important meeting on "Cancer Control in the Cancer Center" by the International Union Against Cancer, the Damon Runyon-Walter Winchell Fund, the Association of American Cancer Institutes, the Association of Community Cancer Centers, and the American Cancer Society. All groups will take an active part in contributing to this important meeting and to its written proceedings. We feel that in the progress against cancer that various phases are to be emphasized and should be updated and made current. The contributions by the representatives in this important two-day meeting are most timely and reflect the advances made in this area. The progress, of course, is national and international, as well as institutional. There are many new phases of work in the field of cancer control that have not received due and adequate evaluation or attention. Therefore, this meeting is a most timely and effective means of transmitting this information to various societies, including organizations such as the National Cancer Institute, as well as to individuals. We thank all of you for your cooperation and participation.

Gerald P. Murphy

Progress in Cancer Control IV: Research in the Cancer Center, pages 1–2
© 1983 Alan R. Liss, Inc., 150 Fifth Avenue, New York, NY 10011

VIEWPOINTS ON CANCER CONTROL

Tim Lee Carter, M.D.
Chairman
National Cancer Advisory Board
Tompkinsville, KY

There has been a great deal of cancer control programming in the last ten years and it is entirely fitting that we take a look at it at this 4th Conference on Progress in Cancer Control. Certainly there has been progress.

I am told that 50% of the women at risk for cervical cancer had had a Pap Smear in 1970 and by 1979 it was 86%. That is certainly progress and you have made a great deal of it in many areas.

At the same time there has been criticism. Part of this criticism may be attributed to confusion in some people's minds about what cancer control is. Part of it has to do with the feeling at the outset of the National Cancer Program that something had to be done awfully quick. But certainly all of us had much to learn and it was inevitable that things did not always go the way we wanted or the way others expected.

Now we are at a turning point. The emphasis is less on immediate application. The new emphasis is more on research to learn how best to proceed. I know that this change in emphasis will mean some professionals who have devoted themselves to applications will not immediately find new roles in research. But I hope this new turn will be productive. And I hope that people who have devoted years to this work will continue to contribute their skills and their efforts.

Problems will arise. They always do. I hope you will stay in touch with the National Cancer Advisory Board. Tell

me and my colleagues on the Board what we need to know to
help improve the program. We always want to hear from you.
I shall be an attentive listener as you move through this
ambitious and interesting program.

Progress in Cancer Control IV: Research in the Cancer Center, pages 3–18
© 1983 Alan R. Liss, Inc., 150 Fifth Avenue, New York, NY 10011

INTERNATIONAL RESOURCES FOR CANCER CONTROL

R. Lee Clark, M.D., President Emeritus
The University of Texas System Cancer Center
M.D. Anderson Hospital and Tumor Institute
Houston, Texas

Cancer Control has been a controversial term, largely because of the varying concepts that conern it as new information about cancer and its management develops. Cancer prevention and diagnosis, treatment and rehabilitation are now accepted in their broader aspects as parts of Cancer Control when applied to the populations of world regions, nations and their subdivisions. Research in Cancer Control is concerned with development of new ideas for application of the modalities of prevention and treatment. This includes methods for the transfer of technology which is so vital in the acceleration from basic science research to application in Clinical Medicine. Many discussions of Cancer Control outline in detail the dissemination of information by means of educational programs distributed from the regional cancer research and treatment center to the community hospitals. This is the so called "outreach" program to the tertiary care center from the Comprehensive Cancer Center as defined by the National Act of U.S.A. in 1971. [1]

"Cancer Prevention" was the topic for discussion of a subcommittee of the Association of American Cancer Institutes in June of 1980[2]. The committee defined cancer prevention as the identification and control, by appropriate interventions of those environmental and hosts factors which influence the occurrence of cancer and its progression to clinical disease. Prevention as applied to infectious and contagious diseases which has been so successful in preventing the death and ravages of mass population, from small-pox (1795) to polio myelitis (1956-60) is a dream of the future as far as cancer is concerned. Even when we know of factors

influencing the occurrence of cancer which have been shown
to have an etiologic role, such as cigarette smoking and
lung cancer, prevention is an unattained goal, because of
the nature of man and the long period between cause and
effect. Control then, while including the hope of prevention, must deal with the actual fact of developing and
existing cancer in humans.

One of the earliest examples of collaboration between
Cancer Centers occurred after World War I. Professor James
Heyman (1882-1956) of the Radium hemmet (Karolinska Institute), Stockholm Sweden, devised several important techniques
for treatment of uterine cancer by internal radium implant
and external irradiation. Heyman was influential in establishing the "Annual Report on the Results of Radiotherapy
in Carcinoma of the Uterine Cervix,[3]" and was editor of
the journal for many years. An initial report sponsored
by the League of Nations Health Organization in 1923 was
the first international attempt at scientific assessment of
therapeutic results.[4]

After Professor Heyman retired, Professor H.L. Kottmeir
continued with the project and editorship. The group of
initial cancer centers cooperating on the study, approximately 5, increased to over 300 in the next 50 years. This
great contribution was and is, perhaps, the most outstanding
example of information and technology dissemination for the
control of one of the most devastating of cancers. The
first report demonstrating less than 20% five year survivals
has progressed through all the great discoveries in regard
to detection and treatment of Cervical cancer to a present
survival rate in most civilized countries of 70% for cancer
of the cervix and up to 95% in Carcinoma in-situ. These
great discoveries cover the whole panorama of supervoltage,
isotope, electron beam and, neutron therapy as well as the
advent of advances in cellular diagnosis and exfoliative
cytology as proposed by George Nicholas Papanicolaou
(1882-1962) in various publications beginning in 1923-28
with animal cytology, progressing to human cytology as
depicted in his book Diagnosis of Uterine Cancer by Vaginal Smear published in 1943.[5]

International organizations of world wide significance
and a long standing history of programs in Cancer Control
are:

The World Health Organization, representing 133 nations (WHO) Geneva, Switzerland.

The International Agency for Research in Cancer, (IRAC) Lyon, France.

The Pan American Health Organization, (PAHO) Washington, D.C.

The International Union Against Cancer (UICC with over 200 members representing 82 nations.

The first three organizations are official governmental agencies, while the UICC is a free-standing voluntary organization.

A long list of International Professional Health Organizations and Associations hold meetings concerned with cancer control on a periodic basis. The purpose of these meetings, generally, is to review progress and to update practices in the various medical specialities which deal with cancer prevention, diagnosis, and treatment. Evaluation of cancer development in at-risk populations includes identification of both environmental carcinogens and genetic abnormalities, as well as recommendations for research into therapeutic modalities which show promise for new horizons in cancer control in the individual patient, (by modifying the host reaction to cancer growth and spread) are considered in the population aggregate as control factors.

International associations of research scientists are seeking to accelerate the control of cancer by investigating factors involved in the etiology of cancer. These groups hold international meetings on a regular basis, usually annually or bi-annually, to exchange ideas for advancement in specialized fields of investigations. Many nations have active scientific research organizations with comprehensive programs, publications, meetings and fellowships. The American Association of Cancer Research, whose objectives are control of cancer by determining its characteristics and etiology, is an example.

All nations of the world have departments of health except emerging countries which are victims of governmental disorganization. These various national health programs were concerned originally with epidemics, infectious diseases, malnutrition, infant mortality and the development of health practices aimed at providing immediate results for the creation of a thriving, long-lived, healthy population.

Degenerative disorders such as heart disease, cancer, stroke, arthritis and senility have been given consideration as international problems, only since bacteria, viral, and parasitic attrition of the population has decreased due to control.

Cancer Control efforts have been an objective of international health efforts largely as a product of twentieth century progress. The national effort toward Cancer Control in the U.S.A. started in 1937 with the establishment of the National Cancer Institute. The initial appropriation for the NCI's annual research and cancer control of one half million dollars grew to approximately one billion dollars by 1982. During almost half a century the NCI's world wide progress in Cancer Control, in its broadest sense, demonstrates the greatest effort ever achieved by any nation in any field of medicine. The N.C.I. has shared its goals and gains in this regard with all peoples of the world.

Within each nation cancer control programs are usually subdivided regionally by provence or state. In addition to official governmental cancer control organizations that participate in world wide cooperative programs, but are nationally based by Country, voluntary organizations such as the American Cancer Society have been established in many countries. The American Cancer Society has served as a model and has been invited to be an active participant in organizing similar voluntary agencies in other countries.

The establishment of international resources for cancer control was an objective under discussion at the UICC International Cancer Congress in Madrid, Spain in 1933. Dr. J.R. Heller was Chairman of the Cancer Control Commission of the UICC which published "Technical Report, Number 1.," on the world wide cancer control efforts in 106 countries. The report was distributed at the 8th Cancer Congress in Moscow in 1962, is recognized as a landmark publication.[6]

The UICC has now held thirteen international cancer congresses, one every four years whenever world conditions permit. The most recent UICC Congress held at Seattle, Washington, September 8th through 16th, 1982, with over eight thousand registrants and some 4100 presentations. The formal programs of the UICC are of a continuous nature and occupy the intervals between Congresses. The UICC is the most comprehensive non-governmental agency engaged in "Cancer Control" world-wide. Its seven programs were changed to nine by the assembly and council of the UICC at the XIII Congress. These original seven programs were:

    -Epidemiology
    -Voluntary Cancer Leagues and Societies
    -International Collaborative Activities
    -Experimental Oncology
    -Clinical Oncology
    -Fellowships and Personnel Exchange
    -Cancer Education

The New Programs and Chairmen are:

    -Detection and Diagnosis   U. Veronesi (Italy)
    -Tumor Biology   M. Burger (Switzerland)
    -Epidemiology and Prevention   T. Hirayama (Japan)
    -Professional Education   S. Eckhardt (Hungary)
    -Campaign, Organization and
        Public Education   J.H. Young (USA)
    -International Collaborative
        Activities - CICA   R. Lee Clark (USA)

    -Fellowships and Personnel
        Exchange   L.G. Lajtha (UK)
    -Smoking and Cancer   N. Gray (Australia)
    -Treatment and Rehab-
        ilitation   I. Elsebai (Egypt)

These changes reflect the flexibility and continuing assessment of the UICC and its mission by its governing body. It is supported by membership dues and gifts and grants from many countries and organizations. A detailed report of the UICC and its activities and publications is contained in article entitled, "The Programs of the International Union Against Cancer", by Gerald P. Warwick, Executive Secretary CICA-UICC, in Progress in Cancer Control, Edited by Mettlin and G.P. Murphy, 1981.

The UICC established the Committee on International Collaboration (CICA) in 1973. Its goal's mobilization of world wide resources for cancer control.[7] A summary report of the CICA program over the past 10 years is presented in the end segment of this paper.

The World Health Organization in their report: [8]
"The Second Ten Years 1958-67" summarizes their early work
in Cancer Control, as follows: In accordance with recommendations made by a WHO scientific group in 1959, organization work on cancer has been directed particularly to
epidemiological and pathological studies: It has also
included activities designed to promote the prevention and
treatment of cancer. A new approach to coordination of research was the establishment in 1965 by the International
Agency for Research in Cancer. The Agency concentrates on
environmental biology (Carcinogenesis) and Cancer epidemiology (etiological aspects) while WHO, per se, is expanding
its activities on cancer control, clinical research and
training and education, both professional and public.

The Program of the WHO in Cancer Control summarized by
L. Dobrossy, WHO Consultant of the Regional Office of WHO,
for Europe to the General Assembly of the Organization of
European Cancer Institutes in Moscow 10-11th, May 1982, is
best expressed in his own words:

"There exists a bilateral relationship between the
Organization of European Cancer Institutes (OECI) and WHO,
which should be mutually supportive: WHO has a role to
play in developing cancer institutes and can assist them in
fulfilling their mission; on the other hand, European cancer
institutes can help WHO in implementing its cancer programmes
in the European Region. The fundamental concept of WHO
cancer-related programmes is the "application of knowledge,"
in other words, the transfer of the existing knowledge provided by basic, clinical and epidemiological research into
policy and practice.

The role of WHO in the field of cancer up to now has
been focused on clinical pathology. Most clinicians and
researchers with a special interest in cancer are aware of
WHO contributions in this field, through the International
Classification of Diseases for Oncology (ICD-0) - (ICD-0)
published in 1975 - see annual report IARC 1978 and the
International Histological Classification of Tumours (IHCT).

During the past year, WHO has re-oriented its programme
to focus on intensifying efforts in the field of cancer
control. I would like to take this opportunity to outline
WHO cancer-related programmes and to point out those areas
and means whereby a long-range cooperation between OECI and

WHO is not only possible, but essential:

1. First, what is WHO policy related to Cancer Institutes?

Who feels that a more systematic approach to a comprehensive, community based cancer control programme is a
need for each country of the European Region. This is why
the overall objective of WHO cancer-related programmes is
to assist Member States in developing cancer control policies
and programmes at the country level. In the implementation
of this programme, the specialized cancer institutes have
an important role to play.

In the first phase of this stepwise process, the Regional
Office convened a working group (Luxembourg, October 1981).
The scope and purpose of this meeting was: (a) to review
the present situation with regard to the cancer institutes
and the ongoing cancer control programmes in the European
Region, and (b) to reconsider what were the respective roles
of cancer institutes in community based cancer control programmes.

As a basis of the situation analysis and when making
recommendations, the working group adopted the concept of
comprehensive cancer centres, elaborated by the UICC Committee on International Collaborative Activities (CICA).
The concept has been a "Magna Carta" for the majority of
cancer institutes represented in OECI.

In its recommendations, the working group emphasized
that cancer centres as an important element of the national
cancer control programme would be included in national cancer
policies. Taking into account the various health infras-
tructures in individual European countries, (Pre-determined
by traditions and other historical, social and economical
factors and by different planning and financing systems), and
in particular, the already existing cancer institutes of
various types established early in this country and mainly
during the past 3 or 4 decades, the working group suggested
that cancer centres may take 2 main forms: (a) comprehensive
centre, providing all aspects of cancer care in a free-
standing, single physical and organizational unit, or (b)
coordinating or "functionally comprehensive" centre coordinating the cancer-related activities of separate institutions
in a geographically defined area.

In full accordance with the CICA concept, we feel that, cancer centres should provide a multidisciplinary approach to patient care, conduct goal-directed research and provide education programmes. But in the WHO concept, the centre is requested to be more than centre of excellence in the field of diagnosis, treatment oncological research and training. In the WHO report on the working group (still in preparation), the necessity for providing a leading role in the community-programmes was also strongly emphasized.

The WHO programme in this respect has taken into consideration the recommendations made by the working group, and accordingly, the Regional Office has decided: (a) to influence Governments in incorporating the "Comprehensive cancer centre" concept into their national cancer policy and in promoting their development. (b) to stimulate the cancer centres in taking their responsibility in the field of community cancer control programmes, and, (c) to assist the cancer centres, by all possible means, in developing and providing cancer control measures at the highest possible level to the largest possible proportion of the population.

To promote community-involvement of cancer centres is the corner stone of WHO policy related to the cancer institutes in the European Region. Two specific objectives of the regional medium-term programme deserve special attention here, because in order to implement these objectives, WHO must utilize the expertise embodied by the cancer institutes represented in OECI and because other institutes can benefit from the implementation.

Both objectives have been given high priority by the Scientific Advisory Committee to the Regional Office, as well as by more than 2/3 of the European countries in their reply to Consultation Letter asking Governmental comments on our programmes. Both objectives aim at promoting improved cancer care.

These objectives have adopted the concepts of "Model Health Care" as well as of "Appropriate Technology" into cancer care and aim at setting up an operational model for systematic planning and implementation of care programmes and technologies which are medically, economically, socially acceptable at the national level." This concept is wholeheartedly endorsed in the program of UICC-CICA.

Since its establishment in 1965 by the WHO and the development of its headquarters at Lyon, France, the International Agency for Research in Cancer has made outstanding contributions in research and publications in the field of Epidemiology, Biostatistics, Environmental Biology, and Chemical Carcinogenesis. The training programs and investigational activities have been of world-wide significance. This information is essential as the basis for the projection of a Cancer Control Program for any given world area. The report "The Impact of Cancer in Texas" is such an example.[9]

Annual reports of the WHO, IARC and UICC are recommended for review by those interested in the details of international resources for cancer control. However, of particular value are fundamental documents which are vital resources in the study of cancer control projects as follows:

1. The International Classification of Disease (Oncology-9) (Ms. J. Nectaux) 1975 Revision, Geneva WHO 1977.
2. The International Association of Cancer Registeries (IACR) Drs. C.S. Muir and Ms. S. Whelan) Annual Report.
3. Cancer Incidence in Five Continents Vol. IV (CS Muir, S. Whelan) Annual Report IARC 1978. Published 1981.
4. Clearing-House for on-going Research in Cancer Epidemiology - C.S. Muir, G. Wagner, C.O. Kohler, 1980 (5th edition). The last of five directories contained 1261 projects from 69 countries and was assisted with support from the international Cancer Research Data Bank of the National Cancer Institute, U.S.A.

HISTORY

In May, 1970, the Xth International Cancer Congress convened in Houston, Texas, U.S.A. During that Congress, the Association of American Cancer Institutes represented by Congress Chairman R. Lee Clark, M.D., hosted a meeting for International Directors of Cancer Institutes and Centers who were attending the Congress. It was evident that there was, among these approximately 90 directors, an active interest in future communication and collaboration. A resolution to the effect passed unanimously. In March, 1972, the AACI submitted a resolution to the UICC Council proposing a Committee for International Collaborative Activities (CICA). The resolution, presented by Dr. R. Lee Clark was approved by the council, and CICA was established as a UICC Committee in May of 1973 with Dr. Gerald Murphy of Roswell Park Cancer Institute as Chairman. In October of 1974, the UICC council conferred full program status to CICA with Dr. T. Symington of the Institute of Cancer Research in London, England as Chairman.

ORGANIZATION

The chairman of CICA is appointed by the council of the UICC. The eleven members are appointed by the UICC Executive Committee. The UICC President and Secretary General are Ex Officio members. These 14 members are voting members of CICA and are responsible to the UICC council and the Executive Committee.

The 12 appointed members of CICA (later increased to 14) are directors of cancer institutes and centers throughout the world. In 1975, Dr. Symington resigned and Dr. R. Lee Clark, President of the UT System Cancer Center, M.D. Anderson Hospital and Tumor Institute succeeded him to serve out Dr. Symington's unexpired term. Subsequently, Dr. Clark was appointed to serve a four year term ending in 1982. He was reappointed for an additional term as Chairman, 1982-86 at the Seattle Congress, with Dr. Ed Scanlon, Chicago, U.S.A. as assistant to the Chairman.

There is an attempt underway to have regional world wide representation on CICA, with the membership rotated on approval by the UICC Executive Committee. For economic reasons, the official committee will be reduced to 10 members, plus the Chairman. The UICC President and Secretary General will be Ex-officio members.

OBJECTIVES

The objectives of the CICA are to:

1. Provide international leadership in the development of collaborative programmes among cancer institutes;
2. Act as the international advisory group the U.S.A. National Cancer Institute for planning the International Cancer Research Date Bank (ICRDB);
3. Foster the exchange of personnel among cancer institutes
4. Foster international development of the comprehensive cancer centre concept;

5.   Organize and develop 7 - 10 associations of the Cancer Centers throughout the world, such as the Association of American Cancer Institutes (AACI), for facilitating the exchange of technology and cooperation in cancer control, research and education on a global basis.

The CICA program to date has been an official approved program of the UICC, made possible by a Grant from the ICRED of the NCI, U.S.A.

I.   ANNUAL MEETING

An annual meeting is held in a different cancer establishment whose director is a member of the CICA and listed in the UICC International Directory, in conjunction with a scientific meeting presenting cancer-related activities of the host country or region. Stockholm, Moscow, Budapest, Bordeau, Houston and Cairo are meeting locations where the host centre paid all of the per diem costs of the meeting. However, work on the details of the program proceed on a continuing basis, through the Chairman and among members by mail and telephone telex. Communication by satellite has been demonstrated and is undergoing further study.

II.   INTERNATIONAL CANCER RESEARCH DATA BANK OF THE NCI, (ICRDB)

The CICA serves an an International Consultant of the ICRDB assisting the Chairman and Executive Secretary, Dr. Gerald P. Warwick, in carrying out a continuing program of promotion, interpretation, education and collection of data through their various international regions.   Advisory, consultative, and liaison services in support of the ICRDB of the NCI are of the highest priority. All 14 members of CICA have carried out a continuing program of promotion at their own expense in their country and world region. Great progress in scientific, technological and communications concepts have been achieved world wide through the various mechanisms of the ICRDB. "Clin-Prot" is now changing cancer treatment around the world. The World Health Organization (WHO) and the Pan American Health Organization (PAHO) have been of much assistance. Encouragement of member nations of the UICC to contribute information on current cancer research projects and clinical trials to the ICRDB, "CanProj and ClinProt," is being continued. The committee is assisting in identifying more efficient methods

for collecting abstracts appearing in current cancer-related
publications for inclusion in the "CANCERLINE" program of the
ICRDB.

III. THE INTERNATIONAL DIRECTORY OF SPECIALIZED CANCER
      RESEARCH AND TREATMENT ESTABLISHMENTS (Produced by
      the UICC)

Compilation of this international directory has been a
successful achievement of CICA through the continuous help
of the entire staff of the Geneva office of the UICC. First,
Mr. David Reed, then Dr. Gerald P. Warwick, with the
assiduous editing capabilities of Mr. Luder, have completed,
updated and published three editions. The third edition
contains detailed profiles of 678 cancer establishments in
82 countries. Updated names and addresses of over 9000
members of the staffs of the institutions are available
from the UICC office in Geneva. The cost of publishing was
paid by a loan from the UICC Foundation and was repaid from
sales of the directory.

IV. INTERNATIONAL CANCER RESEARCH WORKSHOPS AND THE INTER-
     NATIONAL CANCER RESEARCH TECHNOLOGY TRANSFER ICREW
     AND ICRETT

The CICA role has been one of the encouragement of more
active participation in the ICRDB programs, ICREW and ICRETT.
Dr. B. Gustafsson (Sweden), Chairman: Fellowships and
Personnel Exchange Program, has done an outstanding job of
reviewing over 600 applications for participation in the
program, with assistance of Dr. L.G. Lajtha, (UK) Chairman:
Cancer Research Campaign International Fellowships; and
Dr. J. Ponten (Sweden) Chairman: ICRETT Financial support
for ICREW has been withdrawn by the NCI and that for ICRETT
has been greatly restricted. Some support for the latter
has come from other countries and is detailed in the
Fellowship Program of the UICC. Initially 5 workshops were
held by CICA and the proceedings published by the UICC.

V. INTERNATIONAL CANCER PATIENT DATA EXCHANGE SYSTEM, (ICP
    DES)

Coordinated by Dr. Vincent F. Guinee, for the Data
Committee of the CICA.

The program was started in 1977 with 14 institutions

in 8 countries, (2 more recently accepted), reporting 35,000
patients. Three editions of a data manual have been completed. This manual is compatible with the data sponsored
by WHO (ICD-09), the UICC (TNM) SEER and CCPDS. Also a
report of the patient acquisitions in five anatomic sites
including 25,000 patients has been made as an official UICC
publication. In furthering the goals of and participation
in the ICPDES an annual report is published. Emphasis is
placed on self-funding of all participating institutions.
It is agreed to proceed with the reporting of all sites and
"follow-up" reporting of all sites and "follow-up" reporting
as a requisite for participation.

VI. GUIDELINES FOR DEVELOPMENT OF A COMPREHENSIVE CANCER
    CENTER

    In promotion of the comprehensive cancer center concept
and encouragement of the team approach to cancer research,
treatment and education, the development of guidelines were
essential. A publication was sponsored by the CICA, with
the committee serving as an editorial committee under the
chairman, (2000 copies, 1978). An updated second edition
was completed in 1981. This volume was a best seller among
UICC publications at the XIIIth International Cancer Congress
in Seattle, Washington in 1982. A supplement to the
"Guidelines," has been prepared by 10 members of CICA and
Dr. A. Smart, Executive Director of the Cancer Commission
of the American College of Surgeons. This supplement con-
siders the impact of the CCC on other cancer control
institutions and organizations both voluntary and official.
Advisory and consultative services to the nations or regions
wishing to build comprehensive centers are available through
CICA and have already been carried out on request in some
dozen instances, at the expense of those assisted.

VII. REGIONAL ASSOCIATIONS OF WORLD CANCER CENTERS

    Encouragement for the formation of regional organization
of cancer centers and cancer institutions began with the
development of the Association of American Cancer Institutes,
(AACI). This association with 12 tasks has invited international collaboration of cancer control, education and
research activities. To further international collaboration
and the exchange of personnel and cancer training activities,
a pattern for regional organizations of cancer centers and
institutions have been prepared. There are now such organ-

izations as the Association of Latin American Cancer
Institutes, the European Organization of Cancer Institutes,
and others in the Middle East, France, and Communist Europe.
Two more are under discussion including India, Japan and
China and other Far Eastern Countries. All of these will
be a part of the UICC-CICA program and will furnish a maximum of contact, (through regional association presidents)
for projects, such as publication in the director or its
supplement listing training facilities and programs in
oncology throughout the world in conjunction with the Cancer
Education Program of the UICC, Chairman, Dr. S. Eckhardt
(Hungary).

VIII. ESTABLISHMENT OF CANSAT - A Cancer Education and
       Technological Transfer Program Transmitted Between
       Institutions World-Wide Via Satellite

The technology for such a program is currently on the
global market "CICA Satellite Primer" is available at cost
on request at UICC-Geneva Office. One thousand copies of
the primer were published by a grant from the Mike Hogg
Fund, Houston, Texas, U.S.A. The publication acquaints
those interested with the background information necessary
to proceed with installation of Satellite communication
facilities. One hundred eighty eight Satellite Earth
stations exist in over 136 countries. Consequently, every
cancer institute has the opportunity to participate when
funds are available and the laws regulating communication
via satellite in their country permit. A model for a down
link satellite communications receiver is being prepared as
a kit. The University of Texas M.D. Anderson Hospital in
conjunction with CICA made an initial demonstration of such
live global satellite broadcast, reaching four continents
via the INTELSTAT Atlantic and Indian Ocean satellites. The
90 minute TV program was viewed by an estimated 20 million
people in November, 1981, as the culmination of the UT Anderson Cancer Center 40th Anniversary Celebration Colloqium,
termed Cancer: 1981-2001. Sixty presentations of selected
proceedings were recorded on videocassettes and are available
for commercial distribution, at cost through CICA.

IX. STANDARDIZATION OF THE TERMINOLOGY FOR CANCER ETIOLOGY

Consideration of collaboration among editors of cancer
journals for standardization of the terminology for cancer
etiology has been requested of CICA.

X. CANCER OVERVIEW BY NATION MEMBERS - UICC

    An outline has been completed for the publication by
each nation   of an overview of the cancer-related activities within that nation such as prevention, epidemiology,
detection/screening treatment, education, etc. Twelve
countries have been included in a demonstration program
during the past six years.

XI. THE INTERNATIONAL ACADEMY OF ONCOLOGY

    An International Academy of Oncology is now being con-
sidered and carefully studied as a means of establishing
international criteria of excellence in Oncology treatment,
research and education throughout the 82 member nations
of the UICC. The program can provide basis for individual
membership in the UICC if it appears feasible. The interim
meeting of the UICC in Japan in 1984 should see a definitive
report of progress on this challenging and intriguing
proposal.

REFERENCES

1. Public Law 92-328, 92nd Congress, D. 1828, December 23,
    1971 and Public Law 93-352, 93rd Congress, S. 2893,
    July 23, 1974.

2. Progress in Cancer Control, Curtis Mettlin and Gerald
    P. Murphy, Alan R. Liss, Inc., New York, 1981.

3. Fletcher, Gilbert H., Annual Report on the Results of
    Radiotherapy in Carcinoma of the Uterine Cervix, The
    University of Texas System Cancer Center M.D. Anderson
    Hospital and Tumor Institute, 1982.

4. The Cancer Bulletin, Vol. XIII No. 2, March-April 1961-
    p. 22.

5. Papanicolaou, George N., and Trout, Herbert, Diagnosis
    of Uterine Cancer by the Vaginal Smear, New York, The
    Commonwealth Fund, 1943.
    Papanicolaou, George N., Atlas of Exfoliative Cytology,
    New York, The Commonwealth Fund, 1954.
    The Cancer Bulletin Vol. XIV No. 4 July - Aug. 1962,
    p. 72.

6. Pamphlet - International Union Against Cancer - Commission
    on Cancer Control - Cancer Control Throughout the World -
    This special report is prepared for distribution to the
    members of the International Union Against Cancer atten-
    ding the 8th International Cancer Congress, Moscow,
    U.S.S.R. July, 1962 - J.R. Heller, M.D., Chairman Cancer
    Control Commission, Mildred E. Allen, American Cancer
    Society, Incorporated - Technical Report 1, 1982.

7. Cancer Bulletin, Vol. X, No. 3, August, 1982.

8. World Health Organization, The Second Ten Years
    1958-67, Geneva, 1968.

9. Impact of Cancer on Texas, Second Edition, University
    of Texas System Cancer Center, M.D. Anderson Hospital
    and Tumor Institute, 1980.

Progress in Cancer Control IV: Research in the Cancer Center, pages 19–27
© 1983 Alan R. Liss, Inc., 150 Fifth Avenue, New York, NY 10011

CANCER CONTROL RESEARCH PROGRAMS OF THE NATIONAL CANCER
INSTITUTE

Jerome W. Yates, M.D.
Peter Greenwald, M.D.
Carlos E. Caban, Ph.D.
National Institutes of Health
National Cancer Institute
Division of Resources, Centers, and Community
Activities

Cancer control is "the reduction of cancer incidence,
morbidity and mortality through an orderly sequence from
research on interventions and their impact in defined
populations to the broad, systematic application of the
research results." This new definition of cancer control
reflects the major changes in direction of the National
Cancer Institute's cancer control program: the emphasis on
research with specified interventions; and the categorization
of cancer control research into phases. Many prior cancer
control programs were uncontrolled "demonstration projects"
often not providing a clear evaluation or interpretable data
on efficacy. In an effort to avoid repeating many of these
past problems in cancer control, a rigorous intradivisional
planning effort in cancer control is underway.

To reinforce the definition of cancer control, emphasis
on the words _research_ and _interventions_ serves to delineate
this from past cancer control definitions as well as conventional epidemiology. In the phases of cancer control
research, the first phase is hypothesis development or the
collection of existing ideas to develop a hypothesis which
subsequently is going to be tested (see table 1). Phase II
encompasses the development of methods, including situations
where intervention-related descriptive, cross-sectional,
methodological research will all be necessary to acquire
adequate information before the implementation of Phase III
or Phase IV trials. Examples of Phase II cancer control
research would include the testing of survey instruments

for reliability and validity.

TABLE 1

PHASES OF CANCER CONTROL RESEARCH

Phase   I   Hypothesis Development
Phase   II   Methods Development
Phase III   Controlled Intervention Trials
Phase   IV   Defined Population Studies
Phase   V   Demonstration and Implementation

The third phase is that of the controlled intervention trials. These may include cancer control versions of case control studies, where one starts with the outcome and then looks backward to see what type of "intervention exposure" was experienced by individuals in the groups with and without the outcome of interest. Phase III studies may also include cohort studies where delineated populations are followed with and without "intervention exposures" until they develop the outcome of interest. This can include experimental trials where the "intervention exposure" of interest is a treatment controlled by the investigator and the participants may be randomized, or alternatively, controlled for in other ways. A population of patients would generally be appropriate for Phase III studies, but might have difficulty meeting the requirements as a defined population. Phase III studies tell you primarily about the efficacy of a cancer control intervention. Phase IV includes defined population studies or those studies in which a specified population over time (denominator) is available, along with the ability to determine the outcomes of interest (numerator). Examples of this situation would be areas with regional cancer registries or specific geographic areas having isolated or low mobility populations, in combination with the ability to follow the population for the outcomes of interest. Phase IV studies should be generalizable to the target population thus allowing an estimation of potential impact from a cancer control intervention. A Phase V study would be the demonstration and implementation of interventions which have already proven beneficial through previous research. With these Phase V studies, there is an expectation of assessing the practicality, efficiency and the impact of the interventions selected for the demonstration project in a wider population setting.

The highest priority in future cancer control efforts will go toward the cancers causing the greatest morbidity and mortality in the United States, for which effective interventions are available. Existing prevention and management techniques for cancers are limited in number, and a continuing effort to develop innovative approaches as well as to access current "optimal" prevention and management techniques is desirable. Through the consensus of experts, acceptable approaches to many aspects of prevention and management of specific cancers may be outlined, and comparisons of these activities with existing efforts should provide new insights as to the relative value of aggressive cancer control programs. In the area of diagnosis and treatment, the baseline standard management may be represented by well designed clinical research protocols or by locally developed management guidelines. An attempt to facilitate community physician participation in protocol studies, and the development and evaluation of the effectiveness of local management guidelines has evolved in many communities.

In the area of prevention, individual exposures preventing cancer (as in the case of some dietary factors) and also the causes of cancer, both require accurate description before the cancer control linkage of interested community and governmental health agencies can be accomplished. In an effort to develop an effective National program for cancer control, qualified personnel are necessary, and those with experience and training in the disciplines of epidemiology, biostatistics, disease control management, and oncology must all interface to achieve a smooth and effective reorganized approach to cancer control by the National Cancer Institute.

The Division of Resources, Centers, and Community Activities, soon to become the Division of Cancer Prevention and Control, has undergone a variety of changes over the past year. Dr. Peter Greenwald joined the Division from the New York State Health Department. Dr. Joseph Cullen came from Los Angeles to become the Division Deputy Director and is supervising the Cancer Control Applications Program. Dr. William DeWys came from the Division of Cancer Treatment to take over the Prevention Program. Dr. Jerome Yates came from the University of Vermont to manage the Centers and Community Oncology Program. A variety of other individuals with demonstrated expertise in cancer control have joined the Division, and this has changed its internal complexion.

As part of new Division operational initiatives, we are reviewing past programs to assess their effectiveness in the areas of diet and cancer, cancer screening, occupational cancer, education, behavioral medicine, and the Centralized Cancer Patient Data System. We are expanding efforts in the areas of chemoprevention, diet and cancer, smoking and health, the community clinical oncology program, the cancer control research units, and the cancer control science programs.

The organization has three major program areas: The Cancer Control Applications arm, headed by Dr. Cullen, the Centers and Community Oncology program, headed by Dr. Yates, and the Prevention area, headed by Dr. DeWys (see Figure 1).

Figure 1

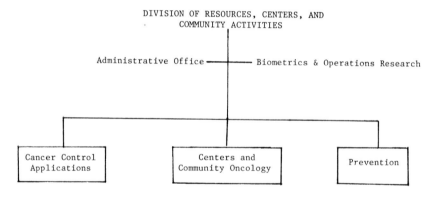

DIVISION OF RESOURCES, CENTERS, AND
COMMUNITY ACTIVITIES

In the Cancer Control Applications Program there is a Cancer Control Science Branch under Dr. Caban which includes the cancer control research units and the cancer control science program (see table 2). The Behavioral Medicine Branch is headed by Dr. Levy, the Education Branch is headed by Dr. Gigliotti, the Cancer Training Branch is headed by Dr. Lepovetsky, and the Cancer Development Branch is headed by Dr. Burnight.

TABLE 2

CANCER CONTROL APPLICATIONS PROGRAM

Cancer Control Science
Behavioral Medicine
Education
Cancer Training
Career Development

The Centers and Community Oncology Programs include Cancer Centers, Community Oncology, continuing care and rehabilitation (see table 3). Also included in this program are the Organ Systems Branch headed by Dr. Chiarodo, which includes the prostate, bladder, colorectal, pancreas, and breast sites, and the Research Facilities Branch headed by Dr. Fox, which is charged with responsibility for renovations and new construction.

TABLE 3

CENTERS AND COMMUNITY ONCOLOGY PROGRAM

Cancer Centers
Community Oncology and Rehabilitation
Organ Systems
Research Facilities

In the Prevention area, the Cancer detection and occupational cancer branches have been joined by many new prevention activities (see table 4). New initiatives in chemoprevention are underway. A variety of efforts in the area of chemoprevention are coming to maturation with the funding of concepts to take place later this year.

TABLE 4

PREVENTION PROGRAM

Cancer prevention studies
Chemoprevention
Diet and Cancer
Occupational Cancer
Cancer Detection

Divisional resources including cancer control can be seen in figure 2. The allocation of the 57 million dollar cancer control budget may be seen in figure 3.

Figure 2

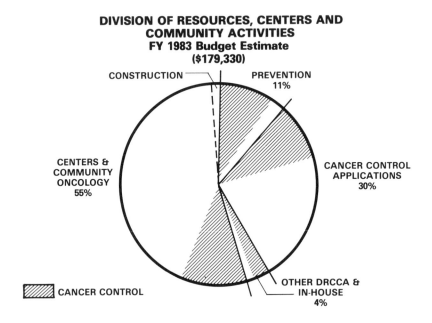

DIVISION OF RESOURCES, CENTERS AND
COMMUNITY ACTIVITIES
FY 1983 Budget Estimate
($179,330)

CONSTRUCTION

PREVENTION
11%

CENTERS &
COMMUNITY
ONCOLOGY
55%

CANCER CONTROL
APPLICATIONS
30%

CANCER CONTROL

OTHER DRCCA &
IN-HOUSE
4%

The potential interdigitation of some community and cancer center activities in the future is great. If one looks at the clinical cancer centers, they are charged with regional cancer control responsibility, and interest in cancer control varies greatly as one goes from center to center. The new Community Clinical Oncology Program will link some community clinical oncology programs with centers in a common effort.

The community programs have evolved from the community oncology programs developed in the mid seventies, where the primary focus was on patient management guideline development by community hospital physicians; this gave impetus to the later Community Hospital Oncology Program (CHOP). The initial planning activity by 23 CHOP groups was later reduced to 17 who would carry out the implementation and monitoring of the use of the management guidelines.

Figure 3

DIVISION OF RESOURCES, CENTERS AND COMMUNITY ACTIVITIES
FY 1983 Budget Estimate — Cancer Control
($57,000)

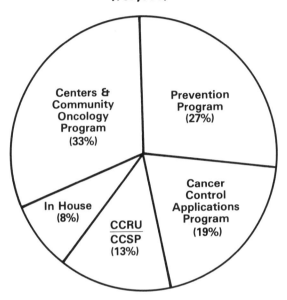

At about the same time as the original community oncology programs were trying the development of guidelines in the community, the Cooperative Group Outreach Program was initiated. This program was designed to involve community physicians in clinical research activities, and involved participants from all areas of the United States. The majority of physicians participating in the Cooperative Group Outreach Program contribute fewer than 10 patients per year to clinical research studies.

The new Community Clinical Oncology Program (CCOP) has a requirement for accession of a minimum of 50 patients a year per group to studies; therefore, it is aimed at participants with greater accrual capability than generally has been the experience in the Cooperative Group Outreach Program.

Cancer centers around the country are primarily focused in the large metropolitan areas of the country. The cooperative members, supported by the Division of Cancer Treatment are found largely in the northeast with some on the west coast. We have received 191 applications for the Community Clinical Oncology Program (CCOP) and these applications come from most States in the United States. A composite of all of these NCI funded clinical research and control activities demonstrate activities in every State in the United States (see figure 4). These activities are and should serve to diffuse advances in clinical research and impacting cancer management in communities throughout the nation.

Figure 4

Distribution of clinical research activities funded by the National Cancer Institute through the Cancer Centers, Cooperative Groups and potential Community Programs

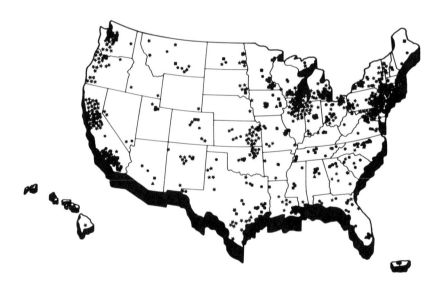

Community oncologists are working together with cancer centers and clinical cooperative groups in these dynamic NCI sponsored programs (1). Patients throughout the country have an opportunity to participate in clinical studies in their own individual communities. The participation by community physicians in clinical trials affords an important educational activity and assures up-to-date patient management. This cooperative venture links the research centers of the National Cancer Institute and community oncologists, and should provide new insights into patterns of care and technology diffusion, which are key ingredients toward the effort of reducing cancer morbidity and mortality. With the evolution of this network, it is anticipated that other cancer control efforts will be added to the existing clinical trial participation in many communities.

References

Begg CB, Carbone PP, Elson PJ and Zelen M: Participation of community hospitals in clinical trials - Analysis of experience in the Eastern Cooperative Oncology Group. New Engl. Journal Med., 306:1076-1080, 1982.

Progress in Cancer Control IV: Research in the Cancer Center, pages 29–35
© **1983 Alan R. Liss, Inc., 150 Fifth Avenue, New York, NY 10011**

CANCER PREVENTION AND CONTROL BY THE AMERICAN CANCER SOCIETY

Alfred Goldson, M.D.
Howard University Cancer Center
Washington, D.C.   20060
Diane J. Fink, M.D.
American Cancer Society
New York, NY   10017

We know that the disease cancer is a very old one.
Evidences of it stretch back to antiquity. And yet, for
centuries men and women faced the disease with fear, with
silence, and with bitter resignation -- not at all the
reaction one would expect from the race which defied nature
by building pyramids and then suspension bridges; by
conquering the sea and then the air. Against the broad
movement of time, cancer prevention and detection efforts
are actually recent undertakings. And it is remarkable to
note how much has been done in those relatively few years.

The American Cancer Society, which itself will soon be
70 years old, a relative patriarch in the health care field,
looks with pride at its own prevention and detection programs.
Through the years we have been as bold and thorough and
innovative as we knew how to be. And it would be a very
pleasant task for me to stand here this morning and tout the
accomplishments the ACS has earned over the years. However,
there is a truth which cannot be ignored, a simple although
somewhat contradictory truth, and one that we've all
felt. "We have done everything we could; we have not done
enough. There still is so much of this work to be done; so
much more about this disease we need to understand".

We would like to share with you brief
accounts of ACS prevention and detection efforts; successful
programs from our past, but most importantly those which are
shaping our future.

At first glance we may seem a diverse and complex

organization since we involve ourselves in research, education (both public and professional), and service and rehabilitation, while maintaining fund raising efforts as well. But in fact, the diversity of the American Cancer Society has a single and unifying purpose: to control cancer whether in the research lab, the treatment center, or the schools, work places, and homes of our communities.

One of our first and most successful cancer detection efforts also gave us an early taste of controversy. Forty years ago, the American Cancer Society began supporting a doctor who had developed a test which could detect uterine cancer in its early stages. Surprisingly the public reaction was hesitant and the medical reaction was sometimes resistence. To our modern sensibilities their reactions and reasons seem incomprehensible, and yet they are an historical reminder of how much fear and mystery surrounded cancer, even in the medical field.

So the ACS took its message to the people, as it always has; more specifically, to the American woman, and we waged an enormous public education campaign. Women all over America and then all over the world began to ask for the test. And doctors relented, of course; not so much because the American Cancer Society wields clout. But because Truth and Hope wield clout. As a result of the Pap Test there has been a 60% reduction in the death rate from uterine cancer in women. More positively put, with early detection, the survival rate of women with uterine cancer is now over 80%.

A yearly Pap Test became one of the ACS' recommended guidelines for good health and early detection of cancer. And as new detection techniques for other cancer sites were developed, the ACS adopted them and added them to its guidelines for a cancer-related checkup, a recommended part of one's annual health checkup. We believed that these recommendations were urgently needed and appropriate to their time; however new technology, improved detection techniques, plus rising health costs, and an attendant rising public concern and interest in health matters dictated a re-examination. That re-examination led to the revision of the ACS guidelines for the cancer-related checkup. In making the new recommendation the ACS had four main concerns: first there must be good evidence that each test or procedure recommended is medically effective in reducing morbidity or mortality; second the medical benefits must outweigh the risks; third the cost of each test or procedure must be reasonable compared to its expected benefits; finally the recommended actions must be practical and feasible.

With these criteria in mind we looked again at our stands on the nine tests and procedures we had hitherto endorsed: sputum cytology, chest x-ray, digital rectal examination, sigmoidoscopy, stool occult blood test, Pap test, mammograph, breast physical examination and breast self-examination.

For the purposes of an example, the Pap smear is now recommended every 3 years instead of every year. Research indicated that the transit time between the development of precancerous lesions and invasive carcinoma of the cervix is a long one -- perhaps as much as five to fifteen years. Therefore as long as a woman tests negatively 2 years in a row a tri-ennial smear should suffice for asymptomatic women who are not at special risk.

Changes in other recommendations were based upon this type of research as well. Public and professional reaction, however, flew in the face of the old axom about building a better mousetrap. People beat a path to our door with questions, concern, and sometimes anger. Some thought we were stepping back from our very strong, and we consider, leadership role in cancer detection efforts. Of course, we are not. We still believe that detection, and especially early detection is our best defense against a disease which we cannot yet prevent or predict. Obviously the most effective detection program would be one administering these tests and procedures every day. Just as obviously this is impractical in every way. A pragmatic schedule had to be devised. Some doctors felt that without impetus for a yearly cancer checkup, patients would then start to neglect their general annual checkup. Although this must be true in some cases, we still believed that our responsibility was to make recommendations which more truly reflected the state of cancer research, the state of detection technology, and the economic realities, as well.

Will our guidelines change again? It is possible. As we learn more and learn how to be more effective, our early detection recommendation will certainly reflect our best thinking and the newest discoveries.

Other means of early detection are currently being investigated. Cancer cells produce characteristic substances which can sometimes be detected by chemical analysis or immunological testing. There are now in existence several blood and skin tests which will diagnose cancer in about ninety percent of the cases. Unfortunately, this is not good enough, for both false positive and false negative results will cause considerable harm. Furthermore, many of these tests are not organ specific, so that a positive test in an asymptomatic patient will require considerable testing which still may not demonstrate a very early cancer. We need more and better tests before these blood and skin tests will have a practical application.

One of the most exciting developments at present is the work on monoclonal antibodies. An antigen is some substance that is foreign to the body and which provokes an immune response from the host. The antigen may be a virus, a bacteria, a pollen, a foreign body, or a cancer cell. A part of the immune response of the body to these antigens, and here we are particularly concerned about the cancer cell as an antigen, is the development of specific antibodies. These antibodies are made by a specific type of white blood cell called the lymphocyte. Unfortunately, the lymphocyte is short-lived, perhaps a matter of a few weeks, while at the same time the cancer cell is virtually immortal and continues to grow and divide indefinitely. The cancer cells may be held in check for a while by the antibodies, but as time passes the cancer cells may become too numerous. It was thought that perhaps by using genetic engineering that a specific antibody-producing lymphocyte could be fused to a cancer cell from either an animal or a human, and that the lymphocyte might then have the life expectancy of the cancer cell. This hybridization has been done, and in fact, it works. The cells produce specific antibodies against the patient's cancer cells, and they are harvested and given to the patient, which is expected to enhance the patient's immune defense. If radioactive materials are attached to this antibody after the antibody has sought out and fused with the antigen, a Geiger counter will indicate the location of even microscopic amounts of cancer within the body. Furthermore, this is a mechanism by which radiotherapy can be delivered to the specific cancer cell without irradiating surrounding normal cells.

The future of cancer detection is filled with promise.

And yet this promise is not enough to offset the general impatience when it comes to cancer. In recent years that impatience has manifested itself strongly in the public's concern for cancer prevention. It seems suddenly that the complexities of life we once took in stride and with nonchalance have come back to disturb and distress us.

When the public hears that 70-90% of cancers are related to our environment, it evokes anxiety and frustration since there are relatively few specific environmental elements which have been identified as carcinogenic agents, with the exception of tobacco, asbestos, alcohol, and certain chemicals. Therefore, people become suspicious about various things in their homes, food, clothing, schools, workplaces, and recreational areas. Alarm is sounded almost weekly about a new potential hazard, and this profound public anxiety and frustration about life style, the environment, and cancer provoked us to embark on Cancer Prevention Study II, an American Cancer Society Study of Environmental and lifestyle factors related to cancer.

As you may remember, the Cancer Prevention Study I was conducted for 1959-1965 and then reactivated to extend to 1972. It provided a wealth of evidence about human health and disease; and among the most significant was the documentation of the dose-related risk of cigarette smoking for lung cancer. Since the completion of CPS I, we have identified new problems, new concerns, and new questions to be answered. And we expect CPS II will be even more timely and more inclusive than its predecessor.

80,000 ACS volunteers will again reach over 1 million people in family groups with at least one member over 45 years of age, and follow them every other year for 6 years. The new study will investigate among other things, the long-term effects of oral contraceptives and estrogens, various common medications such as antihypertensive drugs, tranquilizers, anti-acids, caffeine, also occupational and environmental exposure, the long-term effects of low dose radiation, air and water pollution, artificial sweeteners, vitamins, various foods and methods of cooking, and the influence of low tar and nicotine cigarettes on lung cancer rates.

But the Cancer Prevention Study is only one part of the ACS cancer prevention efforts. One other we will

continue to focus on is our all-out assault on the number
one most preventable and avoidable form of cancer -- lung
cancer related to cigarette smoking. Fifty-three million
Americans still smoke and 350,000 of them will die of
smoking related disease each year. In more graphic terms
this means that this year we would lose the entire
population of Stockton, California. Next year Spokane,
Washington would become a ghost town; and the year after
that, Augusta, Georgia would go up in smoke. We feel that
plans like our Target 5, a 5-year program to reduce the
number of adult smokers by 50% through intensifying public
awareness and increasing local antismoking programs and
specific events like our Great American Smokeout, have been
enormously successful.

Nevertheless, a recent survey shows that there are still
20 million Americans who do not admit in any way, shape, or
form that there is any correlation at all between smoking
and lung cancer. Maybe you're asking yourself where have
these people been for the last 2 decades. We are asking
ourselves how we get to them? How can we convince them,
scare them, cajole them that they are surely killing
themselves by continuing to smoke.

The National Conference on Smoking and Health initiated
and underwritten by the American Cancer Society, was co-
sponsored by 21 national organizations. As a result of
recommendations by participants, the American Cancer Society
has joined with the American Lung and American Heart
Associations to form a strength-sharing coalition in
Washington, D.C. Together we three organizations hope to
provide a single, clear voice to the American Congress
about smoking. Whether it means new, higher excise taxes
on cigarettes, rotating warnings on packages, or simply
pricing a package of cigarettes so high it loses its appeal,
we will make certain that necessary legislation is passed
reflecting the will of the majority of Americans instead of
the wishes of special interests.

Most of the cancer detection and prevention efforts
discussed highlight the true strength of the
organization -- its 2 million volunteers -- the men, women,
and child-power we need to launch public education, public
information campaigns or perform the invaluable time-consuming
research involved in CPS II.

Now to touch briefly on one other way the ACS expresses its commitment in these areas. We award special institutional 5-year grants for the study of various environmental cancer links. With these grants the ACS hopes to compile solid data based on extensive, long-term research in cancer cause and prevention; to establish a number of cancer prevention research centers capable of immediate investigation of any new suspected carcinogen; and to create a "network" approach to this research, where a number of centers could collaborate on a single project.

As indicated at the beginning of this, today, we are a diverse and complex organization, but with a simple and direct goal: a world free from cancer; a world safe from cancer.

Progress in Cancer Control IV: Research in the Cancer Center, pages 37–46
© **1983 Alan R. Liss, Inc., 150 Fifth Avenue, New York, NY 10011**

CANCER CONTROL RESEARCH IN AMERICAN COLLEGE OF SURGEONS
APPROVED PROGRAMS

Charles R. Smart, M.D.

Latter Day Saints Hospital, Salt Lake City, Utah
Commission on Cancer, Chicago, Illinois

The multidisciplinary Commission on Cancer of the
American College of Surgeons currently has approved 994
Hospital Cancer Programs that evaluate or treat over 513,000
new cancer cases annually. The hospital program requires
identifiable multidisciplinary active leadership, a clinical
program aimed at improving cancer patient management and a
two phased evaluation program - patient care evaluation
audits - and the registration, life-time follow-up and
survival evaluation of all cancer patients. The following
presentation, after a brief historical review of cancer
registration in the College, will describe the efforts at
research in cancer control carried out through the Commission
on Cancer.

In August, 1920, Dr. Ernest Codman sent a letter to
every fellow of the College, seeking information on the
living cases of bone sarcoma. This later developed into a
cancer registry including breast, lung and several other
sites. In 1930, standards for cancer clinics were developed
at the request of the American Society for the Control of
Cancer (American Cancer Society) and in 1931 the first
hospitals were surveyed for approval. In 1952, the American
Cancer Society popularized hospital cancer registries and in
1956 the College made registries a requirement for having
an approved program. In 1964, Dr. R. Lee Clark transformed
the cancer committee into the multidisciplinary Commission
on Cancer and set as one of the goals for the 60's the
computerization of data from the approved hospitals.
Unfortunately, at the time the task was too formidable and
expensive.

In 1976, Dr. Gerald Murphy initiated national site-
specific patient care evaluation studies gathering a limited
number (25 or 50) sequential cases from two time periods,
the current year as well as a period starting six years
prior, to allow analysis of trends in management as well as
determining survival. These studies were initiated for a
two-fold purpose (1) to assist hospital cancer committees
meet their patient care evaluation audit requirements and
(2) to provide national data on trends in current management.
Hospital registries were helpful in identifying the cases
and the follow-up for the survival analysis for the long-
term audits, however, this did not obviate the necessity
of obtaining the hospital record for carrying out the
short-term (process)studies. These audits of management
included information not reasonably expected in a tumor
registry abstract such as presenting symptoms, specific
physical examinations, initial laboratory studies and
diagnostic x-rays and procedures.

These national site-specific surveys have been some
of the largest patient management reports ever published,
each covering anywhere from 5,000 to 50,000 cases (Table
1) and have resulted in numerous publications (1-26). Each
participating hospital received not only the analysis of
the total but also received individual comparative reports
showing their results contrasted with the total for each
item in the survey. An example of the magnitude and
importance of these studies is demonstrated by the Long-term
and short-term Surveys of Patterns of Care of the Female
Breast in American College of Surgeons' Approved Cancer
Programs, October, 1982. In the long-term survey, 27,442
consecutive cases before 1976 were reported from 565 hospitals
and in the short-term survey, 19,981 patients diagnosed and
treated in 1981 were reported from 756 hospitals, making a
total of 47,423 cases in this study of breast cancer. The
age distribution was the same as seen in Surveillance,
Epidemiology and End-Results (SEER) Program of the National
Cancer Institute. Fifty-two per cent of the cases in both
the long and short-term studies were diagnosed in the
localized stage of disease and less than 3% had in-situ
cancers. Remarkable changes occurred in treatment, with
radical mastectomy going from the major treatment 10 years
ago to 3.1% in 1981, being replaced by the modified radical
mastectomy (Table 2). Wedge excision went from 3.1% in 1976
to 7.5% in 1981. While adjuvant radiation therapy had
dropped from 1972 to 1976 and chemotherapy had increased,

both plateaued between 1976 and 1981 at about 20% (Figure 1). The five year relative survival trends improved for patients with regional and distant disease between 1972 and 1976 (Table 3).

TABLE 1

PATTERNS-OF-CARE SURVEYS OF THE AMERICAN COLLEGE OF SURGEONS BY CANCER SITE, YEAR, NUMBER OF INSTITUTIONS PARTICIPATED AND TOTAL NUMBER OF PATIENTS

Site	Year	No. of Institutions Reporting		No. of Patients		No. of States Represented	
		Short Term	Long Term	Short Term	Long Term	Short Term	Long Term
Liver	1976	*	477	*	543	*	49
Colon	1977	491	327	11,655	38,621	50	46
Breast	1978	626	498	15,488	24,136	50	47
Rectum	1979	716	441	7,023	20,371	50	46
Prostate	1980	659	414	14,079	20,166	50	50
Carcinoma In Situ of the Cervix	1981	*	392	*	9,468	*	48
Melanoma of Skin	1981	614	*	4,816	*	48	*
Breast	1982	756	565	19,981	27,442	50	49
Endometrium	1982	564	*	7,200	*	47	*
Hodgkin's Disease	1983						
Prostate	1984						
Soft Tissue Sarcoma	1984						

TABLE 2

DISTRIBUTION OF PATIENTS WITH BREAST CANCER FROM THE LONG- AND SHORT-TERM SURVEYS OF THE AMERICAN COLLEGE OF SURGEONS ACCORDING TO THE TYPE OF SURGERY

Surgery	Long-term		Short-term	
	N	%	N	%
Biopsy Only	1471	5.4	1198	6.2
Wedge excision (Lumpectomy)	840	3.1	1461	7.6
Total mastectomy only	2210	8.2	1001	5.2
Total mastectomy with low axillary dissection	1340	5.0	997	5.2
Modified radical with full axillary dissection	14051	51.9	13981	72.3
Radical mastectomy (Halsted type)	6905	25.5	605	3.1
Radical mastectomy with internal mammary node biopsy	255	0.9	94	0.5
TOTAL	27072	100.0	19337	100.0

N = Number of patients
% = Percent of total
Long-term = 1976
Short-term = 1981

TABLE 3

COMPARISON OF 5-YEAR (ACTURARIAL) SURVIVAL RATES BY STAGE
BETWEEN THE 1972 AND 1976 LONG-TERM BREAST CANCER SURVEYS
OF THE AMERICAN COLLEGE OF SURGEONS

	Year			
	1972		1976	
Stage	Percent	N	Percent	N
In-Situ	98.8	455	97.5	685
Localized	89.6	11664	90.6	13861
Regional to:				
Adjacent tissue	70.8	922	72.7	855
Axillary nodes	62.5	8923	70.9	9519
Distant	16.4	1592	22.3	1980

N = Number of patients

Figure 1

ADJUVANT THERAPY

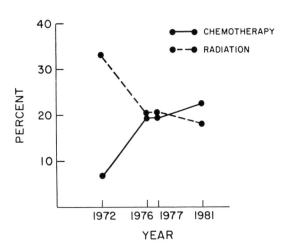

The second attempt to utilize the date from the Approved Hospital Cancer programs for cancer control research was the development of the Annual Hospital Activity Report. This report summarized the chief components of the program and included an audit of the last seven years of their registry files, recording by year the number of alive and dead cases registered for each site. Cancer in most cases being a deadly disease, the ratio of living to dead for each time period over 7 years made it relatively accurate and easy to compare these ratios against a standard set of data wherein all of the factors were known, allowing the development of a formula for estimating survival curves for each site. These estimated survival curves for each site were then compared against the total merged site experience and were returned to each participating hospital. While some statisticians frowned upon the technique, many clinicians felt it had merit and encouraged its continuation.

One of the interesting studies which came from the Annual Hospital Activity Reports was the merging of the hospital data with the American Hospital Associations computer tape containing bed size, type of hospital, type of facilities available, training programs etc. Studies were then carried out on the types of cancer seen in different categories of hospitals as well as estimates of their survival in University, General Acute Community Hospitals, V.A. Hospitals and Children's Hospitals (Table 4). This demonstrated well the unique nature of the different types of hospitals and their special clientele such as the V.A. Hospitals with three out of the five most frequent cancers being smoking related as compared to the University and the Community and Children's Hospitals.

TABLE 4

COMMISSION ON CANCER OF THE AMERICAN COLLEGE OF SURGEONS
1.9 MILLION CANCERS FROM 719 HOSPITALS
FROM THE 1979 HOSPITAL ACTIVITY REPORT BY TYPE OF HOSPITAL

	Community	University	VA & Military	Childrens
# Hospitals	555 (84%)	28 (4%)	67 (10%)	9 (2%)
# Cancers	1,420,213 (82%)	196,483 (11%)	114,639 (7%)	14,292 (1%)
5-Yr. Estimated Survival	37%	36%	30%	45%
Most frequent cancer sites:	Breast	Lung	Lung	Leukemia
	Lung	Breast	Head & Neck	CNS
	Colorectal	Cervix	Prostate	Soft Tissue
	Prostate	Colorectal	Colorectal	Bone
	Cervix	Lymphoma	Bladder	Kidney

TABLE 5

COMMISSION ON CANCER OF THE AMERICAN COLLEGE OF SURGEONS

Five-Year Relative Survival Rates

Type	* NCI study 1965 - 69	** COC study 1973 - 79
Ten most frequent cancers:		
Lung	9%	11%
Breast (female)	65%	73%
Colon	46%	50%
Prostate	57%	68%
Corpus uteri	75%	84%
Bladder	62%	70%
Rectal	42%	49%
Stomach	13%	15%
Cervix (invasive)	57%	65%
Pancreatic	2%	3%
Other types:		
Multiple myeloma	16%	22%
Acute leukemia	3%	18%
Acute leukemia in under age 20 years	36%	50%
Chronic leukemia	32%	40%
Bone	32%	49%
Soft tissue sarcomas	42%	54%
Hodgkins disease	54%	72%
Testicular embryonal ca	50%	63%
Testicular malig. teratoma	60%	77%

* Cancer Patient Survival, Report No. 5, 1976, U.S. DHEW. These rates are for the white population, which gives slightly higher survival rates than if blacks were included. The rates also exclude in-situ carcinomas.

** These rates include all races and in-situ carcinomas, except in cervix.

The third and most important project in cancer control research was a by-product of a further effort to provide the Community Hospital with comparative statistical data from its registry. Appreciating the fact that 75% of hospitals and manual registries, central registries with computerized data from their (coded) participating hospitals were invited to submit coded data, and comparative statistical reports would be provided free to those hospitals that wished to participate. The merged data from 22 central registries covering 921,000 cancer cases was analyzed and reports were prepared based upon the 468,288 cases from 1973-1979 for 645 hospitals. Comparing this information with the survival data priore to 1973 and with published population based reports, it became evident that in many sites cancer control was being accomplished at the community level resulting in encouring improvements (Table 5). There was also noted a considerable variation in over-all and site specific survival from one geographic area to another possibly based upon the stage of disease at diagnosis or on more effective treatment, demonstrating an opportunity through public and through professional education to improve cancer control at the community level.

In conclusion, the Hospital Career Program of the American College of Surgeons has provided a valuable source of data on the impact of cancer measures in the community. The large base of data deriving from the fact that approximately sixty percent of cancer patients in the United States are treated in the participating institutions may provide a perspective on trends in care and treatment effectiveness achievable by no other means. Future studies may build upon those already completed and the resources of the hospital tumor registry may provide reference points against progress in cancer control may be assessed.

REFERENCES

Murphy GP (1977). ACS Commission on cancer survey supports suggested association between oral contraceptive usage and liver tumors. Bulletin of the American College of Surgeons 62(4): 28-33.

Vana J, Murphy GP, Aronoff BL and Baker HW (1977). Primary liver tumors and oral contraceptives. Results of a survey. JAMA 238(20): 2154-2156.

Vana J, Bedwani R, Nemoto T and Murphy GP (1978). Preliminary Report: American College of Surgeons Committee on Cancer, long-term patient care evaluation study for carcinoma of the female breast. Bulletin of the American College of Surgeons, October.

Evans JT, Vana J, Aronoff BL, Baker HW and Murphy GP (1978). Management and survival of carcinoma of the colon: Results of a national survey by the American College of Surgeons. Ann Surg 188(6): 716-720.

Vana J and Murphy GP (1979). Primary malignant liver tumors. Association with oral contraceptives. New York State J Med 79(3): 321-325.

Vana J, Murphy GP, Aronoff BL and Baker HW (1979). Survey of primary lover tumors and oral contraceptive use. J Toxicol and Environm Hlth 5(2-3): 253-273.

Nime F, Pickren JW, Vana J, Aranoff BL, Baker HW, and Murphy GP (1979). The histology of liver tumors in oral contraceptive users observed during a national survey by the American College of Surgeons' Commission on Cancer. Cancer 44(4): 1481-1439.

Vana J, Murphy GP, Aronoff BL and Baker HW (1979). Survey of primary liver tumors and oral contraceptive use. In: Liver Carcinogenesis, L. Lapis and J.V. Johannessen (eds.), Hemisphere Publishing Corp., Washington and New York, pp. 85-103.

Nemoto T, Vana J, Bedwani RN, Baker HW, McGregor FH, and Murphy GP (1980). Management and survival of female breast cancer: Results of a national survey by the American College of Surgeons. Cancer 45(12): 2917-2924.

Rosner D, Bedwani RN, Vana J, Baker HW and Murphy GP (1980). Non-invasive breast carcinoma: Results of a national survey by the American College of Surgeons. Ann Surg 192(2): 139-147.

Vana J, Bedwani R, Mettlin C and Murphy GP (1980). Trends in diagnosis and management of breast cancer in the U.S. From the Surveys of the American College of Surgeons. Cancer 45: 2917-2924.

Mettlin C, Mittelman A, Natarajan N, Murphy GP, Schmitz RL and Smart CR (1981). Trends in management of adenocarcinoma of the rectum in the United States. Results of a national survey by the American College of Surgeons. Surg Gynec & Obst 153: 701-706.

Nemoto T, Vana J, Natarajan N, Bedwani R, Mettlin C (1981). Observations on short-term and long-term surveys of breast cancer by the American College of Surgeons. In: International Advances in Surgical Oncology, G.P. Murphy (ed.), Alan R. Liss, Inc., New York, Vol. 4: 209-239.

Bedwani RN, Vana J, Rosner D, Schmitz R, and Murphy GP (1981).

Management and survival of female patients with "minimal" breast cancer: As observed in the long-term and short-term surveys of the American College of Surgeons. Cancer 47: 2769-2778.

Mettlin C and Natarajan N (1981). Studies on the role of oral contraceptive use in the etiology of benign and malignant liver tumors. J of Surg Oncol 181: 73-85.

Mettlin C, Natarajan N, Mittelman A, Smart C, and Murphy GP (1982). Management and survival of adenocarcinoma of the rectum in the United States: Results of a national survey by the American College of Surgeons. Oncology 39: 265-273.

Murphy GP, Natarajan N, Pontes JE, Schmitz RL, Smart CR, Schmidt JD and Mettlin C (1982). The national survey of prostate cancer in the United States by the American College of Surgeons. J Urol 127: 928-934.

Mettlin C, Natarajan N, Murphy GP (1982). Recent patterns of care of prostate patients in the United States: Results from the surveys of the American College of Suregons' Commission on Cancer. In: International Advances in Surgical Oncology, G.P. Murphy (ed.), Alan R. Liss, Inc., New York, 5: 277-321.

Nemoto T, Natarajan N, Bedwani RN, Vana J, Murphy GP (1983). Breast cancer in the medial half. Results of 1973 National Survey of the American College of Surgeons. Cancer 51(8): 1333-1338.

Nemoto T, Natarajan N, Mettlin C, Murphy GP (1982). Patterns of breast cancer detection in the U.S. J of Surg Oncol 21: 183-188.

Huben R, Natarajan N, Pontes JE, Mettlin C, Smart CR and Murphy GP (1982). Carcinoma of the prostate in men less than 50 years old: data from a national survey by the American College of Surgeons: Urology 20(6): 585-588.

Mettlin C, Mikuta J, Natarajan N, Priore R, Murphy GP (1982). Treatment and follow-up study of squamous cell carcinoma in situ of the cervix uteri. Surg Gynec & Obst 155:481-488.

American College of Surgeons' Commission on Cancer, Patient Care and Research Committee Audit of Current Management of Malignant Melanoma of the Skin in the United States. April 14, 1982.

Balch CM, Mettlin C (1982). Symptoms and treatment of melanoma in the United States. Bulletin of the American College of Surgeons, September, 1982.

American College of Surgeons' Commission on Cancer, Long-term and Short-term Surveys of Patterns of Care of the Female Breast in American College of Surgeons' Approved

Cancer Program, Report to the Commission on Cancer Patient Care and Research Committee. October 22, 1982.

Balch CM, Karakousis C, Mettlin C, Natarajan N, Donegan WL, Smart CR and Murphy GP (1983). Management of cutaneous melanoma in the United States. Results of the American College of Surgeons' melanoma survey. Surg Gynec and Obst (in press).

Progress in Cancer Control IV: Research in the Cancer Center, pages 47–54
© 1983 Alan R. Liss, Inc., 150 Fifth Avenue, New York, NY 10011

OCCUPATIONAL CANCER AND CANCER INSTITUTES

ANDERS ENGLUND, M.D.

INTERNATIONAL UNION AGAINST CANCER

GENEVA, SWITZERLAND

The control of occupational cancer is mainly a primary preventive action. The role of the cancer institute in controlling occupational cancer will accordingly also, to a great extent, be on the primary prevention level. A few words will be spent in the end on the early diagnostic and treatment aspects of cancer control, where the role of the cancer center is more easily identified.

I. PRIMARY PREVENTION

Primary prevention in occupational cancer control has three elements - identification of the risk, elimination of that risk, and monitoring of the effect of the intervention.

I.1 Risk Identification

The components necessary to identify a possible risk in the work environment are data on exposure and disease. Only the latter one is generally available to health professionals such as those in the cancer centers. Without the additional information on exposure from people outside the cancer center, in the factories an association between exposure and disease is impossible to assess. The awareness of individual open-minded doctors have identified most of the cancer hazards in industry known to us today. This applies all the way back to Rammazini and to Pott with his chimney sweepers and up till today to Esme Hadfield, a British ENT physician in High Wycombshire (outside London). There, she observed

that a substantial number of cases with adenocarcinomas of
the nasal sinuses appeared among furniture makers. Her
findings have later been confirmed in large case-control
and cohort studies. The recognition in a certain population,
of an unexpected pattern of diseases - including cancer - is
in my opinion the primary role of the health establishments.
Frequently, a certain geographical area has gotten a predominant industrial structure. Accordingly, it might be
likely that an aggregation of a large number of occupationally induced cases of a certain tumour will occur. This happened
to Dr. Haddfield, who lived in the center of the English
furniture making area. A cancer center should have as one of
its tasks to continuously monitor the cancer pattern in its
captive population. More sophisticated techniques for information retrieval and analysis are certainly available today
than 200 or even 20 years ago - to refer back to Pott or
Haddfield. Dr. Smart talked yesterday about the patient data
banks which are so nicely used for follow-up of treatment
performance in the medical centers. I would propose to go
even a step further and use them for etiological research
purposes. A cohort study approach is natural for the occupational health physician who has his/her population at risk well
defined. That approach will be difficult for the cancer center with its inability to define such a population at risk
The case-control/reference approach will be the natural one
for a hospital based monitoring activity. However, the important question will be how to avoid bias in selecting your
controls. I have seen reports of studies on occupational cancer from Roswell Park, where use has been made of such hospital data. I have understood that follow-up of patient exposure was an ongoing procedure in that hospital. Reports
from that programme have on several occasions contributed to
the accumulated knowledge about cancer risk due to certain
exposures. Such hospital based information might have an outstanding value because the closer you are to the data source,
the more sophisticated your information will be.

In my own native country, Sweden, like a few others,
there are national cancer registries with compulsory incidence
reporting. Recent linkage between such a registry and population census data has been used to search for association between occupation and increased cancer incidence. In principle,
similar models could be applied to hospital based registries.

Your problem, however, will be to identify your denominator. On the other hand, even descriptive epidemiology, showing the cancer pattern of the region related to the socio-economic differences and to the different geographical areas within the total target area of the cancer center, is an important knowledge. Without such information, we will have difficulties when interpreting what other more analytical studies of occupational etiology show. The British Registrar General´s decennial reports on causes of Death by Occupation have nicely shown how some cancers are more frequent in certain occupations than in others, but those cancers were not only related to the occupation as such, but rather to the social groups as a whole. To identify what is "occupationally caused caner" among such cases would not be easy and the responsible factor might as well be a different hygienic, dietary etc, habit. I would like to illustrate what I have said with a few tables based on research, using a patient data base like the cancer registry in Sweden.

Slides of Tables were shown on occupational differences in cancer incidences and mortality. Both proportional figures using occupations registered within the registry and incidence figures per occupation derived through recent linkage between Cancer Registry and population census data were shown. Finally, data from a cohort study of painters, plumbers and insulators were used to illustrate the identification process.Part of the data has previously been reported in: Occup. Cancer and Carcinogenesis Ed. H. Vainio, M. Sorsa K. Hemmiki, Hemisphere Publishing Corporation, Washington N.Y. 1981.

So what about oesophageal cancer among painters ? What about the total cancer pattern among painters ? It is comparable with that of the shoemaker ! (Figure 1)

Figure 1 : CANCER INCIDENCE IN SOME OCCUPATIONAL GROUPS

	DIAGNOSIS (ICD VII)	SMR	NUMBER OF CANCER CASES
PAINTERS (1511)	150	167	32
	155,1-9	202	7
	162,0-1	130	202
	162,2	268	5
SHOEMAKERS (579)	150	171	7
	155,0	187	8
	155,1-9	288	3
	204	156	21

Total number of reported Cancer Cases within brackets.

Is it not likely that they had a similar solvent exposure in the past ? What other occupations show an excess of oesophagus cancer in the same study ? (Figure 2)

Figure 2 : CANCER OF THE OESOPHAGUS (ICD VII 150) IN SOME SELECTED OCCUPATIONS

OCCUPATION IN FOLLOWING TRADES	ICD 150 SMR	NUMBER OF OESOPHAGEAL CANCER CASES	TOTAL NUMBER OF CANCER CASES
RUBBER INDUSTRY	190	11	843
PETROL STATION	213	5	238
CHEMICAL INDUSTRY	212	11	408
SHOES AND BOOT IN-DUSTRY	171	7	579
PAINTERS	167	32	1511

It is unlikely to me that excess intake of alcohol - a usual reason to this particular cancer - should be in excess among these groups only. Could solvent exposure be the common denominator that explains this finding among these trades ?

As an occupational health expert, I need the assistance of a site specialist. Otherwise, the magnitude of the non-occupational influence on the cancer pattern of different occupational groups will be impossible to assess. The inter-action between occupational exposure and personal habit constitutes such a situation. Perhaps the alcohol related disease pattern in the painters is the result of alcohol and solvent exposure together. Does a "normal" alcohol intake give a more severe effect on the body than is seen among non-solvent exposed persons ? The interaction between smoking and asbestos for the development of lung cancer is another example. Still another example would be that of excess stomach cancer observed in certain occupations which might be caused by a different diet habit rather than the occupations themselves.

This review of the role of the Cancer Center in Risk Identification highlighted: 1) the need to use available data sources. 2) but also to identify possible pitfalls before analyses.

I.2 Risk Elimination

I would then like to go to the second step. Use the knowledge you acquired!!!!! Dr. Smart made the same remark yesterday, it is not enough to identify a problem, you have to do something to correct it. Until you have solved the problem the first step was of no real use - only l'Art pour l'Art. The real preventive actions are taken by others than ourselves within the medical profession. An occupational health risk is eliminated by industry itself or after government and union pressure. Should not we as physicians be extremely pleased when dangerous exposures are eliminated ? Is this the case ? To judge from certain issues of the newsletter of this organization this does not seem to have always been the case. To judge from opinions expressed by European and Swedish clinicians, this does not seem to be the case either. Rather than supporting those who want to eliminate unnecessary exposure to asbestos or VCM or other carcinogenic components unnecessarily used, certain clinicians fight against those who stress the view that several occupational exposures are avoidable in nature. They even shed tears for the poor industrialists who have to change their production or trade.

I have always been astonished how this attitude could be
formed among my medical collegues. It is not only that we
should as physicians always be pleased when the hazard is
eliminated, but we are not even those who are able to tell
that the elimination of asbestos or VCM or any other product
is too costly. In fact, the market adjusts itself whenever
the full story gets broadcasted. An interesting difference
was shown between the less than one year needed to eliminate
unnecessary exposure to vinyl chloride monomer and the 31
years needed to eliminate an unncessary exposure to asbestos.
The issue of the interactive role of smoking gives us no
reason not to eliminate asbestos. Both preventive actions
are necessary. My advice to the Cancer Centers is :
- realize that the real preventive measures are not taken
  inside the hospital, but by others outside in the society
  and industry
- encourage such measures to be taken and do not as today
  discourage in a belief that you save society and industry.
  You would then do a disgrace!!!!!
- society and industry are able to adopt themselves if a
  product needs to disappear and cannot remain competitive
  on the market.

Technology can àlways find new ways to achieve necessary performance requirements. The general disappearance of asbestos
in Sweden, or the gradual replacement of it for brake lining
purposes everywhere, the elimination of vinylchloride monomer exposure in production halls as well as from products,
are examples.

I am frequently asked whether I subscribe to the 25%
occupational etiology in cancer causation estimated by some
NIOSH-sources, or to the more frequently cited 4-6% estimate
by Higginson, Doll and others. My reply is that I am not that
much interested in either figure. 4-6% is high enough to do
something whenever possible. It would mean 1'000 males/year
in a country like Sweden.

The concept of WHENEVER POSSIBLE - psychologically,
technically or economically feasible - is a concept that has
to be added to the priority setting parameters in cancer control. Intervention is easy for occupational exposure, but
difficult when changing diet or reproductive habits. You

should not forget that what seems to be a low proportion of
a total figure, might be a substantial number of patients a
year. This is the case with regard to occupationally caused
cancer in the U.S.A. as Doll in fact pointed out in his recent report to the O.T.A. It might also hide a high incidence
figure or attack rate in a certain sub-population for a certain cancer site. The incidence of nasal sinus tumours
among furniture makers in the U.K. was as high as the lung
cancer incidence in the general population, according to
reports by Acheson. We are concerned with the latter and we
combat it. Less concern has been expressed for the former.
In the past, very high attack rates in industrially exposed
populations were not unusual. An example is the β-nafthyla-
mine exposure in dye-stuff workers which lead to an extremely high bladder cancer incidence.

My summary of the role of the Cancer Center in risk
elimination will be:
- Follow Dr. Smart's advice; when you have identified a problem by using your patient data base, then do something
  to get the problem solved -
Do not, as in the past, rather delay preventive action by
taking a passive, society neglecting preservation attitude,
but realize that your center is the sole source of knowledge
and that it's up to both Society and Industry to find solutions to the problems you found.

I.3 Effect Follow-up

The monitoring of the effect of the interventions made
does not differ conceptually from the first identification
step. The same thinking, the same models, the same epidemiological techniques will have to be applied. An example of the
need and value of such a monitoring concept is Sir Richard
Doll's report in 1955 on lung cancer among the employees in
the asbestos textile industry in the U.K. The study was done
to see if the high incidence of asbestosis - a non-malignant
disease of the lung caused by asbestos exposure - seen in
the early decades of this century had declined as a result
of the technical improvements in the factories, forced on
them by new legislation in the early 30's. It was found that
the initially aimed at decline in asbestosis was achieved
but that an unexpected lung cancer problem had appeared.

Similar findings of successful combat of the original enemy,
but unexpected detection of a new one has been the result
of monitoring disease pattern in the British Rubber industry
during the 70's.

II   SECONDARY PREVENTION AND TREATMENT

I said initially that the role of the Cancer Center in
secondary prevention - which would be equivalent to early
detection programmes - is more easily defined.

Programmes have been established for bladder cancer detection - cytology screening or as in the past even cysto-
scopy - Since a long time, such programmes are running in
the rubber industry in the U.K. Asbestos exposed workers
now constitute a target group for respiratory cancer detection
but, what can really be achieved for them ? Early detection
for lung cancer programmes have so far not proven to increase
survival, even in high risk groups.

Mesotheliomas - another asbestos induced malignant disease in the chest, or in the abdomen - is even worse from
an early detection point of view. Of course, Cancer Center
resources should be designed to respond to the needs of the
surrounding community. That community might have a large
number of asbestos exposed persons. A commanding figure is
the number of mesotheliomas expected to appear until the
year 2000, due to previous asbestos exposure. A figure has
been estimated on the basis of past exposures to asbestos -
number and level- dose-response date available and latency
periods known. What can be done for these people ? It is a
problem for the Cancer Centers to attack, both in terms of
diagnostic and treatment models. I understand that NCI and
NIEHS are concerned about that problem, but they need the
involvement of the treatment facilities.

The occupational cancer patient as such does not con-
stitue another treatment and rehabilitation demand than any
other cancer patient. It is rather the special sites or
histological types that might be expected due to the industrial structure in the area, that should be watched carefully
in terms of planning of treatment resources within a Cancer
Center.

Progress in Cancer Control IV: Research in the Cancer Center, pages 55–66
© **1983 Alan R. Liss, Inc., 150 Fifth Avenue, New York, NY 10011**

LIFESTYLES AND CANCER PREVENTION

Guy R. Newell, M.D.

Department of Cancer Prevention
UT M. D. Anderson Hospital and Tumor Institute
Houston, Texas

The desire to deal with cancer by prevention undoubtedly goes back as far as Pott (1775) and beyond. During more recent times, the preventability of cancer by changes in lifestyle and other environmental factors was reviewed by an expert committee of the WHO in 1964 (13). They equated the scope of cancer prevention to the proportion of human cancers in which extrinsic factors are responsible. These ... "collectively, account for more than three-quarters of human cancers. It would seem, therefore, that the majority of human cancer is potentially preventable." The committee presented two classifications of cancer prevention. The first was "excluding" and consisted of:

"(1) prevention of the carcinogenic process from arising in the first place;

(2) prevention of the tumor from eventually developing;

(3) forestalling the development of the tumor by appropriate detection methods and treatment."

The second they called "interfering" and was:

"(1) removal of the causative factor

(a) at the start (avoiding initiation), or

(b) subsequently during the latent period
(avoiding promotion);

(2) interfering with the evolution or development of
the carcinogenic process by modifying factors
(including therapy) during the latent period.

(3) forestalling the development of the tumor by
appropriate detection methods and treatment."

Note that neither of these descriptions adheres to
the more classical definition of prevention which included
primary, secondary and tertiary. The committee listed 14
etiological factors that they considered susceptible to
control. The list, published 19 years ago, contains all
of the factors we recognize today and some that we would
not. The report is of further interest in that it spells
out a teaching program and a pilot scheme for cancer
prevention in a city of 100,000.

In 1967, Sir Richard Doll presented The Rock Carling
Fellowship lecture entitled "Prevention of Cancer,
Pointers from Epidemiology" (4). In his presentation of
practical steps to prevention, he states:

"In the case of cancer, our lack of knowledge
of the intimate mechanism by which the disease is
produced stands in the way of attempts to prevent
it. When we know how the body normally regulates
cellular proliferation and understand the nature of
the molecular changes that result in the breakdown
of this mechanism, it may be possible to develop a
simple and effective programme for preventing the
disease in all its manifestations."

What better admonition supporting research as part
of cancer control could one have?

Sir Doll goes on to point out that even for known
causes of cancer, practical prevention involves interface
with government and often requires the participation of
society as a whole. He then presents some of the ways in
which it may be possible to influence personal behavior.
He sums up by saying we might now be able to prevent about
40% of cancer deaths in men and about 10% in women. In
addition, a large proportion of the remaining types is

preventable with continued research.

A sustained interest in cancer prevention related to lifestyle and individual risks was kindled by a conference convened by the NCI and the ACS in Key Biscayne, Florida, December 10-12, 1974 (7). MacMahon, in his overview of the presentations on environmental factors noted the great variety that exists (9). Physical, chemical and biologic agents are all represented. Several modes of action are known - genetic mutation, aberrations during anatomic development, changes in physiologic development, and action as true carcinogen or through several mechanisms. Substances can exert their actions during a variety of ages - ancestral times for genetic determinants, in utero, early childhood or at any age in childhood and adult life. The same agent may act at different ages, such as DES. Regarding the implications for research, he states that environmental causes of cancer must be far more numerous than those identified at that time. The complexity of the situation presents another argument for continuing support of the individual investigator with imagination and initiative to explore new fields.

During that same conference, Shimkin proposed a new specialty, Preventive Oncology (11). He suggested three tasks:

"(1) The acquisition and validation of knowledge regarding prevention through research and field trials,

(2) The transmission of such knowledge, through education, which also needs research and validation,

(3) The use of knowledge, through development of motivation and compliance with health practices and procedures. This task also needs research, and the feedback of validation."

Note that all three tasks require research, whether in acquisition, transmission, or use of knowledge for preventing cancer.

So far, I have tried to lay the foundation for two themes - the almost desperate plea for more research related to cancer prevention, and the necessary involvement of government, society, and the individual to successfully act on knowledge gleaned from the research. The two must go forward together.

The most comprehensive lists of conditions associated (does not necessarily imply causation) with cancer was published by Fox in a monograph Cancer: The Behavioral Dimensions (6) (Table 1). The two major arms of cancer prevention are the identification of the contributors to the cause(s) of cancer, and the action taken in response to this knowledge. The former is the function of the researcher, the latter is usually enacted by legislative control or preferably by voluntary actions taken on the part of concerned individuals. It is a sobering fact that we could possibly know the cause of every cancer and, at the same time, not prevent a single one of them. Cullen and Gritz wrote "What individuals do with this knowledge, how they perceive, accept, and act upon it, will determine whether cancer prevention is achievable. What really counts is behavior modification, or agent change, whether in the environment, the medical care system, or the individual" (2).

TABLE 1

Conditions associated with cancer

Conditions	Range of confidence[a]	Site[b]
I. What people are, or what happens to them personally.		
A. Psychological characteristics		
1. Personality	3-4	Nonspecific
2. Transient or newly occurring states		
a. Mental illness, especially schizophrenia	4	Nonspecific
b. Depression	4	Nonspecific pancreas, blood
c. Neurologic symptoms	3-4	Nonspecific
d. Specific life stresses		
(1) Hypotheses: low male hormone; high blood corticosteroids; conditioned immunosuppression	4	Stomach, nonspecific
(2) Experimental stress in animals	3-4	Nonspecific
B. Physical characteristics		
1. Somatotype	4	Nonspecific
2. Specific body dimensions		
a. Structure	4	Breast, nonspecific
b. Obesity	3	Endometrium
c. Height and weight	3-4	Breast, cervix
3. Hair color	4	Breast
4. Complexion and eye color	1-3	Skin
C. Congenital and genetic traits		
1. Age at menarche	3	Cervix, breast
2. Age at menopause	4	Breast
3. Family history of cancer	1-4	Breast, various nonspecific
4. Congenital deficiency or abnormality	1-4	Various
D. Other diseases and pathology		
1. E.g., cirrhosis of liver, skin keratoses, kidney or bladder stones	2-4	Various
2. Traumata, scars, burns	2-4	Skin, esophagus
3. Communicable diseases	2-4	Bladder, blood
4. Irritation of tissues	3-4	Nonspecific
E. Demographic and social characteristics		
1. Sex	1	Various
2. Age	1	Nonspecific
3. Socioeconomic level	1-4	Nonspecific

Conditions associated with cancer

Conditions	Range of confidence[a]	Site[b]
4. Marriage	2-4	Breast, cervix
5. Race	1-4	Various, nonspecific
6. Religion	1-4	Various
7. Ethnicity	1-4	Various
8. Geographic location		
a. World (ozone, ultraviolet)	1-4	Various
b. Country region	1-4	Various
c. Urban-rural	1-4	Various

Conditions associated with cancer

Conditions	Range of confidence	Site
d. Rainfall	4	Nonspecific esophagus
9. Culture	2-4	Nonspecific
II. What People Do to Themselves		
A. Habits		
1. Drinking	1	Mouth, throat, larynx, liver, esophagus
2. Tobacco use		
a. Smoking, chewing, snuff-dipping	1-3	Lung, mouth throat, larynx, esophagus, bladder
3. Coffee	4	Nonspecific
4. Marijuana	4	Nonspecific
5. Narcotics (reduced risk)	4	Cervix
B. Customs and cultural behavior		
1. Cultural behaviors		
a. The sun cult	2	Skin
b. Breast feeding	4	Breast
c. Age at marriage	2-4	Breast, cervix
d. Size of family	4	Leukemia
e. Circumcision	2-4	Penis, cervix
f. Sick pets	4	Leukemia
g. Eating habits	4	Esophagus
2. Hygiene		
a. Washing, douching	4	Cervix
b. Mouth cleanliness	4	Oral
c. Trichomonas infection	1-3	Cervix
3. Intercourse		
a. Early, several partners	1-3	Cervix
b. Many other variables	2-4	Cervix

Conditions associated with cancer

Conditions	Range of confidence[a]	Site[b]
III. Diet		
A. Natural components and lacks		
1. Amount eaten	2-4	Nonspecific
2. Fat, protein	4	Colorectal
3. Vitamin deficiencies	3	Esophagus, other
4. Carcinogens	2-4	Various
B. Processing effects		
1. Refined foods and lost bulk	3-4	Colorectal
2. Preservatives and colorants	3-4	Nonspecific
3. Purification of water	4	Various
IV. What is Done to People		
A. Environmental pollution		
1. Pesticides, herbicides	4	Liver, nonspecific
2. Air pollution	2-4	Lung, nonspecific
3. Water pollution	4	Nonspecific
4. Ionizing radiation	1-4	Leukemia, thyroid, other
B. Occupation		
1. Carcinogen known		
a. Some examples: X-ray, uranium, asbestos, arsenic, polyvinyl-chloride, certain organic compounds, sun, benzo[a]pyrene	1-4	Various
2. Dangerous nonbehaviors	2-3	Various
C. Possible iatrogenic effects		
1. Drugs	1-4	Various
2. X-ray-therapy and diagnosis	1-4	Various
3. Irritation by prosthetics	3-4	Various
4. Immunosuppression (e.g., transplantation medication)	1-4	Various
Conditions associated with cancer		
5. Errors in diagnosing precancerous states	2-4	Various
6. Errors in diagnosing precancerous states	4	Hodgkin's disease

[a]Range of confidence that the condition is associated with higher or lower risk of cancer (personal judgment): (1) certain, (2) high to moderate, (3) moderate to low, (4) suspicion or not enough data.

[b]Site(s) that has been associated with the variable.

From Fox, BH. Cancer - The Behavioral Dimensions, pp 12-14, 1976. Reprinted with permission from Raven Press.

I will not reiterate the specific lifestyles determined to contribute to the causation of cancer or to their preventability whether described as feasible, potential, and/or practical. The recent work by Doll and Peto does this (5). The contributions of environmental and lifestyle factors to cancer causation have long been established. Controlling those factors is the problem at hand.

(1) The implementation of intervention designed to prevent cancers from known or proven causes, and (2) the verification of highly suspected causes of major types of cancer between now and the year 2,000 will be the two biggest challenges for the cancer research establishment. In the first category the proof that tobacco use, especially cigarette smoking, causes between 35% and 40% of all malignancies is established. Even though past efforts directed toward smoking cessation may have caused a decrease in use of cigarettes by some segments of society, deaths due to lung cancer and other tobacco-related sites continue to increase unabated, now in women as well as in men. Knowledge that tobacco products cause 35% to 40% of all cancers has not led to the successful prevention of smoking-related cancers by anyone's criteria (12). The American Cancer Society together with other voluntary health groups have shown a renewed interest in this public health problem (1). It is doubtful that the public or the health establishment will respond with any more enthusiasm or vigor than it has in the past.

The second challenge will be verification of the increasing suspicions that dietary habits resulting in certain nutritional milieus actually cause cancer and that changes in such dietary habits will, in fact, result in a decrease in cancer incidence. Doll and Peto (5) estimated overall that 30% of cancers may be caused by various dietary factors with a wide possible range of 10% to 70%. The National Research Council endorsed previous positive associations between dietary habits and cancer, and offered interim guidelines consistent with good nutritional practices (3). It was disappointing, however, that they stopped short of making quantitative estimates of the contribution of diet to cancer, and that they would not predict the percent reduction in risks that might be achieved by dietary modifications.

The prevention of cancer will eventually be implemented by the government exercising its regulatory authority, or by individuals exercising their personal lifestyle choices. Neither has been successful with regard to cigarette manufacture, subsidy, promotion, sales, and consumption. The latter method is, however, preferable to the former. The individual usually requires encouragement, guidance, and continuing involvement of the health professional. I believe the practitioners of cancer prevention in the future will be the physician, mostly as the provider of primary health care, together with the individual as its recipient.

The physician, either formally practicing epidemiology as a science, or practicing good bed-side medicine can continue to make etiologic observations. Identifying the causes or predisposing risk factors for cancer is essential for future potential for cancer prevention. The practicing physician in the community should be the first line of defense in the ultimate prevention and control of cancer (10). In addition to making etiologic observations, he/she is obligated to assess patient's risks for developing cancer, usually related to lifestyles, and to educate patients for changing harmful lifestyle practices (8). The third place where primary care physicians interface with cancer prevention is in screening and detection for early cancer while it is still treatable and often curable.

Traditionally, the clinician's training has been oriented toward the symptomatic patient, rather than to the care of well people. Only in the relatively recent past has the concept of disease prevention, as practiced by the public health specialist, been adopted by the clinical practitioner and incorporated into comprehensive patient care. The reason is simple. The primary care physician assumed responsibility for maintaining the health of his or her patients as well as the responsibility for treating their diseases. This will eventually change the role of the family physician into one of more participation in clinical research and more history taking oriented toward risk factors for cancer. This will lead to individual health-risk appraisals with recommendations for constructive change on the part of the patient.

In closing, I would like to impart several messages.

First, cancer prevention is a positive action or series of several positive actions. Taken together they are greater than the sum of their individual components. Second, cancer prevention has not one but two natural constituencies - primary care physicians, whose responsibility is now to keep people well, and those people who have more financial resources and leisure time to devote to staying well. Working together, this combination can create an enormous positive force. Third, everything does not cause cancer, but those things which do should be considered extremely seriously. Those things which might cause cancer (usually transmitted by the media from incomplete information) should be considered, but not excite overreaction. Those things that are not proven to cause cancer should be considered with guarded skepticism because our scientific knowledge is woefully incomplete. Fourth, basic, fundamental research is still required and should be supported with enthusiastic vigor by the public both in concept and with financial resources. Fifth, cancer is not one disease, but hundreds of diseases each with a personality and endurance of its own. However, three kinds of cancer account for 46% of all human cancer - lung, breast, and large bowel cancer. If every individual adopted prudent anti-cancer lifestyles, we could begin reducing the toll of cancer among Americans tomorrow, if not today. These include primary prevention by abstinence from tobacco consumption and adherence to proper diet, coupled with a program of secondary prevention for early detection of breast cancer in women and bowel cancer in men and women.

Many well-meaning and respected individuals have asked, "What, other than the cigarette smoking problems, can really be done to prevent cancer?" The answer to that question is not simple. Even if all cigarette smoking could be decreed to cease, there would still be cases of lung cancer occurring into the next century. If all individuals would change their dietary habits beginning today, it would take at least a generation if not two, for the resultant decrease in breast and colon cancers to be appreciable. In short, there is no "magic bullet" for preventing cancer just as there has not been one for treating it. Success will be measured in small increments both by individuals who have made a personal commitment to staying as healthy as possible, and by primary care physicians who have made the commitment to help them.

References

1. American Cancer Society (1981). Proceedings of the National Conference On Smoking Or Health, New York, November 18-20.
2. Cullen JW, Gritz ER (in press). Behavior modification for cancer prevention. In Newell GR (ed): "The Practice of Cancer Prevention in Clinical Medicine", New York: Raven Press.
3. Diet, Nutrition and Cancer (1982). Committee on Diet, Nutrition and Cancer. Assembly of Life Sciences, National Research Council. Washington, D.C: National Academy Press.
4. Doll, R (1967). Prevention of Cancer, Pointers from Epidemiology. The Rock Carling Fellowship. The Nuffield Provincial Hospitals Trust, 1967. London: The Whitefriars Press, Ltd.
5. Doll R, Peto R (1981). The causes of cancer: Quantitative estimates of avoidable risks of cancer in the United States today. JNCI 66:1191-1308.
6. Fox BH (1976). The psychosocial epidemiology of cancer. In Cullen JW, Fox BH, Isom RN (eds): "Cancer: The Behavioral Dimensions" New York, Raven Press, pp 11-22.
7. Fraumeni JF Jr (ed) (1975). "Persons at high risk of cancer. An approach to cancer etiology and control." New York: Academic Press.
8. Isom RN (1980). Cancer education: a professional responsibility. The Cancer Bull 32:154-156.
9. MacMahon, B (1975). Overview: Environmental Factors. In Fraumeni JF Jr (ed): "Persons at High Risk of Cancer. An approach to Cancer Etiology and Control," New York: Academic Press, pp 285-290.
10. Newell, GR and Webber, CF (in press). The primary care physician in cancer prevention. Family and Community Health.
11. Shimkin MB (1975). Overview: Preventive Oncology In Fraumeni JF Jr (ed): "Persons at High Risk of Cancer. An Approach to Cancer Etiology and Control," New York: Academic Press, pp 435-448.

12.   U.S. Department of Health and Human Services (1982).
      The Health Consequences of Smoking. Cancer. A
      report of the Surgeon General Public Health
      Service. Office of Smoking and Health.
      Superintendent of Documents. Washington, D.C.
      20302. U.S. Government Printing Office.
13.   World Health Organization (1964). Prevention of
      cancer. Geneva: WHO, (Technical Report Series
      276).

Progress in Cancer Control IV: Research in the Cancer Center, pages 67–81
© 1983 Alan R. Liss, Inc., 150 Fifth Avenue, New York, NY 10011

LINKING RESOURCES: CANCER CENTERS AND HEALTH DEPARTMENTS

Dwight T. Janerich, DDS   Kathleen Carlton, BA
Edward Fitzgerald, PhD   Philip C. Nasca, PhD
New York State Department of Health
Empire State Plaza
Albany, New York 12237

Cancer Control is a broad term that includes primary, secondary and tertiary prevention measures. Primary prevention involves preventing disease occurrence. Secondary prevention is designed to prevent mortality from cancers which have already occurred, and tertiary prevention focuses on effective treatment that enhances survival of advanced disease. Although health departments conduct cancer control activities which span the entire range of prevention, their programs can be most effective when focused on the former end of the spectrum.

In an earlier era, health departments worked effectively in conjunction with microbiology laboratories to bring about the control of infectious diseases. In our current era the focus is on chronic disease prevention with a special emphasis on cancer control. A mission similar to the one which lead to the control of infectious diseases can be accomplished through a partnership between health departments and cancer centers. The examples presented here are selected to illustrate areas where such a partnership offers the potential for effective cancer control.

In New York State, we are working towards linking the cancer control activities of three Comprehensive Cancer Centers with those of the State Department of Health. This provides a mechanism for extending the scientific and clinical expertise of the cancer centers out to the entire population which is the responsibility of the State Health Department. Integrating the activities of four major New York institutions can provide a comprehensive approach to conducting cancer control research within a population-based setting, and provides for more efficient utilization of limited resources.

The audience is probably more familiar with those programs conducted in the cancer centers than with those of a health department. Therefore, concentration will be given to describing the cancer control activities conducted by the New York State Department of Health.

TABLE 1
DEVELOPMENT AND IMPLMENETATION
OF DISEASE CONTROL MEASURES

I SCIENTIFIC INVESTIGATION

II PROPOSAL FOR PREVENTIVE STRATEGY

III LIMITED TRIAL

IV GENERAL CHANGE IN CLINICAL PRACTICE OR IN
PUBLIC HEALTH REGULATIONS

V MONITORING FOR EVIDENCE OF POPULATION EFFECT

Table 1 presents an outline of a strategy for development and implementation of disease control measures. Phases I and II are generally the focus of programs conducted by the cancer centers. The Limited Trial Phase (III) may be handled by either a health department or a cancer center, while the final phases are often the province of health departments.

DES

The New York State Department of Health is actively involved in many specific cancer control programs at various levels of development and implementation. I would like to begin with the Department's DES program. This program is an example of a Phase V disease control measure.

Diethylstilbestrol (DES) is a synthetic non-steroidal estrogen that was first produced in 1938. In 1948, its use during pregnancy was recommended to prevent miscarriages and premature births and to treat diabetes and toxemia. There was extensive use of DES in pregnancy during the late

1940's and early 1950's. However, a controlled clinical
trial in 1955 concluded that DES did not reduce the incidence of miscarriage, prematurity, post-maturity, perinatal
mortality, or toxemias. Although there was a decline in the
use of DES during pregnancy following this report, common
use did continue until 1971 when the FDA banned its use
during pregnancy.

The New York State Department of Health conducted
investigations which confirmed an association between pre-
natal exposure to DES and the subsequent development of
clear cell vaginal adenocarcinoma (Greenwald, et al, 1971).
Although the risk of clear cell adenocarcinoma among DES
exposed female offspring (DES daughters) is low (1 in
10,000), a much larger proportion of the DES offspring, male
and female, have urogenital abnormalities associated with
exposures. While these abnormalities are noncancerous,
they are adversely affecting fertility and reproductive outcomes. In addition, there is still concern that DES exposed
mothers, daughters and sons may be at higher risk of developing other cancers as they age. In 1978, the New York State
Legislature passed a bill to establish a DES program to
deal with the adverse health effects associated with DES
exposure for the estimated 300,000 DES exposed persons in
New York State. The objectives of this program are:

1. To identify individuals exposed to DES.
2. To inform exposed individuals of their increased
   risk of adverse health effects, including clear
   cell adenocarcinomas of the vagina.
3. To assure proper medical care for the diagnosis
   and treatment of these adverse health effects for
   those who cannot otherwise afford it.

In order to accomplish the first two goals, a multi-
media, state-wide educational campaign was conducted for a
year and a half. A volunteer confidential DES registry was
also established via a toll free "DES Hotline." The purpose
of the registry is two-fold; 1) to alert registrants to any
new developments regarding DES exposure and 2) to carry out
long term follow-up and research into the adverse health
affects associated with DES exposure. The toll free number
is 1-800-462-1884.

To accomplish the third goal, seven DES Screening
Centers are being funded around the state to provide con-

sultation and screening. These centers are located in
major medical facilities and have the resources available
to deal with any other adverse health effects that may
arise as this exposed population ages.

TRENDS IN FEMALE CANCER

Another major cancer control function of the New York
State Department of Health involves the monitoring of cancer
morbidity and mortality rates. This is accomplished via the
data set maintained by the State's Cancer Registry. The
Registry can report incidence and mortality data on the
county level. By examining site-specific cancer rates by
county, or by other subgroups, researchers are able to
identify high risk groups which may benefit from the initiation of a screening program. The Registry also provides a
mechanism for monitoring changes in cancer mortality. For
example, breast cancer has been the leading cause of cancer
mortality among women in New York State, but analysis of
Registry data shows that during 1983 lung cancer will become
the leading cause of cancer death among women (Figure 1)
(Greenwald, Polan 1979). In addition, further analysis
demonstrates that shortly after the year 2000, female deaths
due to lung cancer will equal those of men (Figure 2).

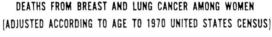

**DEATHS FROM BREAST AND LUNG CANCER AMONG WOMEN
(ADJUSTED ACCORDING TO AGE TO 1970 UNITED STATES CENSUS)**

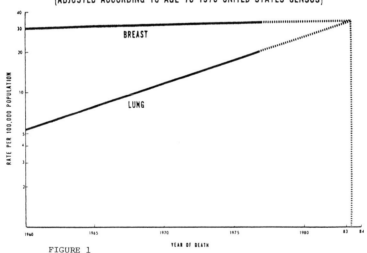

FIGURE 1

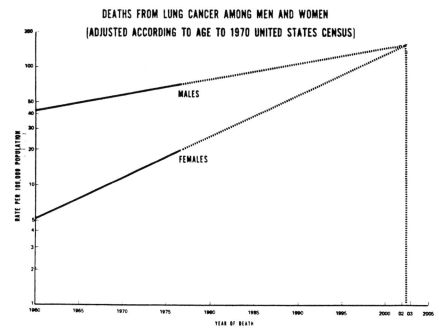

DEATHS FROM LUNG CANCER AMONG MEN AND WOMEN
(ADJUSTED ACCORDING TO AGE TO 1970 UNITED STATES CENSUS)

- THE DATA ARE FOR NEW YORK STATE, EXCLUDING NEW YORK CITY, FOR THE PERIOD 1960 TO 1977.
- THE DASHED LINES SHOW PROJECTED TRENDS.

FIGURE 2

Analyses of data from a recent study of female breast cancer mortality (Upstate New York, 1970-77) show that while the mortality rates for white females did not change, the mortality for nonwhites increased (Notani, et al, 1982). Increased mortality for nonwhites was evident at all age groups over 30 years, whereas for whites an increase was observed only for women over 80 years. These data were also analyzed by county for differences in mortality rates. Nassau, Suffolk and Erie counties had the highest rates (Notani, et al, 1982). The significantly elevated rate in Nassau County has resulted in the initiation of a scientific investigation. The aim of this project is to identify groups of women who are at high risk of breast cancer. This information will be then utilized to develop a cost-effective intervention strategy.

The Pap smear is a cytologic method used to detect precursor lesions of the cervix (Papanicolau and Trout, 1943). It has been widely used for decades as a screening

technique for cervical cancer, but randomized clinical
trials were never conducted to rigorously test its effectiveness (Shapiro, 1975; Bailar, 1979). Such a trial is no
longer ethical, since the Pap smear is such a commonly
accepted, effective cancer control procedure. Its role in
reducing cervical cancer incidence and mortality must therefore be evaluated from non-experimental studies. Many of
these investigations have been reviewed elsewhere (Guzick,
1978). These are frequently mass screening programs, and
their results generally support the conclusion that the
Pap testing for cervical cancer is efficacious.

Another method to assess the effectiveness of screening
for cervical cancer is to examine its distribution by stage.
The rationale is the belief that if screening is successful,
more cases will be detected in the earlier in situ stage
than in the later invasive stage. The ratio of invasive to
in situ carcinoma should therefore be an indicator of Pap
smear testing effectiveness, with a relatively low ratio
suggestive of more successful screening and a comparatively
high ratio indicative of less effective screening.

A preliminary investigation of this issue was conducted in upstate New York (Ellish, 1982; Janerich, et al,
1982). Using data supplied by the New York State Cancer
Registry, the ratio of invasive to in situ cases of cervical
cancer was calculated for the 57 upstate New York counties
for 1974-1976. The counties were then ranked by descending
order of the ratio and divided into terciles. They were
labelled as "poor," "medium" or "good" concerning effective Pap screening, depending on whether the ratio was high,
medium, or low, respectively.

As shown in Table 2, the overall ratio for upstate
New York was 0.47. In other words, there were approximately
half as many cases of invasive cancer as in situ cases. As
the ratio decreased from the average value of 0.76 for "poor"
to 0.32 for "good" counties, the crude incidence rate for
invasive cervical cancer declined from 16.3 to 11.6 per
100,000. The crude incidence rate for carcinoma in situ,
however, was inversely related to the ratio, since it
increased from 21.6 for "poor" to 36.4 per 100,000 for
"good" counties. The crude annual mortality rates, calculated for the three year intervals 1974-1976 and 1977-1979,
exhibited a pattern similar to that observed for invasive
incidence, i.e., it was positively associated with the ratio.

As with invasive incidence, the largest difference in mortality rates was that between the "poor" and "medium" counties. For the "medium" and "good" counties, mortality rates were very similar. For all three groups, the mortality rates for 1977-1979 were lower than those for 1974-1976.

These preliminary data show an apparent difference by county in screening effectiveness as measured by the ratio of invasive to in situ cervical cancer and this ranking, in turn, is related to cervical cancer mortality experience. The counties in the "poor" category had the highest ratio, lowest in situ incidence, highest invasive incidence, and highest mortality. The "medium" and "good" categories differed primarily in their incidence of in situ cases, with the "good" counties having a higher incidence. Invasive cervical cancer, as measured by incidence and mortality rates, may exhibit a threshold effect, since it is reduced to a certain extent by effective screening, but a level is reached beyond which screening has no impact.

TABLE 2

CRUDE ANNUAL INCIDENCE RATES (1974-1976) AND MORTALITY

RATES (1974-1979) PER 100,000 FEMALE POPULATION FOR

CERVICAL CANCER IN UPSTATE NEW YORK

	COUNTY GROUPS*			
	POOR	MEDIUM	GOOD	TOTAL
NUMBER OF COUNTIES	19	19	19	57
RANGE OF RATIOS*	3.00-.62	.62-.43	.42-0.00	3.00-0.00
GROUP RATIO*	.76	.50	.32	.47
INVASIVE CERVICAL CANCER INCIDENCE RATES	16.3	12.1	11.6	12.7
CARCINOMA IN SITU INCIDENCE RATES	21.6	24.4	36.4	27.2
MORTALITY RATES (1974-76)	6.0	4.6	4.7	4.9
MORTALITY RATES (1977-79)	5.6	4.1	3.9	4.3

*BASED ON THE RATIO OF INVASIVE TO IN SITU CASES OF CERVICAL CANCER

Table 3 presents the female population, the number of in situ and invasive cases, and the number of cervical cancer deaths by county. As Table 3 indicates, 21 deaths from cervical cancer in New York State could have been prevented if the lowest mortality rate prevailed. The implication is that these lives may have been saved if a more intensive screening program was employed in the other groups of counties. Furthermore, it is likely that more effective procedures, even in the "good" counties, could lower mortality even further.

TABLE 3

FEMALE POPULATION (1975), ANNUAL NUMBER OF CASES OF INVASIVE AND

IN SITU CERVICAL CANCER (1974-1976) AND ANNUAL NUMBER OF CERVICAL

CANCER DEATHS (1974-1979) FOR UPSTATE NEW YORK

COUNTY GROUPS*

	POOR	MEDIUM	GOOD	TOTAL
FEMALE POPULATION	1,005,269	2,919,127	1,519,746	5,444,142
Number of cases of invasive cervical cancer	164	354	176	694
Number of cases of carcinoma in situ	217	713	553	1483
Annual number of deaths (1974-76)	60	134	71	265
Annual number of deaths (1977-79)	56	120	60	236
Expected deaths** (1977-79)	40	115	60	215
Excess deaths (Observed minus expected)	16	5	0	21

*Based on ratio of invasive to in situ cases of cervical cancer

**Expected based on 1977-1979 mortality rate for "Good" counties

It should be noted that these results are preliminary. Adjustments must be made for age and hysterectomy, since unequal distribution of these two variables throughout the state could affect incidence and mortality rates. Other risk factors which can influence cervical cancer, such as socioeconomic status, may also be considered. The results nevertheless suggest that more effective screening in certain upstate New York counties can further reduce the incidence and mortality rates for invasive cervical cancer.

LOVE CANAL

The New York State Department of Health has also conducted a study of cancer incidence in the Love Canal area (Janerich et al, 1981). This activity differs from those previously discussed. The Love Canal study has implications for prevention, but was primarily a scientific investigation assessing whether exposure to toxic wastes was related to the development of cancer. The purpose of including it in this discussion is to demonstrate how a state health department may be involved in the full range of disease control measures, e.g., etiologic as well as applied research and epidemiologic study in addition to health education and promotion.

Over eighty chemicals have been identified in the Love Canal dumpsite. They include benzene and trichlorethylene, compounds which are carcinogenic in humans or animals. To determine if the contamination of the Love Canal area with these chemicals resulted in excess cancer among its residents, data from the New York Cancer Registry were used for the years 1955 through 1977. This period spans the interval between the time the dumping stopped (about 1953) and the point public concern about health hazards associated with buried wastes began (early 1978).

During these years, the population of the census tract surrounding the Love Canal grew rapidly. According to the 1970 census, the tract contained 4,897 persons. Approximately 700 individuals lived on or near the dumpsite. Population data were also available from the 1960 decennial census and a special census in 1967. Linear interpolation or extrapolation were used for the other years of the study to obtain denominator data for the calculation of incidence rates.

Standardized incidence rates (SIR's) were calculated for each cancer site by dividing the observed number of cancer cases in the Love Canal tract by the number expected (Lilienfeld 1976). The expected number was derived by applying the annual age-, sex-, and site-specific incidence rates for upstate New York to the Love Canal population. Statistical significance was assessed by the Poisson distribution.

Table 4. Reported Cases of Liver, Lymphoma and Leukemia
Comparisons of Observed and Expected Numbers
Love Canal Census Tract
1955-1965 and 1966-1977[a]

Time Period/Cancer (ICD 9th Revision)	MALES				FEMALES			
	Obs.	Exp.[b]	5% Sig. Limits[c]	SIR[d]	Obs.	Exp.[b]	5% Sig. Limits[c]	SIR[d]
1955-1965								
Liver (155)	0	0.4	0-2	0.0	2	0.3	0-1	6.7
Lymphomas (200-202)	3	2.5	0-5	1.2	2	1.8	0-4	1.1
Leukemias (204-208)	2	2.3	0-5	0.9	3	1.7	0-4	1.8
1966-1977								
Liver (155)	2	0.6	0-2	3.3	0	0.4	0-2	0.0
Lymphomas (200-202)	0	3.2	0-6	0.0	4	2.5	0-5	1.6
Leukemias (204-208)	1	2.5	0-5	0.4	2	1.8	0-4	1.1
1955-1977								
Liver (155)	2	1.0	0-3	2.0	2	0./	0-2	2.9
Lymphomas (200-202)	3	5.6	2-11	0.5	6	4.3	1-8	1.4
Leukemias (204-208)	3	4.8	1-9	0.6	5	3.5	0-7	1.4

[a] Cases by year of report for 1955-1965; by year of diagnosis for 1966-1977.

[b] Computed by applying age-specific rates for Upstate New York to the population estimated for the Love Canal Census Tract

[c] Five percent, approximately, of sample values fall outside of these limits in a Poisson distribution with a mean equal to the stated expected value. For example, for females in the 1955-65 period, the two cases of liver cancer are outside of the 0-1 limits and are statistically significant at the five percent level. This five percent is entirely in the upper tail when the expected value is 3.6 or less.

[d] Ratio of observed number to expected number (age-standardized).

The results are shown for liver cancer, lymphoma, and leukemia in Table 4. These cancers are the most likely neoplastic outcomes if chemical contamination at the Love Canal resulted in actual human exposure, given studies of the effects of benzene and halogenated hydrocarbons (Lemen et al, 1978; Popper, 1979; McConnell and Moore, 1979). There was no evidence of any elevated risk for lymphoma or leukemia. For liver cancer, the SIR was statistically significant only for females from 1955 to 1965. None of these liver cancer patients lived in close proximity to the dumpsite.

Table 5 gives SIR's for other selected cancer sites. None showed statistical significance except the respiratory system, which was elevated for both sexes. This finding was examined in greater depth by comparing the SIR for Love Canal with those for the 24 other census tracts which compromise the city of Niagara Falls. As Table 6 illustrates, seven other census tracts, as well as the city in general, had statistically significant SIR's for respiratory cancer among men. One other tract also had a significantly higher SIR for female respiratory cancer. The street addresses of these respiratory cancer patients, however, indicated no tendency for cases to be located in close proximity to the dumpsite, nor were they clustered in any other pattern that suggested an association between the cancers and the location of the chemical wastes.

Although the SIR's for respiratory cancer in the Love Canal area were higher than the city averages, the rates for Love Canal did not differ significantly from those for the 24 other census tracts. In other words, instead of being Love Canal-specific, the elevated risk of lung cancer in that tract may simply reflect a high rate for the entire city of Niagara Falls. The magnitude of the increased frequency is within the range of those that have been associated with factors such as cigarette smoking. The design of the study, however, precluded the testing of such a hypothesis. Other important factors which could not be examined include migration and latency periods. These limitations are common restrictions in any investigation of occupational and environmental hazards. The study nevertheless demonstrates how the resources of a state health department may be employed to empirically address issues of public health significance.

Table 5. Reported Cases of Selected Cancer Sites
Comparisons of Observed and Expected Numbers
Love Canal Census Tract - 1966-1977[a]

Site (ICD 9th Revision)	MALES				FEMALES			
	Obs.	Exp.[b]	5% Sig[c] Limits	SIR[d]	Obs.	Exp.[b]	5% Sig[c] Limits	SIR[d]
Buccal Cavity & Pharynx (140-149)	2	2.7	0-6	0.7	1	1.1	0-3	0.9
Digestive Organs (150-154) (156-159)	13	15.7	8-24	0.8	15	13.8	7-22	1.1
Respiratory System (160-165)	25	15.0	8-23	1.7	9	4.6	1-8	2.0
Connective Tissue, Bone, Skin & Breast (170-172) (174-175)	2	2.1	0-5	1.0	27	21.2	13-31	1.3
Genital Organs (179-187)	13	7.9	3-14	1.6	8	12.5	6-20	0.6
Bladder, Kidney, Ureter (188-189)	7	6.0	2-11	1.2	1	2.4	0-5	0.4
Liver, Lymphoma, Leukemia (155, 200-202, 204-208[e])	3	6.3	2-12	0.5	6	4.7	1-9	1.3
All other (190-199, 203)	6	5.1	1-10	1.2	4	5.1	1-10	0.8
All Sites (140-172, 174-208)	71	60.8	46-77	1.2	71	65.4	50-82	1.1

a) Cases by year of diagnosis.

b) Computed by applying age-specific rates for Upstate New York to the population estimated for the Love Canal Census Tract.

c) Five percent, approximately, of sample values fall outside of these limits in a Poisson distribution with a mean equal to the stated expected value. The five percent is entirely in the upper tail when the expected value is 3.6 or less.

d) Ratio of observed number to be expected number of (age-standardized).

e) See table 4 for details.

Table 6.   Reported Cases of Cancer of the Respiratory System[a]
Comparisons of Observed and Expected Numbers
By Census Tract, Niagara Falls, N.Y.
1966-1977[b]

Census Tract	MALES				FEMALES			
	Obs.	Exp.[c]	5% Sig. Limits[c]	SIR[a]	Obs.	Exp.[c]	5% Sig. Limits[c]	SIR[a]
Love Canal	25	15.0	8-23	1.7	9	4.6	1-8	2.0
A	24	29.5	19-41	0.8	16	8.2	3-14	2.0
B	13	10.5	5-17	1.2	2	3.0	0-6	0.7
C	13	9.7	4-16	1.3	0	2.6	0-5	0.0
D	14	14.6	8-23	1.0	5	4.4	1-9	1.1
E	28	22.7	14-32	1.2	10	7.8	3-14	1.3
F	18	16.5	9-25	1.1	10	5.0	1-10	2.0
G	26	22.4	14-32	1.2	5	6.3	2-12	0.8
H	8	7.8	3-14	1.0	3	2.1	0-5	1.4
I	32	20.1	12-29	1.6	7	5.7	2-11	1.2
J	28	26.5	17-37	1.1	5	7.0	2-13	0.7
K	23	20.3	12-30	1.1	8	6.6	2-12	1.2
L	18	21.6	13-31	0.9	3	6.7	2-12	0.4
M	18	20.7	12-30	0.9	10	5.8	2-11	1.7
N	34	17.6	10-26	1.9	3	4.9	1-10	0.6
O	34	19.9	12-29	1.7	4	5.2	1-10	0.8
P	26	13.7	7-21	1.9	2	3.4	0-7	0.6
Q	28	18.5	11-27	1.5	5	5.3	1-10	0.9
R	19	14.0	7-22	1.4	8	3.7	1-8	2.2
S	15	6.2	2-12	2.4	2	1.6	0-4	1.3
T	27	16.5	9-25	1.6	6	4.5	1-9	1.3
U	19	13.7	7-21	1.4	1	3.4	0-7	0.3
V	27	25.6	16-36	1.1	7	7.1	2-13	1.0
W	17	18.2	10-27	0.9	9	5.4	1-10	1.7
X	13	10.5	5-17	1.2	1	2.7	0-6	0.4
Niagara Falls City	547	432.1	391-473	1.3	141	123.2	102-145	1.1

[a] ICD 9th, 1975 160-165.

[b] Cases by year of diagnosis.

[c] Computed by applying age-specific rates for Upstate New York to the population estimated for the census tract.

Five percent, approximately, of sample values fall outside of these limits in a Poisson distribution with a mean equal to the stated expected value. The five percent is entirely in the upper tail when the expected value is 3.6 or less.

Ratios of observed number to expected number (age-standardized).

CONCLUSION

    The major tools for cancer control activities are found mainly in clinical practice and are usually conventional in major cancer centers. The resources for strategic deployment of these tools are concentrated in health departments and in other population based centers. Optimum use of the tools for cancer control can be achieved by linking the resources of both types of facilities in order to identify the subgroup of the population which can receive the greatest benefit from cancer control resources and to monitor the results of the strategic application of these tools.

    We have presented selected examples of areas where health department resources, particularly data from cancer registry reports and vital records, have been used to identify specific needs or to target the application of cancer control measures. Program efficiency and economies of scale from large population based activities are the major benefits that can be produced by linking the resources of cancer centers and health departments, but there are also ethnical and social benefits that can accrue from programs that are capable of assuring that "hidden" or overlooked segments of the population receive their fair share of benefits of the cancer control capability that is evolving from the cancer research community.

    Cancer centers are often not involved with individuals until they have, or are suspected of having, cancer. Health departments on the other hand are involved with an entire population throughout their lifetime. Therefore, early intervention, like that required for primary or secondary prevention of cancer, can be effectively routed to the entire population by being attached to existing health department programs. In this way significant efficiency can be gained by linking the resources of cancer centers and health departments.

Bailar JC (1979). The case for cancer prevention. J Natl Cancer Inst 62:727.

Ellish NJ, Janerich DT (1982). Cancer screening - A state health department prospective. In Mettlin C, Murphy GP (eds): "Issues in Cancer Screening and Communications," New York: Alan R. Liss, p 67.

Greenwald P, Barlow JJ, Nasca PC, Burnett WS (1971). Vaginal cancer after maternal treatment with synthetic estrogens. N Engl J Med 285:390-392.

Greenwald P, Polan AK (1979). Lung cancer deaths among
women (Letter). N Engl J Med: 274.

Guzick DS (1978). Efficacy of screening for cervical
cancer: A review. AJPH 68:125.

Janerich DT, Ellish NJ, Howe HL, Greenwald P (1982). Pre-
vention and early detection. In "Proceedings of the
Third National Conference on Cancer Nursing/1981,
"American Cancer Society, Inc., p 6.

Janerich DT, Burnett WS, Feck G, Hoff M, Nasca P, Polednak
AP, Greenwald P, Vianna N (1981). Cancer incidence in
the Love Canal area. Science 212:1401.

Lemen RA, Brown DP, Rinsky RA, Mernhardt TJ (1978). Health
problems associated with selected petrochemicals: Benzene,
chlorinated hydrocarbons, and styrene-butadiene rubber.
In Nieburgh HE (ed), "Prevention and Detection of Cancer,"
New York: Decker, p 1879.

Lilienfeld AM (1976). "Foundations of Epidemiology."
New York: Oxford University Press, p 62.

McConnell EE, Moore JA (1979). Toxicopathology characteristics of the halogenated aromatics. Ann NY Acad Sci
320:138.

Notani PN, Varma AO, Leske MC, Janerich DT (1982). Breast
cancer in New York State. Trends in female mortality
1970-1977. NYS J Med 82:1044-1049.

Papanicolaou GN, Trout HF (1943). "The Diagnosis of Uterine
Cancer by the Vaginal Smear." New York: The Commonwealth
Fund.

Popper H (1979). Hepatic cancers in man: Quantitative perspectives. Environ Res 19:482.

Shapiro S (1975). Screening for early detection of cancer
and heart disease. Bull NY Acad Med 51:80.

I. PATIENT AND PUBLIC EDUCATION ABOUT CANCER

Progress in Cancer Control IV: Research in the Cancer Center, pages 85–89
© 1983 Alan R. Liss, Inc., 150 Fifth Avenue, New York, NY 10011

MEETING THE EDUCATIONAL NEEDS OF ADOLESCENTS WITH CANCER

Barbara D. Blumberg, Sc. M.

Office of Cancer Communications
National Cancer Institute
Bethesda, Md. 20205

Adolescence is a relatively short period in which a number of developmental tasks are typically accomplished against a backdrop of rapid physical growth. Review of the literature in medicine, nursing, and the behavioral sciences (Blumberg, Flaherty 1980; Kellerman, Katz 1977; Moore, Holton, 1969), along with interviews with experts in the field, established that adolescents are confronted with special developmental tasks that are different than those of younger children or adults. These include: establishing independence from parents and other adults, entering into mature relationships with peers of both sexes, and beginning to plan for the future. When the adolescent has cancer, these tasks are compounded by the realities of the disease and its treatment -- hospitalization, disruption of schooling and other activities, separation from peers, side effects of treatment, and dependence on parents and caregivers. However, despite the peculiar needs of this audience, little or no information was available to help them cope.

To fill this gap, the National Cancer Institute (NCI) and Adria Laboratories undertook a project whose objective was the development of educational materials for adolescents with cancer. It was anticipated that materials developed would help adolescents cope with the disease, its treatment, and the impact of these on the developmental tasks confronting them. Throughout the project, adolescents with cancer were viewed as normal teenagers whose development was complicated by the diagnosis of cancer and concomitant treatment.

In order to develop materials that had the potential of

meeting the information and psychosocial needs of this
audience, a research project was designed to identify issues
of concern and confirm these through data collected from
adolescents and caregivers. The methodology chosen was
pretesting, a type of formative evaluation that allows for
the assessment of comprehension, attitudes, and other
perceptions of target audience members to concepts and draft
materials in early stages of planning and development. It
also provides for the systematic gathering of reactions to
materials before their final production (National Cancer
Institute, 1981).

Pretesting is a qualitative, not quantitative methodology.
It does not yield results reportable in terms of their statistical significance. The diagnostic or formative information
gleaned from pretesting can lead to improvements in materials
while revisions are still possible and affordable. Although
pretesting will not guarantee successful finished products,
it can help reduce some of the uncertainty and risk of
producing materials that may be misunderstood or misinter-
preted.

In total, 89 responses were collected from patients at
four treatment centers: St. Jude Children's Research Center,
M.D. Anderson Hospital and Tumor Institute, Cardinal Glennon
Hospital (St. Louis, Mo.), and Memorial Sloan-Kettering Cancer
Center. Respondents were between the ages of 13 and 19.
Participating institutions were chosen based on patient
population and interest expressed by treatment center staff.
Informed consent forms satisfying both the NCI and specific
center requirements were signed by all patients and by
parents for those under age 18.

All patients were either currently on treatment or had
been on treatment while teenagers; 62% were male and 38%
were female. Diagnoses included: leukemia, non-Hodgkin's
lymphoma, Hodgkin's disease, Ewing's sarcoma, osteosarcoma,
brain tumors, and rhabdosarcoma.

Fifty-three health professionals who work with adolescent
patients also participated. They represented the four institutions already mentioned plus Georgetown University Hospital,
Vincent T. Lombardi Cancer Center, Roswell Park Memorial
Institute, and the Mayo Comprehensive Cancer Center.
Respondents represented the following disciplines: nursing,
medicine, social work, psychology, recreational therapy,

physical therapy, pharmacy, and pastoral counseling.

Pretesting was conducted in two stages. During the first stage, short discussion papers addressing psychosocial ramifications of cancer and its treatment were developed and used as a forum for target audience response. The objectives of this stage of research were to:

- determine whether the information addressed in the papers was relevant and complete;
- obtain tips or suggestions for coping with cancer, treatment, and accompanying problems;
- gather anecdotal experiences and colloquial language for incorporation into materials to be developed; and
- obtain direction for appropriate media for materials development.

Data were collected via one-to-one interviews with patients and self-administered questionnaires with health professionals.

The stage one pretest confirmed that adolescent patients had little or no access to written or audiovisual information about their cancers. Overall the issues identified and discussion of them were found to be valid. Points of interest included observations that:

- patients almost uniformly urged that progress in cancer treatment be stressed;
- patients reacted negatively to anything implying that they were different from others;
- although patients had little to say about loss of friends, caregivers indicated this to be a problem;
- caregivers felt that patients would respond favorably to the information and that they would provide it to patients; and
- a combination of a written piece and an audiotape seemed to be the preferred media.

Based on these findings, a 64-page booklet and a one-hour audiotape of radioplay-style dramatizations for patients, and a user's guide for health professionals were developed.

Before producing these materials in final form, a second pretest was conducted with a different group of patients and health professionals. The purpose of this pretest was to assure that the materials contained accurate, appropriate, and useful information, and were in a form that adolescents and caregivers would use. Mock-ups of potential covers and formats were also developed for testing.

Data were collected via a combination of one-to-one and group interviews and self-administered questionnaires with patients and self-administered questionnaires with professionals.

The second pretest of the audiotape showed that, with the exception of one dramatization, adolescents found the stories and issues reasonable, but felt the music and characters to be overly dramatic and unbelievable. Responses to the dramatization concerning a young woman's decision to marry and have a child following cancer treatment showed that adolescents, and particularly males, did not identify with the story and its main character. Specific reactions to this and the other dramatizations provided information on where characters and plot were believable and whether main points were communicated.

Revisions to the booklet included modifying quotes by patients and adding puzzles and games to create a more magazine-like format. A new cover photo showed adolescents with cancer and their friends and siblings.

Pretest finding indicated that both professionals and patients felt that sexuality and reproduction should be addressed, but on an individual basis. As a result, a note was added to the user's guide recommending personal discussion of these topics.

As a result of the formative research described, a unit of materials for adolescents with cancer and health professionals was produced. This unit, entitled, "Help Yourself - Tips for Teenagers with Cancer", consists of three parts.

1. A 36-page booklet discussing reactions to diagnosis, life at the clinic or hospital, changes in physical appearance, relations with family and friends, continuation of schooling, recurrence, and the future. The booklet emphasizes maintenance of positive attitudes and a sense of control, developing coping skills, and self-help techniques.

2. A 45-minute audiotape containing four radioplay-style dramatizations on issues adolescents with cancer face,

including accepting a diagnosis, sharing feeling between patient and family, adjusting to treatment-induced changes, and relating to friends.

3. A 4-page user's guide for health professionals containing a summary description of the booklet and tape. Discussion topics for each dramatization are also provided.

The health professional package consists of the booklet, audiotape, and user's guide. The patient package consists of the booklet and audiotape.

This approach to materials development can be utilized in other settings and with other populations. Pretesting materials or programs allows for the organized collection of input from the target audience to methods and materials before they are produced in their final form.

The qualititive methodology used in the preparation of these materials has the potential of increasing their acceptance by and usefulness to adolescents with cancer. This methodology is recommended to others developing educational materials.

References

Blumberg B, Flaherty M, Lewis J, eds. (1980). "Coping with Cancer: A Resource for the Health Professional". National Cancer Institute, pp. 72-77.

Kellerman J, Katz EB (1977). The Adolescent with Cancer: Theoretical, Clinical, and Research Issues. J Pediatr Psychol 2(3): 127-31.

Moore DC, Holton CP, Martin GW (1969). Psychologic Problems in the Management of Adolescents with Malignancy. Clin Pediatr 8(8): 464-73.

National Cancer Institute (1981). "Pretesting in Health Communications", pp. v. 1.

Progress in Cancer Control IV: Research in the Cancer Center, pages 91–97
© 1983 Alan R. Liss, Inc., 150 Fifth Avenue, New York, NY 10011

PROJECT CHOICE: EVALUATING A SCHOOL-AGE CANCER PREVENTION
AND RISK-REDUCTION CURRICULUM

David Docter; Terry Janicki, Ph.D.; Connie Hansen

Fred Hutchinson Cancer Research Center
1124 Columbia Street
Seattle, WA 98104

Project CHOICE is a comprehensive, grade-sequential
cancer prevention and risk-reduction curriculum for grades
kindergarten through senior high school. Developed by staff
of the Fred Hutchinson Cancer Research Center Cancer Control
Program in cooperation with the Superintendent of Public
Instruction in Washington state, Project CHOICE has been
evaluated statewide, and soon will be available for general
distribution.

Frequently, school curricula are purchased by education
specialists and placed in schools without specific evidence
that the new curriculum will be effective in achieving its
stated learning objectives. If the teachers enjoy teaching
the program and the students respond, the curriculum is
accepted and becomes a regular part of the school year.
Assuming that the students score reasonably well on an end
of unit knowledge exam, the curriculum's impact goes
unquestioned (Bartlett 1981).

Current literature has shown that knowledge change is
not sufficient to engender behavior change, thus creating
serious questions about health curricula; in particular,
about those that are designed to bring about behavioral
change, but which, in fact, can only be shown to increase
knowledge.

In this respect, then, it should no longer be acceptable
in school health education to merely accept teacher and
student enthusiasm, and knowledge gain, as evidence of a
curriculum's worth; nor should we be so willing to equate

the success of any public education; i.e., cancer control programs, with the number of people who attend the programs, how many brochures are distributed, and how many people tell us how much they liked the program.

What follows will be a brief rendition of how a comprehensive cancer education program has been developed, and how, once developed, its impact was formally evaluated. While it would be presumptuous to claim that the developmental and evaluation processes for Project CHOICE are the only means by which health education programs can be deemed valid, the process may provide a model from which we can learn to be more demanding when we proclaim the worth of programs. For health education to gain its proper place along side medical research, it must adopt stringent requirements for proof of effectiveness similar to those imposed upon new drugs before they reach the marketplace.

Project CHOICE resulted, importantly, from a community request rather than from a research institute office. At the request of statewide educators who attended a cancer center-sponsored education program, a grant was successfully submitted to the National Cancer Institute to develop a school education curriculum to meet what the educators saw as a vacuum in health education materials. By forming a cooperative liaison between the worlds of school education and health science, the project got off to solid beginnings.

Over the next 18 months, Project CHOICE received input from teachers and students who allowed the project into their classrooms to test the developing curriculum ideas and activities. With added input from the state supervisor for health education, statewide curriculum specialists and members of the Hutchinson Center's medical and scientific staffs, the curriculum took shape cognizent of teachers' and students' needs, and at the same time, accurate both medically and epidemiologically. As considerable controversy exists in several areas of cancer etiology, care had to be taken in what the curriculum materials said or implied. Designed to be taught by the regular classroom teacher, particular care had to be taken that delicate concepts of risk and causation not be overstated or exaggerated.

Project CHOICE began with the identification of two basic goals:
    1) That students will institute behaviors to minimize

the risk of getting cancer; and knowing that complete cancer prevention currently is not possible,

2) That students will institute behaviors for early detection and appropriate treatment of cancer.

The curriculum activities were designed to teach cancer information and to develop the attitudes and skills to help students evaluate health information, and take responsibility for and make decisions for their own health. Teachers, curriculum specialists and a youth advisory committee provided constant input to staff during the course of initial program design and development. Specific learning objectives were developed to provide the directional focus to activities and materials.

Eight broad areas of cancer risk are addressed in the curriculum at varying grade levels: Host Factors; Drugs--including alcohol and tobacco; Occupational Hazards; Stress; Environmental Factors--including radiation exposure; Nutrition; Sexual and Reproductive Behavior, and Sun Exposure. While some of these topics represent well-established causal links to cancer, others are only beginning to show possible relationships. The difference is meticulously explained in the activities and in the teacher resource materials.

Upon completion of the first prototype units, pilot sessions were carried out in several school districts. Each lesson at each grade level was observed by staff as it was being taught in the classroom; and teachers and students were invited to contribute their comments. This initial process evaluation led to curriculum revisions. The revised results were also piloted in school classrooms before the final prototype units were prepared.

It was at this point that Project CHOICE sought additional funds to formally evaluate the impact of the curriculum: Though the curriculum was observed to be accepted and liked in the schools, the true question remained as to whether it achieved its goals and made a difference in not only knowledge, but as well, in attitudes, and in health decision-making skills

With the addition of an evaluation design specialist/ statistician to the staff, plans were developed for a statewide formal evaluation. The study design and the

selection of sample population had to take into account both
the requirements of an evaluation and the realities of working
with school districts and classroom schedules and composition.
Individual contact was made with each school district
superintendent, principal and teacher once the selections
were made by program staff. Seven geographically distinct
school districts were selected to participate, three of
which doubled as experimental and control districts. The
sample represented urban, suburban and rural parts of the
state; ranged in size from large metropolitan area to small,
isolated farm community; and consisted of several SES strata.
Several ethnic populations were also well-represented. All
districts were eager to participate in the study. Schools
which were to serve as controls were told they could use
the curriculum kits at the completion of the study.

An experimental versus control, pre- post- and retention-
test design was used. One experimental classroom per grade
from each of the seven school sites participated (i.e., seven
distinct experimental classrooms per grade). One matched
control classroom per grade from three of the seven school
sites participated (i.e., three distinct control classrooms
per grade).

All evaluation instruments were developed to measure
skills or knowledge taught in the curriculum. Test items
were formulated on the basis of the Student Learning
Objectives (SLO's) for each grade. The instruments were
developed by program staff because no appropriate standardized
tests exist. All tests and items were pilot-tested with
teachers and students, and reviewed by a panel of experts
for content and readability. An item analysis was performed
on the pilot data to determine final test composition.

Nine separate Knowledge tests were developed - one per
grade level - based on the curriculum SLO's (K, 1, 2, 3, 4,
5, 6, Jr., Sr.).
Two versions of an Attitudes Toward Cancer test were
developed (Grades 4-6 and Jr.-Sr.).
One version of a Health Locus of Control test was
developed (Grades 5-Sr.), with two subscales: Personal
Control and Luck.
One version of a Health Decision-Making test was
developed (Grades Jr.-Sr.).

Note that not all test instruments were given for the

lower grade levels/younger students.

Tests were administered and data collected by 12 trained field monitors. The testing schedule included a pre-test given immediately prior to the curriculum intervention; a post-test given immediately following the two-week curriculum intervention; and a retention-test given 30 days following the completion of the curriculum intervention. The field monitors, who were recruited from each individual community, served to document the fidelity of the implementation by in-class observations of all lessons at each grade level. The students' responses to the activities were recorded in detailed observation forms which have been summarized.

All curriculum instruction and evaluation testing took place from February to June 1982. Complete data was collected from approximately 1,500 experimental students and from 650 control students who participated in the statewide evaluation.

Data analysis has shown the following results:

Experimental students have statistically significant positive gains over control students at post-test and retention-test for <u>Knowledge</u> (except retention-test, first grade);
Experimental students have positive gains over control students at post-test and retention-test for <u>Attitude</u> (fifth grade and above; N.S. for fourth grade);
Experimental students have positive gains over control students at post-test and retention-test for the <u>Personal Control</u> component of <u>Cancer Locus of Control</u> (fifth grade and above);
Experimental students have **negative** gains over control students at post-test and retention-test for the <u>Luck</u> component of <u>Cancer Locus of Control</u> for sixth grade and junior high school (N.S. for fifth grade and senior high school);
Experimental students have positive gains over control students at post-test and retention-test for <u>Health Decision-Making</u> for junior high school (N.S. for senior high school).
Analysis of the observational data at each grade has shown a consistently high (>90%) student on-task percentage for each of the curriculum components: Teacher Review; Lecture/Discussion; Filmstrips; Small Group Discussions; Manipulative Activities; Individual Seatwork, and Teacher

Summary at the end of a lesson.

While the curriculum has been shown to have a
statistically significant positive impact on students for
the various measures at most grade levels, a more important
gauge may be the curriculum's practical significance. The
use of effect size, defined as the difference between mean
experimental and control scores divided by the control
standard deviation, has been suggested to determine the
real practical impact of the curriculum (Cohen 1969). Using
this measure, Project CHOICE has had a high (as defined by
Cohen) effect on student Knowledge at all grade levels
except first grade (in the 1.1 to 2.4 standard deviation
range). The curriculum has had a medium effect on
Attitudes Toward Cancer for sixth grade and junior and senior
high school (in the .54 to .76 range). A medium effect
size was shown for junior high school for the Personal
Control component of Cancer Locus of Control and for Health
Decision-Making (.69 to .77 range).

Bartlett (1981) and others have concluded that knowledge
is a "basis for behavior change although it is generally not
sufficient for behavior change." Many health curriculum
evaluation designs have been content to measure knowledge,
therefore leaving unknown how those programs may predict
future behavior and behavior change (McAlister 1979). By
looking at additional measures such as attitude, cancer
locus of control, and health decision-making skills the
Project CHOICE evaluation has attempted to measure what are
thought to be better determinants of behavioral change. The
medium effect sizes Project CHOICE has shown for several of
these other measures at various grades is a more convincing
argument that the behavior changes desired in a prevention
and risk-reduction curriculum are likely to occur.

The other important component in the Project CHOICE
evaluation design was the classroom observations. These
observations have documented that the curriculum was
correctly implemented (important to the evaluation) and
provided useful information to the project development
staff. With these minute-by-minute snapshots of how the
teachers and students responded to each lesson, staff were
able to determine that the activities were appropriate for
each age level.

Project CHOICE evaluation data currently is being used to develop state validation and national Joint Dissemination and Review Panel (JDRP) accreditation applications which will assist disseminating the program nationwide. Arrangements also are being finalized for the curriculum to be produced and marketed by a Washington state-based non-profit organization.

Bartlett, EE (1981). The contribution of school health education to community health promotion: What can we reasonably expect? Am J Public Health 71 (12): 1384-1391.

Cohen, J (1969). "Statistical Power Analysis for the Behavioral Sciences." New York: Academic Press.

McAlister AL, Perry C, Maccoby N (1979). Adolescent Smoking: Onset and Prevention. Pediatrics 63: 650-658.

Progress in Cancer Control IV: Research in the Cancer Center, pages 99–102
© 1983 Alan R. Liss, Inc., 150 Fifth Avenue, New York, NY 10011

PHARMACISTS' ROLE IN SMOKING PREVENTION AND CESSATION

Nancy McCormick-Pickett, M.A.*, Sharon Natan-
blut, MPA, Pamela W. Gelfand, MBA, A. Gerald Franz**
Office of Cancer Communications
National Cancer Institute
Bethesda, Maryland 20205

Let me begin with a story. Mrs. Ketchum, a two-pack-
a-day smoker, enters her local pharmacy to pick up her oral
contraceptives. As she nears the pharmacy counter, she
notices a poster that reads, "If you really want to quit,
our pharmacists can show you the way." She then looks at
the wall to her right and sees another poster showing different types of medication. This poster says that if you're
taking certain medications, ask your pharmacist why you
shouldn't be smoking cigarettes.

At this point, the pharmacist walks to the counter to
give Mrs. Ketchum her medicine. Remembering that oral contraceptives were one of the medications in the poster, she
asks the pharmacist to explain why she shouldn't smoke. He
proceeds to tell her that smoking may increase the risk of
strokes, heart attacks, and blood clots. Next, he offers
her a free "How to Quit Smoking" packet. Appreciating the
time he has taken to counsel her, Mrs. Ketchum thanks him,
takes the information, and promises to review it when she
gets home.

The above scenario illustrates how the "Helping Smokers
Quit" program is designed to work.
"Helping Smokers Quit" is the first program developed
in the United States for pharmacists to help patients who
want to quit smoking. Sponsored by the American Pharmaceutical Association and the National Cancer Institue, "Helping

---

**Natanblut, Gelfand and Franz are associates with Porter,
Novelli & Associates in Washington, D.C.

Smokers Quit" is modeled after two programs developed for physicians and dentists. However, unlike these programs, "Helping Smokers Quit" focuses on an issue of special concern to pharmacists---smoking and drug interactions.

The "helping Smokers Quit" kit is divided into three components---display materials, pharmacist materials, and patient materials:

Display materials---Two posters and a counter card encourage patients to ask their pharmacists about quitting smoking and to learn about potential smoking and drug interactions. The posters and counter card can be displayed in several different ways in the pharmacy.

Patient materials--"How to Quit Smoking" packet:
o "Why Do You Smoke" helps smokers understand their reasons for smoking;
o "Clearing the Air" presents a wide variety of quitting tips;
o "Life As A Nonsmoker" provides 30 nonsmoking maintenance tips;
o "What You Should Know About Smoking and Drug Interactions" provides a simplified version of the information included in the pharmacist's guide.

Pharmacist materials---"Helping Smokers Quit: A Guide for the Pharmacist" describes the program and provides up-to-date information on smoking and drug interactions. The pharmacist's side of the counter card summarizes the information on smoking and drug interactions in a chart.

At the conclusion of the program, the pharmacists receive a certificate of participation (Hansten, McCormick-Pickett, Natanblut 1982).

This report presents details of an evaluation of a "pilot test" version of the program (A Summary Report on a Pilot Test of A Pharmacists' Smoking Cessation Program 1982). A "pilot test", consists of assemblying all components of the program in a form as close as possible to its final form to try to obtain a realistic assessment of market reaction. In this way, changes may be made before more extensive, more costly steps are undertaken. The pilot test is not meant to assess the impact of the program; rather, it is designed to uncover any negative elements or potential problems before expanding to a more quantitative assessment.

The pilot test evaluation had a two-fold purpose: to pretest prototype program materials in the pharmacy setting and to pretest the process of involving pharmacists in the smoking program.

The pilot study was conducted with nine pharmacists in Los Angeles and eight pharmacists in the Baltimore metropolitan area. Each of these pharmacists was committed to program participation for a 4-week period in July 1982. The program was designed so that patients would be more likely to initiate an interaction in which the pharmacist would provide counseling and materials related to smoking cessation. Once again, the program materials consisted of: display items to generate patient interest; printed pieces for the pharmacist, to aid in counseling; and take-home smoking cessation printed pieces for patients.

PROGRAM RESULTS

The pilot test seemed to indicate that the smoking cessation effort was a viable program for the participating pharmacies. Pharmacists were able to participate in the program with minimal interference in their schedules. The pharmacists liked the program materials, and they felt that their patients liked the materials, too.

CONCLUSIONS/RECOMMENDATIONS

The following conclusions and recommendations are based on the findings of the pilot test study.

o On a basic operational level, the program functioned well, and pharmacist support for the program concept was still strong after completion of the 4-week test period.

o NCI and APHA should consider developing mass media support for the program. The participating pharmacists strongly felt that media support could improve program credibility and increase public awareness.

o The pharmacists' instructional materials should say that the pharmacist allow the patient to initiate an interaction; however, the materials should also say it is OK for the pharmacist to begin the conversation.

o   NCI and APhA should incorporate into the patient take-
home materials some kind of encouragement (e.g., a post-
card) to stay in touch with pharmacists and keep them
informed of progress in quitting.

o   Some modifications to program materials should be made to
strengthen the program. Included among these modifications are changes to the pharmacist's guide, the counter
card display piece, and the pharmacist's certificate of
participation.

o   NCI and APhA should consider the merits of developing
highly targeted materials for subsegments of the smoking
population (e.g., Spanish speaking individuals), giving
attention to the costs of such development.

Based on these results, as well as numerous requests
for kit materials generated by an article in APhA's American Pharmacy journal, NCI and APhA are considering the
possibility of going national with the program.

Once again, the developmental stages of this program
were supported by the American Pharmaceutical Association.

Thank you for the opportunity to share the information
about this new NCI health communications program.

Special Note: Richard P. Penna, Pharm.D., Director of Professional Affairs and Dorothy S. Smith, Pharm.D., Director
of Clinical Affairs of the American Pharmaceutical Association were consultants to the Office of Cancer Communications,
National Cancer Institute in the developmental stages of the
"Helping Smokers Quit" program.

Hansten P, McCormick-Pickett N, Natanblut S (1982) Smoking
and Drug Interactions, News For Your Smoking Patients.
Am Pharm NS22, No 9.

Office of Cancer Communications, National Cancer Institute
(1982). A Summary Report on a Pilot Test of A Pharmacists'
Smoking Cessation Program.

Progress in Cancer Control IV: Research in the Cancer Center, pages 103–112
© 1983 Alan R. Liss, Inc., 150 Fifth Avenue, New York, NY 10011

CANCER PREVENTION/DETECTION BEHAVIOR BY THE PUBLIC:
LESSONS FROM THREE SURVEYS

Gary D. Murfin, Ph.D.
David A. Wagstaff, Ph.D.
Cancer Center of Hawaii, Univ. of Hawaii - Manoa
1236 Lauhala Street
Honolulu, HI 96813

INTRODUCTION

A five-year community cancer program was completed in
Hawaii on July 31, 1982. This demonstration project was
designed to show that greater cancer control could be
achieved by implementing a coordinated, community-based
approach to the solution of cancer problems. One objective
of the program was to increase the public's knowledge of
cancer through education and information activities and
thereby affect knowledge and behavior. This was consistent
with the objectives of five other community-based control
programs operational in other states. As part of the
national approach to the evaluation of these cancer control
efforts, community surveys were employed to ascertain
program impact. In Hawaii, three Health Awareness Surveys
were conducted.

The survey was conducted initially in 1978 as a joint
effort between the Community Cancer Program of Hawaii (CCPH)
and the American Cancer Society (ACS), the organization most
responsible for CCPH education and information activities
through 1979. It was designed to provide the baseline statistics necessary for determining changes in the public's
cancer knowledge and their detection and prevention practices. The survey was fielded for the second time in 1980
and was used to assess knowledge and behavior changes occurring during the two-and-one-half year period following the
administration of the baseline survey. The survey was
fielded finally in 1982, providing a third set of data.

SURVEY METHODOLOGY

Questionnaire Design and Content: The baseline survey
instrument developed in 1978 had four major sections which
assessed the public's knowledge and detection/prevention
behaviors with respect to cancer of the lung, breast,
cervix/uterus, and colon/rectum. While women respondents
completed sections dealing with female cancer sites (breast,
cervix-uterus), most sections were administered by a trained
interviewer. The questionnaire was reviewed by survey firm
staff and professors from the University of Hawaii's School
of Public Health and School of Social Work. The questionnaire went through the customary pretesting and revision
before it was fielded by trained volunteers from the
American Cancer Society and paid interviewers.

Prior to fielding in 1980 and 1982, some changes were
made in the questionnaire, but these changes did not alter
significantly the content, format or design.

Sampling Procedure: Respondents were defined as all
non-military individuals who were twenty years of age or
older and who lived on the island of Oahu, Maui, Kauai, or
Hawaii. Members of this population were randomly sampled
from a computer listing of all households in the state
obtained through the cooperation of the Hawaii Cooperative
Health Statistics Program.

The survey samples were stratified random samples with
the four islands forming the strata. For the 1978 baseline
survey, the sample was allocated in proportion to each
island's household population. To allow more meaningful
comparisons between males and females living on the less
populous islands, disproportionate allocation was used for
the two follow-up surveys. A comparison of the stratum
sampling fractions with the proportion of the State's population living on each island is provided by Table 1.

For the 1980 and 1982 surveys, staff would randomly
select a household from their listing. Using this randomly
selected starting point, a five-household sampling unit was
assigned to an interviewer, who was then required to
complete interviews with two population members living in
two different households. If the interviewer did not
complete any interview or completed only one interview,
Health Statistics Program staff identified an alternate

starting point within the same census tract. This process was repeated until the entire sample was drawn.

Table 1. Comparison of 1978, 1980, and 1982 Stratum
Sampling Fractions with 1980 Census Statistics

| | | SURVEY | YEAR | | |
ISLAND	1978	1980	1982	1980 CENSUS	*
Oahu	.714	.589	.560	.784	
Maui	.090	.144	.145	.070	
Kauai	.064	.114	.125	.043	
Hawaii	.132	.153	.169	.103	

*Source: Research and Economic Analysis Division, Department of Planning and Economic Development, State of Hawaii, The Population of Hawaii, 1980: Final Census Results, Statistical Report #143, 18 March 1981.

DESCRIPTION OF THE SURVEY SAMPLES

The three survey samples are quite comparable with respect to age, sex, ethnicity, education, and nativity. This is attributable to a relatively stable population in Hawaii.

1978 Baseline Survey: The average age of the 1,035 respondents was 44.5 years. Approximately 40.6% of the respondents had attended high school while 46.6% of the respondents had attended a trade or business school, college, or graduate school. Only 12.2% of the respondents had never attended high school. The annual household income was reported at less than $15,000 for 35.6% of the respondents. Only 20.1% of the respondents earned annual household incomes of $25,000 or more. Females accounted for 55.5% of the respondents. Japanese, Caucasians, Hawaiians and part-Hawaiians, and Filipinos accounted for 31.3%, 30.9%, 13.9% and 8.4%, respectively, of the respondents. Finally, 63% of the respondents were born in the State while 12% of the respondents were born in a foreign country.

1980 Survey: The average age of the 1,616 respondents was 43.6 years. Some 41.9% of the respondents had attended high school while 47.2% of the respondents had attended a trade or business school, college, or graduate school. Only 10% of the respondents had never attended high school. In contrast to the baseline sample, only 30% of the respondents earned annual household incomes less than $15,000. Roughly 28% of the respondents earned household incomes of $25,000 or more. Females accounted for 57.5% of the respondents: Japanese, Caucasians, Hawaiians and part-Hawaiians, and Filipinos accounted for 29.3%, 31.9%, 15.6%, and 10.3%, respectively, of the respondents. The 1980 respondents did not differ from the baseline respondents with respect to nativity.

1982 Survey: The average age of the 1,403 respondents was 44.4 years. Some 43.8% of the respondents had attended high school; 46% of the respondents had attended a trade or business school, college, or graduate school. Only 9.9% of the respondents had never attended high school. Some 38% of the respondents earned annual household incomes less than $15,000, while 33% of the respondents reported earning $25,000 or more. Females accounted for 57.7% of the respondents. Japanese, Caucasians, Hawaiians and part-Hawaiians, and Filipinos accounted for 28.4%, 34.4%, 15.1% and 9.5%, respectively, of the respondents. Roughly 61% of the respondents were born in the State while 12% of the respondents were born in a foreign country.

To assess the degree to which the samples were representative of the State's population, Health Awareness Survey (HAS) data were compared with data collected for the Health Surveillance Program (HSP), Department of Health. Staff from the HSP periodically survey 2% of the State's non-institutionalized population. The latest survey was conducted in 1980.

The HSP sample size is several times larger than the combined size of the three HAS samples. Furthermore, the HSP sample is obtained with a more rigorous sampling procedure. The HSP estimates of population sizes (e.g., the number of Japanese) are, as a result, obtained through a weighting procedure.

In general, the HAS and HSP samples are remarkably similar. This observed similarity is important in two respects. First, it suggests quite strongly that the HAS samples are indeed representative of the larger population from which they were drawn. Second, and more importantly, it suggests that it is unlikely that any change in cancer knowledge or behavior subsequent to the 1978 survey is due to a difference in the statistical composition of the survey samples.

SURVEY QUESTIONS

A number of questions pertaining to personal cancer prevention and detection activity were asked of each respondent. These questions fell under one of two headings: questions about specific actions taken by the respondent (e.g., practice BSE), or questions about specific actions requested through their physician (e.g., asking their doctor for a chest x-ray). For the cancer sites of breast and cervix-uterus, these questions were asked only of the female respondents. For the colon-rectum and lung, all respondents were questioned. Described below are the questions for each site.

Breast: Women were asked if they had learned how to examine their breasts, if they examined their breasts, if a doctor had examined their breasts, if they had asked a doctor to teach them BSE, and if they had asked their doctor to examine them for breast cancer.

Cervix-Uterus: Women were asked four behavior questions designed to determine if the female respondent had ever asked a physician to examine her for cervical cancer (not a pap test), asked a physician to examine her for uterine cancer (not a pap test), had a pap test, and had a pap test regularly.

While these questions appeared in all three survey years, there is not total comparability since changes were made in national guidelines for mass screening and these guidelines formed the basis for the questions asked in 1980 and 1982.

Lung: Respondents were asked if they had ever had a chest x-ray and if they ever had a chest x-ray taken specifically for lung cancer.

Colon-Rectum: Four detection behavior questions were asked to find out if the respondent had ever asked his/her physician to examine him/her for colon/rectal cancer, had an annual colon/rectal exam, a rectal exam with a prostoscope or a test for hidden blood in the stool, had only a proctoscopic exam, and given a stool sample for testing for hidden blood.

DISCUSSION OF SURVEY RESULTS

A review of all response patterns for the three surveys provides several sets of observations.

1) For those cancer sites which are distinctly female-oriented and are associated with simple tests/procedures, there is a high proportion of women respondents who carried out prevention/detection behavior. This was true for questions on direct respondent behavior as well as for questions on requests made to a physician. The contrast between site results is observable in the raw percentages presented in Table 2 on the questions related to BSE practice, breast examination and on lung and proctoscopic exams shown in Table 3.

TABLE 2

Prevention/ Detection Behavior	1978	1980	1982	Trend
WOMEN ONLY				
Practice BSE	82.9%	86.1%	85.4%	Incr.
Have Breast Exam	58.2%	41.6%	44.0%	Decr.*
Ask Doctor to Teach BSE	32.6%	48.5%	45.6%	Incr.*
Ask Doctor for Breast X-Ray	18.5%	24.3%	25.8%	Decr.*
Had Pap Test	87.9%	69.9%	66.6%	Decr.*
Have Pap Test Regularly	79.5%	81.2%	74.5%	Decr.
Ask Doctor for Uterine Exam	35.5%	14.2%	13.5%	Decr.*
Ask Doctor for Cervix Exam	35.5%	27.5%	25.1%	Decr.*
ALL RESPONDENTS				
Had Chest X-Ray	20.5%	14.8%	12.8%	Decr.*
Ask Doctor for Chest X-Ray	6.4%	15.5%		
Have Rectal Exam		28.5%	22.5%	Decr.
Have Procto Exam	28.8%	20.3%	22.4%	Decr.*
Give Stool Sample	24.7%	18.4%	22.4%	Decr.
Ask Doctor for Colon/ Rectal Exam	12.1%	16.5%	19.0%	Incr.*

*Difference between '78 and '82 Significance P < .001

2) A second observation stems from the contrast

appearing between the results for the predominantely female
sites and the results on the sites common to male and female
respondents; colon-rectum and lung. In this case, there is
no situation in which a high proportion of males are seen to
be carrying out prevention/detection actions. In addition,
on these sites females show correspondingly low percentages
in terms of actions carried out. This is true for direct
behaviors such as having a lung x-ray and for the indirect
behavior of asking a physician to carry out some type of
examination.

TABLE 3

COMPARISON OF BEHAVIOR FOR LUNG AND COLON-RECTUM:

MALES AND FEMALES

	1978		1982	
	YES %	NO %	YES %	NO %
CHEST X-RAY				
MALES	25	75	15	85
FEMALES	19	81	11	89
ASK DOCTOR FOR				
COLON-RECUM EXAM				
MALES	30	70	23	77
FEMALES	29	71	15	85
HAD PROCTO EXAM				
MALES	16	84	22	78
FEMALES	17	83	20	80
GAVE STOOL SAMPLE				
MALES	55	45	25	75
FEMALES	57	43	22	78

The fact that a large proportion of female respondents
in all three surveys did take certain prevention/detection
actions for breast and gyn cancers may be attributable to
two factors: 1) the simplicity of the tests or procedures
involved and 2) the high visibility given to these cancers
in public information/education efforts in general (locally
and nationally).

In the case of many of the questions asked, there was a
statistical significance for the difference between the
years 1978 and 1982. However, as shown in Table 1, the raw
percentages remained fairly stable over the three survey
periods, not changing by more than 10 percentage points in
the case of 10 of the 14 questions.

It is noteworthy that the greatest decreases
(1978-1982) were observed for the questions on breast exami-

nation, having a pap test and having a cervix or uterus exam. This may be related to the fact that by 1980, the Breast Cancer Detection Demonstration Program and the Cervical Cancer Screening Program ceased operation on the island of Oahu and both programs had many clients.

In summary, survey results indicate that the proportion of persons taking personal prevention/detection action between 1978 and 1982 declined for the cancer sites of cervix-uterine, colon-rectum and lung and declined for breast examinations, too. For the breast cancer site, there was an increase in the proportion of women practicing BSE, asking a doctor to instruct them in BSE and asking a doctor to provide a breast x-ray.

CONCLUSIONS

At a level relative to findings on specific site questions the following may be said. Efforts have been successful in maintaining a high level of prevention/detection behavior among women in Hawaii, especially for breast cancer, and, cancer education/information efforts for the sites of colon-rectum and lung have not led to any increases in participation. There has been a consistently low percentage of people taking appropriate prevention/detection behavior for the sites of colon-rectum and lung.

There is another important conclusion to be drawn from the survey results which may be relevant to other programs attempting to assess such efforts. This conclusion pertains to the objective of the surveys to ascertain changes in prevention/detection behavior relative to cancer control efforts in the community. To some degree, this assessment of behavior and knowledge was accomplished; however, the linkage of these areas to programmatic impact is less well determined.

In some cases, the impact of a specific program was observable in survey results, but not for the questions on behavior. This was true in terms of public awareness of the operation of the Cancer Information Line and the Maui and Kauai Breast Cancer Screening programs. Each of these programs was new to Hawaii, consequently, any mention of their existence by respondents was an indication that the program was recognized in the community. This was a case of a project going from a zero level to an observable level of activity.

To be thorough in the analysis of program effect, results also were examined on an island-by-island basis. Particular attention was paid to the islands of Maui and Kauai where Breast Cancer Screening Programs were in operation for 18 months and 30 months, respectively. Survey results on breast cancer for the two islands were compared for the years 1978 (pre-program) and 1982 (post-program). The findings, as shown in Table 4, indicate that for the behaviors of practicing BSE, having a breast exam/x-ray, and asking a doctor to provide instruction in BSE, there was little or no change that was significant statistically between 1978 and 1982.

TABLE 4

BREAST DETECTION/PREVENTION BEHAVIOR COMPARISON BY

ISLAND BETWEEN 1978 AND 1982 RESULTS

PRACTICE BSE

	1978 *	1982 **	x^2, p
OAHU	82%	88%	6.15, p<.01
KAUAI	88%	81%	.44, p -
MAUI	80%	78%	.13, p -
HAWAII	85%	88%	.26, p -

HAVE BREAST EXAM

	1978 *	1982 **	x^2, p
OAHU	60%	75%	16.7, p<.0001
KAUAI	51%	38%	2.0, p -
MAUI	55%	48%	.78, p -
HAWAII	56%	42%	4.3, p<.03

ASK FOR BSE INSTRUCTION

	1978 *	1982 **	x^2, p
OAHU	34%	50%	22.5, p<.00003
KAUAI	23%	41%	4.19, p<.03
MAUI	37%	39%	.06, p -
HAWAII	29%	49%	7.8, p<.005

* Pre Breast Program
** Post Breast Program

Based on the observable results, it does not appear that the instruments were able to detect changes brought about by individual cancer programs. This may be an important lesson learned since it points out that program assessments may be more meaningful when conducted among a specifically defined target population. The community in the Community Cancer Program did refer to the State of Hawaii as a whole and the Program did have a number of projects in operation throughout the State. The Program did not have, however, an outreach that really encompassed the state population as a whole and therefore, efforts to assess the impact on the state population were not as meaningful as an evaluation of program impact as originally had been envisioned.

In summary, community-wide surveys may continue to be a valid way to monitor the status of a population and to conduct needs assessments, however, this approach may not be appropriate to the determination of programmatic impacts when such programs are aimed at certain subgroups within the population and not the population as a whole.

REFERENCES

Research and Economic Analysis Division, Department of Planning and Economic Development (1981). "The Population of Hawaii, 1980: Final Census Results."

Research and Statistics Office, Department of Health, State of Hawaii, Health Surveillance Program (1980). "Report on the Health Suveillance Survey - 1980."

Supported in part by NCI Contract Number NO1-CN-75399.

Progress in Cancer Control IV: Research in the Cancer Center, pages 113-122
© **1983 Alan R. Liss, Inc., 150 Fifth Avenue, New York, NY 10011**

COMMUNITY-BASED CANCER EDUCATION FOR THE ELDERLY

Edna Kane-Williams, M.A., Jack E. White, M.D.

Howard University Cancer Center

Washington, D.C. 20060

INTRODUCTION

The question might be asked: why a cancer education program for the elderly? The answer can be found, in part, in the following statement by U.S. Representative Claude Pepper, who spoke of the urgent need for such programs and services:

> Many. . . cancer deaths occur in later life. Persons over 54 years of age constitute 81 percent of all cancer deaths. People over 60 years of age account for 60 percent of all cancer deaths. . . Cancer is on the way to becoming the No. 1 cause of death among the elderly. Whereas a 25 year old has a 1 chance in 700 of developing cancer in the next 5 years, a 65 year old faces a frightening 1 chance in 14. (Select Committee on Aging, 1980)

Age specific cancer mortality rates confirm that cancer death rates increase sharply with age, until about age 75, after which there is a decline. (Levin, et al., 1974) This decline after 75 years of age is due to a rapidly dwindling population in this age cohort--and not a reduction in cancer risk. In terms of incidence rates, approximately 50% of all cancers occur in the 11% of the population over age 65. (Fox Chase Cancer Center, 1980)

In what way is age linked to cancer? There are several theories. Perhaps the most predominant is that which

implicates the decline of immunologic capacity which occurs
with age. As Dr. Robert Good, Vice President of the
Memorial Sloan-Kettering Cancer Center points out:
> The association between immunodeficiency
> and increased cancer incidence is clear
> cut. When a patient is immunosuppressed
> for kidney transplantation, his or her
> cancer risk increases manyfold. Without
> exception, every known genetic or con-
> genital immunodeficiency is associated
> with markedly increased rates of cancer.
> (Good, 1980)

Other theories involving aging and cancer include:
- a time lag between the events initiating oncogenesis
  (the beginning of a cancer) and the actual appearance
  of a clinically recognizable cancer often is substantial, resulting in more disease diagnosed in the
  later stages of life. (Good, 1980)
- the relationship between diet and cancer, i.e., the
  reduction of the intake of calories, especially fatty
  foods. It is thought that since less was known
  about the effects of fatty foods during the earlier
  part of this century, the elderly have probably
  ingested more saturated fats than others in the
  population. (Good, 1980)
- aging may increase the susceptibility of tissue to
  carcinogens. (Good, 1980)
- genetic mutations occurring with age are felt by
  some to lead malignant disease. (Good, 1980)

Whatever theory is used as an explanation, it is
obvious that cancer is an important health concern for the
elderly. A need recognized by Dr. Vincent DeVita, Director
of the National Cancer Institute, and others, is that of
developing and using methods of prevention and treatment of
cancer which are tailored to the special needs of the
elderly. Of critical proportions is the need for more
widely spread instruction in early screening and detections
procedures, particularly in light of the fact that most
elderly don't realize that they are at increased risk of
developing cancer. Such health education activities could
prove to be a valuable tool in impacting overall morbidity
and mortality rates in the elderly due to cancer.

CANCER EDUCATION AND THE ELDERLY

Health Education was defined by the President's Committee on Health Education as a "process which bridges the gap between health information and health practices. Health education motivates the person to take the information and do something with it--to keep himeslf healthier by avoiding actions that are harmful and by forming habits that are beneficial." (Green, 1980) It follows, then, that the discipline's emphasis is on health promotion and disease prevention. Also key is the acknowledgement with that the responsibility for health monitoring lies both with the consumer and the physician.

Health education can involve different levels of prevention, i.e., primary (hygiene), secondary (early detection), or tertiary (therapeutic). A variety of educational strategies have been employed to implement the aims of health education, including:
- audiovisual aids
- lectures
- individual instruction
- mass media
- programmed learning
- educational television
- skill development
- simulation and games
- inquiry learning
- peer group discussion
- modeling
- behavior modification
- community development
- social action
- social planning and organizational change. (Green, 1980)

Historically, there have been few health education programs designed specifically for older populations. Recent years have witnessed a growth in programming for the elderly, although many of these efforts have been initiated on a pilot basis. Few of these programs have dealt with the topic of cancer control.

Cancer is a difficult topic to address because of the negative beliefs and attitudes that exist about the disease. For example, researchers have found the following beliefs

to be major deterrents to participation in programs promoting
early screening and detection:
- belief that cancer is incurable
- belief that professional diagnosis is no better
  than self diagnosis
- lack of belief in the value of early diagnosis
- absence of perceived susceptibility to the disease

(Kegeles, 1976)

Sociocultural factors also can affect attitudes about
cancer prevention activities. Blacks may view the symptom-
atology for cancer differently than do whites. Similarly,
there may be different operational definitions for pain and
cure. (Kegeles, 1976) There certainly are differences in
the level of knowledge about the disease. A recent study of
black American attitudes towards cancer and cancer tests,
conducted for the American Cancer Society, uncovered the
following contrasts in black vs. white knowledge:
- blacks believed that cancer was primarily a concern
  for whites, whereas high blood pressure is a more
  immediate threat to blacks.
- blacks were less aware than whites of the seven
  warning signals of cancer. This difference is
  most pronounced in the lower income groups.
- blacks had less experience with and knowledge of
  screening procedures such as the Guiaic test or
  proctoscopic examinations. (Evaxx, 1981)

Even given these problematic barriers, however, the
need for special programs in cancer education is intense.
The following section details the experiences of the Howard
University Cancer Center in developing and implementing
cancer education programs for the elderly in the District of
Columbia.

"SENIORS TEAM UP AGAINST CANCER"

This project was designed to increase the awareness
among older persons (i.e., persons 60 years of age and
older) of practices which contribute to the early detection
and treatment of cancer. Specifically, breast, colo-rectal
and prostate cancers were targeted due to their relatively
high frequency among the elderly and the efficacy of available detection methods. The key components of this secondary
prevention program were workshop presentations featuring

demonstrations of self-examination techniques, open group discussions and the use of audiovisual materials to convey information about basic cancer concepts. All program activities emphasized behavioral change and skill development. Specific topics addressed included:
- the seven warning signals of cancer
- early detection techniques, e.g.
  1. breast self-examination
  2. use of Guaiac test for colo-rectal cancer
- recognition of myths and misconceptions about cancer, e.g.
  1. cancer is contagious
  2. a bump or bruise causes cancer
  3. surgery causes cancer to spread

Approximately 600 senior citizens throughout the Washington, D.C. area participated in this project.

Evaluation

A pre- and post-test instrument was developed to assist in the evaluation of this project. The instrument consisted of a series of 12 true or false questions, and was intended to measure change in the elderly's knowledge of the myths and misconceptions about cancer, the early warning signals for breast, colon-rectum and prostate cancer, and early detection techniques.

The pre- and post-test instrument was used in a quasi-experimental, "simulated before and after design," as described by Campbell and Stanley (in Experimental and Quasi-Experimental Designs for Research). Two non-random samples were selected from equivalent subgroups of elderly attending area senior centers. These groups were similar in terms of age, race, sex, socio-economic status and physical condition. One sample was chosen to serve as the pre-test group, receiving the questionnaire approximately two weeks prior to the workshop series. The second sample served as the post-test group, receiving the questionnaire approximately two weeks following the workshop series.

The following tables provide a demographic profile of the pre- and post-test groups.

Table 1 Demographic Profile Pre-Test (N=204)					Table 2 Demographic Profile Post-Test (N=63)				
AGE	−Unknown		−	9%	AGE −				
	55	− 60	−	14%		55	− 60	−	10%
	61	− 71	−	35%		61	− 70	−	35%
	71	− 80	−	31%		71	− 80	−	48%
	81	− 90	−	8%		81	− 90	−	5%
		91+	−	2%			91+	−	2%
RACE −					RACE −				
	BLACK		−	85%		BLACK		−	84%
	WHITE		−	6%		WHITE		−	6%
	HISPANIC		−	−		HISPANIC		−	−
	OTHER		−	−		OTHER		−	−
	UNKNOWN		−	8%		UNKNOWN		−	10%
SEX −					SEX −				
	FEMALE		−	69%		FEMALE		−	78%
	MALE		−	29%		MALE		−	22%

Results

The "Seniors Team Up Against Cancer" project is not
being presented as the model of health education intervention in older populations. However, the experiences of
this project can serve as a point of reference for others
interested in cancer control for the elderly. Results of
the pre-test survey illustrate the baseline levels of
knowledge about cancer found in the elderly. And changes
in knowledge between pre- and post-test groups, although not
statistically significant, do provide information as to the
rigidity of certain attitudes and beliefs and areas needing
special emphasis in future programs.

Preliminary analyses of the collected data indicated
the following:

- In most cases, a majority of the elderly pretested responded correctly to questionnaire items. Most were aware of the possibility of cure, the possibility of risk reduction, and the fact that cancer is not contagious. Most older women reported that they practiced breast self examination, and were aware that all breast lumps were not cancerous.
- In the pretest, fewer men were knowledgeable about symptoms of prostate cancer than were women about breast cancer. Overall men scored poorer than women.
- A majority of the elderly pretested believed incorrectly that a bump or bruise could cause cancer.
- A majority of the elderly pretested believed incorrectly that older people are no more likely to get cancer than younger people.
- A majority of the elderly either did not know, or answered incorrectly the question of whether pain is an early symptom of cancer.
- In each instance, the number of elderly responding correctly to questionnaire items increased in the post-test. Increases were notable for the following questions:
  -- cancer contagious?
  -- bump or bruise cause cancer?
  -- blood sign of cancer?
  -- difficulty urinating sign of cancer?
- Even after the workshop series, a majority of the elderly either did not know, or responded incorrectly to the question about older people being more likely to develop cancer.

Specific response percentages for the pre- and post-test surveys are provided in Table 3.

Table 3
Results of Pre-Test, Post-Test Survey

1. Can some cancers be cured if they are discovered early?

	PRE	POST
**Yes	- 83%	84%
No	- 2%	5%
Don't Know	- 12%	11%

2. Is there anything a person can do to reduce their risk
    of getting cancer?

	PRE	POST
**Yes	– 68%	68%
No	– 12%	13%
Don't Know	– 18%	17%

3. Is cancer contagious?

	PRE	POST
Yes	– 22%	8%
**No	– 59%	82%
Don't Know	– 17%	10%

4. Can a bump or bruise to the body cause cancer?

	PRE	POST
Yes	– 72%	51%
*No	– 6%	30%
Don't Know	– 18%	19%

5. (Women only) Do you know how to examine your breasts
    for cancer?

	PRE	POST
**Yes	– 76%	88%
No	– 15%	8%
Don't Know	– 9%	4%

6. (Women only) Do you ever practice breast self examination?

	PRE	POST
**Yes	– 66%	77%
No	– 23%	21%
Don't Know	– 11%	2%

7. (Women only) Do you believe that all breast lumps are
    cancerous?

	PRE	POST
Yes	– 6%	0%
**No	– 77%	94%
Don't Know	– 15%	6%

8. Can blood in a bowel movement be a sign of cancer?

	PRE	POST
**Yes –	58%	70%
No –	11%	14%
Don't Know –	30%	14%

9. (Men only) Can difficulty when urinating be a sign of cancer?

	PRE	POST
**Yes –	47%	66%
No –	21%	6%
Don't Know –	32%	20%

10. (Men only) Do you know where your prostate gland is located in the body?

	PRE	POST
**Yes –	55%	66%
No –	24%	6%
Don't Know –	21%	20%

11. Is pain usually an early symptom of cancer?

	PRE	POST
Yes –	18%	19%
**No –	46%	54%
Don't Know –	38%	27%

12. Do you think that older people are more likely to get cancer than younger people?

	PRE	POST
**Yes –	18%	46%
No –	60%	36%
Don't Know –	20%	14%

---

*Due to missing data percentages don't add to 100% in every case
**Correct response

These preliminary results indicate that, while the sampled elderly appear to have adequate knowledge about basic cancer concepts, future programs should continue to focus on dispelling cultural myths about cancer and the early warning signals. Special targeted efforts should be directed at older men, who have poorer knowledge about cancer in general and specifically about prostate cancer.

The elderly sampled appear to resist acknowledging that they are at high risk for developing cancer. While further analyses are necessary to substantiate this preliminary finding, it would appear that it is less important to convince them of this fact than it is to educate them about early warning symptoms and screening and detection techniques.

REFERENCES

Evaxx, Inc. (1981). "A Study of Black American Attitudes Toward Cancer and Cancer Tests," New York: American Cancer Society.

Fox Chase Cancer Center (1980). "Cancer and the Aging" The Cancer Letter.

Good, Robert (1980). Cancer and Aging, **Hospital Practice** 11:10.

Green, Lawrence, et al. (1980). "Health Education Planning: A Diagnostic Approach, Palo Alto: Mayfield Publishing Company, p. 4.

Kegeles, S. Stephen (1976). Relationship of Sociocultural Factors to Cancer in "Cancer: The Behavioral Dimensions" by J. W. Cullen, et al. (eds.) New York: Raven Press p. 104.

Levin DL, Devesa SS, et al. (1974). "Cancer Rates and Risks," DHEW Publication No. (NIH) 79-691.

Select Committee on Aging (1980). "Research Frontiers in Aging and Cancer: International Symposium for the 1980's" House of Representatives, Ninety-Sixth Congress, Second Session.

Progress in Cancer Control IV: Research in the Cancer Center, pages 123–133
© 1983 Alan R. Liss, Inc., 150 Fifth Avenue, New York, NY 10011

CANCER AND THE ELDERLY: A CANCER CONTROL CHALLENGE*

Barbara Rimer, Dr.P.H.
Wendy L. Jones, Ph.D.
Christine Wilson, M.A.
David Bennett, B.A.
Paul F. Engstrom, M.D.
The Fox Chase Cancer Center
Philadelphia, PA   19111

THE PROBLEM

It is estimated that almost 535,000 older Americans
were diagnosed as having cancer in 1982. (This estimate was
reached by applying SEER rates to the 1982 Cancer Facts and
Figures, published by the American Cancer Society.)
Although cancer is a common cause of disability and death
in the elderly, relatively little attention has been
focused on the special problems presented by cancer in old
age (Petersen & Kennedy 1979), and few cancer control
programs have been developed with a view toward the needs of
older persons. This is a notable deficiency since there are
now 25.5 million Americans over 65, 11% of the population.
And the proportion of the population over age 65 is growing
steadily. By 2000, 20% of the United States population will
be over 65 (German 1978). We use the word "older" to desig-
nate persons over 65. Nevertheless, we recognize that the
over 65 population is not homogeneous and that it may be
more meaningful to talk about the younger-old (65-75) and
the older-old (above 75).

The implications of an aging population for cancer
control are sobering since most cancers are diseases of
aging. Approximately 50% of all cancers occur in the 11% of
our population over age 65, and the risk for most major cancers increases with age. In fact, older age is one of the

*Supported by National Cancer Institute Contract #4010-01.

most important risk factors for cancer. Indeed, risk factors which affect far fewer people have attracted much greater attention.

While a problem of such magnitude should be the subject of public concern and research, at least until recently, this has not been the case. Surprisingly little is known about the biological behavior of cancer in the elderly, the differences in the effects of chemotherapeutic drugs and other treatments on the elderly, or even the psychological and emotional effects of cancer on older people. While far too little is known about the biology of cancer, there have been few efforts to communicate what we do know about cancer to the elderly. Results of a survey done at the Fox Chase Cancer Center indicate that roughly 70% of people over 62 do not know that the risk of cancer increases with age (Rimer et al., in press). Few cancer education programs have been tailored to the educational, physical, cancer risk and lifestyle needs and constraints of the elderly. This is a serious gap since the older person can practice some behaviors that have been related to better cancer outcomes, such as prompt reporting of symptoms and practice of recommended self-examination and early detection techniques, (Wilkinson et al. 1979).

Because older people are at increased risk for cancer, it is important that they follow appropriate self-examination and screening schedules and report potential cancer symptoms promptly. Nevertheless, some researchers have found that older persons not only report symptoms differently, but also seek care at more advanced stages of disease (Ouslander & Beck 1982) and are less likely to seek early detection or practice self-examination behaviors. A number of studies have found older age to be associated with the decreased practice of prevention and early detection behaviors for cancer (Hobbs 1980; Kirscht et al. 1966; Knopf 1976). Kegeles (1982) concluded that older age is a significant risk factor for non-participation of women in a variety of cancer screening activities, including breast examination by a physician and cervical cytology, and he argued that older women represent a critical target population for cancer control behavior change techniques.

Other researchers (Foster 1978) have found lower rates of breast self-examination practice among the elderly. Knopf (1976) found that, in general, the older the woman or the lower her social class, the more likely she is to hold mistaken ideas about cancer causation. And Hobbs (1980) discovered that, when presented an opportunity to undergo screening, very few older (over 60) women referred themselves to do so. Howe (1981) concluded that older women are less likely than younger women to practice breast self-examination. There is also evidence that older people are more likely to delay in reporting symptoms although the data are by no means clear (Antonovsky 1974; Green & Roberts 1974). Hingson (1981) concluded that the older a person is, the more likely he is to delay treatment.

There are at least three other characteristics of older people which exacerbate the problems of cancer control. First, is the problem of co-morbidity. Elderly individuals tend not to suffer from isolated conditions as do the young but frequently suffer from multiple coexistent chronic conditions upon which acute illnesses are superimposed (Ouslander & Beck 1982). This is an important issue for older people already diagnosed with cancer and for the health professionals who care for them. Additionally, older people may have problems communicating with physicians which might either reduce their likelihood of seeking care or their compliance and/or satisfaction when under treatment (Bertakis 1978; Green & Roberts 1974). Finally, the processes of aging, for example diminished hearing and vision and difficulties with memory and concentration, exacerbate other health and communication problems for the older person.

There is a clear need for programs which seek to identify the reasons the elderly are reluctant to undergo screening and early detection and which offer interventions responsive to the concerns and needs of the elderly.

Health education can be an important tool for older persons who suffer from isolation and immobility and tend to ignore early symptoms of cancer and other diseases (German 1981). Moreover, many of the conditions that predispose the elderly to functional dependency are amenable to early intervention. Education and screening programs can be used with great advantage in the elderly to deal with diseases, including some cancers, which can be detected early and treated successfully.

The Fox Chase Cancer Center made a commitment to develop a Cancer Program for Older Citizens (CAPROC). But before a

health education program could be developed, we needed more
data than currently available about what the elderly know,
believe and do about cancer. Toward this end, we conducted
a series of surveys with over 300 older persons. Our findings suggest that the elderly hold some myths about cancer
and negative attitudes toward physicians that may, in part,
explain some of the delay of older people in seeking care
for potential cancer symptoms and their practice of recommended early detection behaviors.

INTRODUCTION

Researchers at the Fox Chase Cancer Center developed a
slide technique (Wilson *et al*. 1982) to collect data from
older persons. Using this survey method, 267 persons
attending Title XX nutrition centers were surveyed. Characteristics of the respondents are described elsewhere (Rimer
et al., in press).

Because nutrition centers attract primarily lower income,
less educated elderly persons, it was essential to test the
efficacy of the questionnaire technique with other elderly
populations. A second series of field tests was initiated,
the first including 67 respondents from a middle income
church group. The results thus far are not significantly
different from those obtained in the nutrition centers.
Characteristics of the respondents are shown in Table 1.

In general, the results must be qualified by emphasizing
that the data were collected using volunteer participants,
not random samples. Thus, generalizability is limited. However, given the size of the sample, we believe that the
technique and the results deserve replication.

RESULTS

In the surveys, we collected data on beliefs the elderly
respondents held about cancer, attitudes toward the health
care system, some health behaviors, and demographic information. The primary purpose of the analysis was to describe
the attitudes and beliefs of the sample with regard to cancer
and to explore associations between their attitudes and
beliefs and demographic variables.

Table 1

Characteristics of Older Persons
in Study Sample as a Percentage of Group Total

Characteristics	Respondents	
	Nutrition Centers[a]	Church Groups[b]
Age		
Less than 65	10	3
65-70	31	34
71-75	24	30
76-80	11	15
81+	24	18
Gender		
Female	63	72
Male	31	28
Unknown	6	0
Race		
White	93	99
Other	7	1
Education		
8 years or less	43	11
9-12 years	39	48
More than high school	8	41
Not ascertainable	10	0
Health Status		
Good or excellent compared to other persons their age	57	82
Fair or poor compared to other persons their age	43	18

[a] $n = 267$

[b] $n = 67$

Beliefs About Cancer

As shown in Table 2, the older people we interviewed manifested some important false beliefs about cancer. For example, more than one-half of the respondents thought that a woman can get cancer from being hit in the breast, that surgery spreads cancer, and that cancer treatments are worse than the disease. Only 38% of the respondents realized that older persons are more likely to get cancer than younger persons. Men were more likely than women to believe in the myths about breast cancer causation (x^2 = 30.26, p = .0008). Women were more likely to believe that the treatments are worse than the disease (x^2 = 19.09, p = .03). Men were more likely to accept (x^2 = 21.4, p = .01) that having chemotherapy or radiation means a person will die soon.

Several implications for cancer control planning can be drawn from these findings. Not knowing that the risk of cancer increases with age may make older people less likely to take early detection measures than would be desirable. Moreover, false beliefs about cancer treatments may further reduce the likelihood that older people will seek early detection and treatment for cancer symptoms. The elderly might delay seeking treatment for potential cancers because they fear that the treatment will be worse than the disease or that the treatment will exacerbate the disease. Unwarranted fears about cancer treatment may cause some older people to reject accepted cancer treatments and seek alternative, unproven treatments. In addition, beliefs in myths about cancer treatments might reduce compliance for some of the elderly people who have consented to treatment. False beliefs about cancer etiology (for example, cancer being caused by a blow to the breast) probably cause unnecessary worry for older people who already fear this disease. Education programs designed for older people could effect important changes in their false beliefs about cancer, for example, to communicate the actual risk status of the elderly and to correct perceptions about treatment.

Attitudes Toward Physicians and the Health Care System

As Table 3 indicates, respondents in both groups displayed negative attitudes towards physicians and the health care system. The majority of respondents believed doctors cause people to worry because they don't explain everything,

Table 2

Acceptance of Cancer Myths by Older Persons

Myths	Number[a] of Respondents in Agreement	
	Nutrition Centers[b]	Church Groups[c]
Age is not related to a person's chances of getting cancer.	78 (30)	44 (66)
Older persons are more likely to get cancer than younger ones.	80 (30)	31 (46)
Surgery spreads cancer.	166 (64)	35 (52)
Cancer treatments are worse than the disease.	143 (55)	34 (51)
A woman can get cancer from being hit in the breast.	160 (61)	38 (57)
Cancer can only be treated by surgery.	39 (15)	3 (5)
Pain is the first symptom of cancer.	31 (12)	8 (12)

[a]Numbers in parentheses indicate percentages.

[b]n = 267

[c]n = 67

Table 3

Attitudes of Older Persons Toward Physicians

Attitudes Toward Physicians	Number[a] of Respondents in Agreement	
	Nutrition Centers[b]	Church Groups[c]
Doctors reject many cancer treatments that could help patients.	116 (44)	20 (30)
Doctors are careful to check everything.	73 (28)	41 (61)
Doctors cause people to worry because they don't explain everything.	209 (80)	52 (78)
If I have a medical question, I can reach a doctor for help without any problem.	157 (60)	48 (72)
I am happy with the coverage provided by medical insurance plans.	111 (43)	39 (58)
It's hard to get an appointment for medical care right away.	183 (70)	38 (57)

[a]Numbers in parentheses indicate percentages.
[b]n = 267
[c]n = 67

and less than one-half of the respondents felt that doctors are careful to check everything. Women were more likely than men to feel doctors cause people to worry (x^2 = 26.76, p = .002). A majority of respondents also thought that doctors reject treatments that could help people. Women were more likely than men to feel this way (x^2 = 23.5, p = .008). A majority of respondents indicated that they have difficulty getting answers to medical questions and securing appointments with physicians. In all cases, the older-elderly (75 and older) were more likely to express negative attitudes toward physicians.

Some programmatic implications can be drawn from the attitude findings. First, if elderly persons feel that doctors reject cancer treatments that could help patients, they may seek unproven cures, such as laetrile, or avoid seeking appropriate care. To overcome the worry caused by inadequate communication, we believe it is necessary to teach the elderly skills for interacting with health professionals, particularly in asking questions. This is consistent with research results which indicate that the elderly have diffi-culty in asking appropriate, strategic questions and in syn-thesizing complex bits of information (Tamir 1979).

Desire for Communication

The older respondents valued communication. Eighty-four percent wished to be told the diagnosis if they had cancer, and 75% of them would want to talk with relatives and friends about the disease if they found they had cancer. These results, in addition to the respondents' attitudes towards physicians, suggest that older people want informa-tion about cancer and would benefit from education programs tailored to their needs.

FUTURE DIRECTIONS

The results of the surveys and information from other sources have been used to design education programs. The aims are to increase the practice of recommended prevention and early detection behaviors among the elderly and the earliness with which the elderly seek medical evaluation for suspected cancer symptoms. These aims will be achieved through the use of educational interventions designed to increase knowledge about cancer and what the elderly can do about it, to reduce false beliefs and to improve the skills the elderly use in communicating with their physicians. The Fox Chase Cancer Center Cancer Program for Older Citizens (CAPROC) will be offered to community groups with memberships consisting predominantly of older people: nutrition centers, churches, synagogues, and other social organizations. Group interventions will be supplemented by one-to-one methods. The program builds on our past success with slide presentations as a method of gathering data, and the components are presented as educational entertainment.

CANCER CONTROL IMPLICATIONS

In view of the aging of the United States population and the demonstrated association between aging and cancer, cancer control researchers should devote more attention to the problems of the elderly. This includes increasing the acceptability of treatment regimens for older persons, improving the means for ameliorating adverse side effects of treatment and refining methods for improving the rehabilitation and continuing care of older cancer patients. Likewise, researchers should develop educational programs that will change false beliefs and negative attitudes, thereby altering behaviors related to delay, early detection and compliance with treatment. Programs that have been designed for younger age groups should be evaluated for their relevance to older persons. As Yancik observed (Cancer Letter 1982), "In less than 50 years, the size of the older aged group will have more than doubled to about 55 million before the population expansion levels off. Cancer may more likely be an even greater health problem for older persons in the future."

REFERENCES

Boyd J (1982). The Cancer Letter October 29, 1982:4.
Foster R, Lang SP, Costanza MC, Worden J, Haines C (1978). Breast self-examination practices and breast cancer stage. New England Journal of Medicine 299:265-270.
German P (1978). The elderly: a target highly accessible to health education. International Journal of Health Education 21:267-272.

German P (1981). "Delivery of Care to Older People: Issues and Outlooks." Rockville, MD: Aspen Systems.

Green L, Roberts B (1974). The literature on why women delay in seeking medical care for breast symptoms. Health Education Monographs 2:129-173.

Hobbs P, George W, Sellwood R (1980). Acceptors and rejectors of an invitation to undergo screening compared with those who referred themselves. Journal of Epidemiology and Community Health 34:19-22.

Howe H (1981). Social factors associated with breast self-examination among high risk women. American Journal of Public Health 71:251-253.

Kegeles S, Grady K (1982). Behavioral dimensions. In Shottenfeld D, Fraumeni J (eds): "Cancer Epidemiology and Prevention," Philadelphia, PA: W. B. Saunders.

Kirscht J, Haefner D, Kegeles S, Rosenstock I (1966). A national study of health beliefs. Journal of Health and Human Behavior 7:242-254.

Knopf A (1976). Women's beliefs about the causes of cancer. In Wakefield J (ed): "Public Education About Cancer," Geneva: UICC, 24:52-61.

Ouslander J, Beck J (1982). Defining the health problems of the elderly. Annual Review of Public Health 3:55-83.

Peterson B, Kennedy B (1979). Aging and cancer management - part 2. Ca - A Journal for Clinicians 29:333-340.

Rimer B, Jones W, Wilson C, Bennett D, Engstrom P (In press). Planning a cancer control program for older citizens. The Gerontologist.

Tamir L (1979). "Communication and the Aging Process." New York: Pergamon Press.

Wilson C, Bennett D, Jones W, Engstrom PF (1982). A technique for administering a questionnaire to a group with low reading ability. In Mettlin C, Murphy GP (eds): "Issues in Cancer Screening and Communications," New York: Alan R. Liss.

Wilkinson G, Edgerton F, Wallace HJ, Reese P, Patterson J, Priore R (1979). Delay, stage of disease and survival from breast cancer. Journal of Chronic Diseases 32:365-373.

Progress in Cancer Control IV: Research in the Cancer Center, pages 135–144
© 1983 Alan R. Liss, Inc., 150 Fifth Avenue, New York, NY 10011

SKIN CANCER/MELANOMA KNOWLEDGE AND BEHAVIOR IN HAWAII:
CHANGES DURING A COMMUNITY-BASED CANCER CONTROL PROGRAM

P.H.King, Ph.D., G.D.Murfin, Ph.D., K.L.Yanagisako, M.P.H.
D.A.Wagstaff, Ph.D., G.L.Putnam, M.S.W., F.L.Hajas, M.S.W.
and S.C.Berger, M.A.
Cancer Center of Hawaii, University of Hawaii - Manoa
1236 Lauhala Street, Honolulu, HI 96813

INTRODUCTION

During the 1977-82 community-based cancer control
program in Hawaii, statewide health awareness surveys (HAS)
were conducted of the public's knowledge and behavior
regarding many cancer sites and topics. The latter two of
the surveys included questions on skin cancer/melanoma.
During 1981, the year between the second and third survey, a
public information/education campaign was implemented, consisting of a June mailing of an educational comic book and
the airing during the period from May through December of
television and radio public service announcements. The
comic book was mailed to 35,000 households with a surname
indicating likely Caucasian ethnicity. Included in these
were all 8,000 homes in a relatively high Caucasian density
target neighborhood. A baseline survey of the target neighborhood was conducted in conjunction with the 1980-81 HAS.
A follow-up survey was conducted in the target neighborhood
in October to assess the impact of the information/education
campaign.

METHODS

Media Campaign: The skin cancer/melanoma media campaign consisted of two components: an educational 16-page
color comic book and television and radio public service
announcements. The comic book stressed risk of skin
cancer/melanoma for all ethnic groups with special emphasis
on Caucasians. It featured a fictional local Caucasian

family and was designed to provide information and motivation so that readers would:

1. Be able to identify risk factors and prevention/detection practices for skin cancer/melanoma,
2. Apply sunscreen lotions of SPF8 or higher prior to exposure to the sun,
3. Avoid unprotected exposure to the sun, especially between 10 a.m. and 2 p.m.,
4. Examine their skins on a regular basis for changes in moles or sores that did not heal within a two-week period, and
5. See a physician immediately if they discover changes in moles or sores that did not heal within a two-week period.

Two television public service announcements and three radio spots were produced and distributed to local television stations in April of 1981. Both spots promoted the use of protective sun screens, and their overall message paralleled that of the comic book, although in less detail and at less length.

Study Design: Figure 1 pictures the media campaign in temporal relationship to the surveys, and the survey sample sizes. The second HAS and comic book baseline survey took place prior to the media campaign; the follow-up survey took place four months after the comic book distribution, and the third HAS took place six months after the distribution. The larger sample sizes for the HAS surveys compared to the target neighborhood surveys reflect the need of the former to adequately sample the entire State. All surveys were conducted face-to-face in respondents' homes.

FIGURE 1. STUDY DESIGN: SC/M MEDIA
CAMPAIGN AND ASSOCIATED SURVEYS

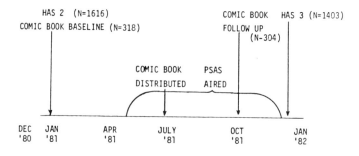

There were four major hypotheses: I: The five study groups will differ significantly in skin cancer/melanoma knowledge and behavior with the HAS 3 group scoring higher than the HAS 2 group, and the comic book readers group more knowledgeable than the other four groups.

II: Knowledge and behavior will be significantly related to respondent characteristics. High levels of knowledge and behavior generally will be positively associated with income level, education level, and Caucasian ethnicity, and negatively associated with age.

III: There will be a positive association between skin cancer/melanoma knowledge and prevention/detection behavior.

IV: Comic book readers will increase their prevention and detection behavior and credit these changes to having read the comic book.

Analysis: Chi-square statistics were used to assess the significance of differences among groups.

RESULTS

Media Campaign Impact: The impact of the media campaign was assessed by measuring the number of sources through which respondents had learned about skin cancer and melanoma. The average number of sources per respondent was greater for the groups measured after the implementation of the campaign (see Table 1). We concluded from this finding that the campaign was successful in reaching the public.

TABLE 1. SC/M INFORMATION: # SOURCES/PERSON

HAS 2	COMIC BOOK BASELINE	COMIC BOOK FOLLOW-UP (READERS)	(NON-READERS)	HAS 3
3.0	2.3	4.5	3.6	3.4

Knowledge: As shown in Table 2, a low percentage of respondents knew that melanoma was the most dangerous skin condition. Even in the group that had read the comic book, fewer than half (48%) of the sample knew the correct answer. A significantly higher percentage of the HAS 3 group than the HAS 2 group knew the correct answer. Similarly, a greater percentage of the follow-up reader group knew the correct answer than the baseline and follow-up non-reader groups. The knowledge level, for this item, while low, increased during the year in which the public information program was implemented and also increased as a function of the complex of factors involved in choosing to read, and reading, the comic book.

TABLE 2. SC/M KNOWLEDGE

GROUP:	HAS 2	HAS 3	COMIC BOOK BASELINE	COMIC BOOK FOLLOW-UP (READERS)	(NON-READERS)
K ITEM					
MELANOMA MOST DANGEROUS	18%	24%	25%	48%	32%
		(p <.001)		(p <.001)	
CAUCASIANS AT HIGHEST RISK	72%	71%	75%	82%	60%
				(p <.001)	
10 am - 2 pm SUN MOST HARMFUL	79%	80%	85%	96%	83%
				(p <.01)	

(PERCENTAGE OF RESPONDENTS KNOWING CORRECT ANSWER)

Overall, a moderately high percentage of respondents knew that Caucasians were the highest risk group for skin cancer. The differences among the three comic book groups were significant. The significance was accounted for by the 22% difference between the follow-up readers and non-readers.

Overall, a high percentage of respondents knew that 10 a.m. to 2 p.m. are the hours in the day at which the sun is most harmful. The follow-up readers group was significantly more knowledgeable than the baseline and follow-up non-readers group.

Behavior: Respondents were asked questions about their behavior in regard to skin cancer/melanoma, prevention and detection. Results are portrayed in Table 3.

The wearing of protective clothing while spending time in the sun did not change as a function of the time between the various surveys nor as a function of comic book reading.

TABLE 3. PREVENTION/DETECTION BEHAVIOR

GROUP:	HAS 2	HAS 3	COMIC BOOK BASELINE	COMIC BOOK FOLLOW-UP (READERS)	(NON-READERS)
BEHAVIOR					
(P) WEAR PROTECTIVE CLOTHING	34%	36%	28%	36%	27%
(P) USE SUNSCREEN	18%	22%	34%	62%	37%
	_____(p<.005)_____			_____(p<.001)_____	
(D) EXAMINE OWN SKIN REGULARLY	58%	53%	68%	72%	61%
	_____(p<.025)_____				
(D) ASKED DOCTOR TO EXAMINE SKIN	21%	18%	31%	24%	25%
	_____(p<.025)_____				

(PERCENTAGE OF RESPONDENTS PERFORMING BEHAVIOR)

Overall, about one-fourth of the total respondents who spent time in the sun used a protective sunscreen. There were substantial differences among the five groups. The HAS 3 group was modestly higher (22% to 18%) than the HAS 2 group. Among the comic book groups, the readers group's sunscreen use ratio of 62% was markedly higher than both the non-readers group and the baseline group. There appear to be three effects here: an increase associated with the passage of time, a higher base level for the comic book samples compared to the HAS samples, and a large increase associated with reading the comic book.

Respondents were asked whether they examined their skin regularly - at least once a year - for changes in warts or moles. There was a decrease in this behavior between the two State-wide HAS groups over time, a finding opposed to the increase in prevention behavior. The comic book readers were again the highest group, but not significantly higher than the baseline and non-readers groups.

As with skin self-examination, asking a physician for a skin examination decreased slightly over the year's duration of the study. This finding is opposite to the hypothesized shift. A possible explanation is that respondents in the groups surveyed later took better care of their skin and therefore developed fewer symptoms than did groups surveyed earlier, or the media campaign gave respondents a greater security in their own examinations and less tendency to seek medical advice.

Knowledge, Behavior and Respondent Characteristics:
Tables 4 and 5 present the association between respondent
characteristics and knowledge and behavior. As predicted,
knowlege was positively associated with education and income
levels, Caucasian ethnicity, and negatively associated with
age for two of the three items.

TABLE 4. SC/M KNOWLEDGE X
RESPONDENT CHARACTERISTICS

K ITEM	SEX (MALE)	EDUCATION	INCOME	ETHNICITY	AGE
MELANOMA MOST DANGEROUS	n.s.	+(.001)	+(.001)	+(.001)	n.s.
CAUCASIANS AT HIGHEST RISK	n.s.	+(.001)	+(.001)	+(.001)	-(.02)
10 am - 2 pm SUN MOST HARMFUL	n.s.	+(.001)	+(.001)	+(.001)	-(.01)

(DIRECTION OF RELATIONSHIP
AND STATISTICAL SIGNIFICANCE)

TABLE 5. PREVENTION/DETECTION BEHAVIOR

X RESPONDENT CHARACTERISTICS

B ITEM	SEX (MALE)	EDUCATION	INCOME	ETHNICITY	AGE
WEAR PROTECTIVE CLOTHING	+(.001)	?	n.s.	?	+(.001)
USE SUNSCREEN	-(.001)	+(.001)	+(.001)	+(.001)	-(.001)
EXAMINE OWN SKIN REGULARLY	-(.01)	+(.001)	n.s.	+(.001)	n.s.
ASKED DOCTOR TO EXAMINE SKIN	-(.05)	+(.05)	+(.001)	+(.001)	+(.02)

(DIRECTION OF RELATIONSHIP
AND STATISTICAL SIGNIFICANCE)

Prevention and detection behavior was also related to
respondent characteristics. Of the four items, three were
positively associated with knowledge, two with income, and
three with ethnicity. Only using sunscreen was negatively
associated with age, as predicted, while both wearing protective clothing and asking a doctor to examine one's skin
increased with increasing age.

Knowledge and Behavior Relationship: Implicit in
public health education/information programs is that
imparting knowledge leads to desired changes in health
related behavior. To test this assumption, responses to
four behavior questions were tabulated with answers to three
knowledge items, yielding 60 discrete knowledge/behavior
comparisons for the five groups. Forty-seven of these
showed positive associations. Table 6 pictures the number
of positive associations out of five possible for each
knowledge/behavior pair. A significant negative relationship appeared twice: both times it involved wearing
protective clothing when out in the sun, a cultural practice
associated with older, less-educated, non-Caucasian respondents, all factors associated with low knowledge scores.

TABLE 6. POSITIVE K/B RELATIONSHIPS

K ITEM:	MELANOMA MOST DANGEROUS	CAUCASIANS AT HIGHEST RISK	10 am - 2 pm SUN MOST HARMFUL
B ITEM			
WEAR PROTECTIVE CLOTHING IN SUN	2/5	2/5	2/5
USE SUNSCREEN	5/5	5/5	4/5
EXAMINE OWN SKIN REGULARLY	5/5	5/5	4/5
ASKED DOCTOR TO EXAMINE SKIN	5/5	4/5	4/5

ITEM PAIR POSITIVE RELATIONSHIPS/
ALL RELATIONSHIPS (TOTAL: 47/60)

These findings of a generally positive relationship
between knowledge and behavior are consistent with the
assumption that imparting knowledge will lead to an increase
in the desired behavior. However, such a conclusion cannot
be drawn with certainty from this analysis, since lack of
experimental control and the self-selection of the readers
and non-readers groups confound the information/education
effect with the pre-existing knowledgeability/motivation
effect.

Effects of Comic Book Distribution in Target Neighborhood: The comic book follow-up groups were asked a
series of questions pertaining to the receipt, reading and
effects of reading the comic book.

Of the 304 households contacted in the post-survey,

respondents in 135 (44%) remembered receiving the skin cancer comic book. Of those recalling the comic book, someone in 122 (90%) of the households had read it. One hundred of the individuals interviewed reported having read the comic book, while 250 others residing in the households had also read it.

Respondents from the 122 households in which the comic book was read were asked if they or other household members had changed various behaviors as a direct result of reading the comic book. As shown in Table 7, the comic book was most effective in motivating individuals to avoid sun exposure between 10 a.m. and 2 p.m., to use a protective sunscreen with SPF "8" or above, to perform self-examination of the skin, and to wear protective clothing. To a much lesser extent respondents reported consulting their physician because of a suspected cancerous condition or calling the Cancer Information Line (CIL) for more information. Comparing responses to this question by respondent characteristics showed that females reported more behavior changes than males in regard to sunscreen use, use of protective clothing, sun exposure, and self skin examinations.

TABLE 7. SELF-REPORTED CHANGES IN READER HOUSEHOLDS

BEHAVIOR	READER HOUSEHOLDS
AVOID SUN 10 am - 2 pm	44%
USE SUNSCREEN (SPF $\geq$ 8)	38%
EXAMINE OWN SKIN	34%
WEAR PROTECTIVE CLOTHING	30%
CONSULT PHYSICIAN	14%
CALL CANCER INFORMATION LINE	2%

The skin cancer comic book appears to have effectively motivated a substantial portion of its readers (30-45%) to make conscious behavior changes in regard to sun exposure, sunscreen use, self skin examinations, and use of protective clothing.

The reported changes in behavior as a result of having read the comic book reflect and are consistent with the differences in behavior among the comic book baseline, follow-up readers and non-readers groups.

The comic book was less effective in encouraging readers to call the Cancer Information Line (CIL) for more skin cancer information or to consult their physician regarding a suspected cancerous condition. However, motivating the reader to contact the CIL was not an objective of the comic book, but rather was a suggestion to the reader in case more information was sought. Similarly, physician consultation was not expected of readers in general, but only the much smaller number with a suspicious physical finding.

The comic book seemed to appeal less to males and older individuals (age 50+). Income and educational levels did not appear to directly affect readership. More Caucasians read the comic book than other ethnic groups, but due to the small numbers involved, it was difficult to compare interest across ethnic groups.

Because only 44% of the residents recalled receiving the comic book (despite a free mailing to each house in this area), it is possible that another means of distribution may be more effective.

DISCUSSION

The comic book was successful in motivating desired behavior change among respondents who had access to it and who chose to read it. The mail delivery mechanism may be improved in effectiveness by personal delivery door-to-door (e.g., via the American Cancer Society's Crusade) and by distribution through pharmacies, grocery stores, schools, health centers, medical offices and other organizations. The comic book format could be modified into a pamphlet to appeal more to older age groups and to men.

Production and distribution costs for the comic book are moderate. Design and production of 50,000 copies cost $16,500, plus staff time. Reprint costs for 50,000 copies were estimated at 12 cents per copy. Mailing costs were 3.5 cents per copy. Costs for personal delivery or distribution through businesses and other organizations could be negligible.

The comic book has been adopted by the Skin Cancer Foundation and widely distributed on the Mainland. This is evidence of its appeal beyond Hawaii and its potential as an educational vehicle in other areas of the country where people are at high risk for skin cancer and melanoma.

Unresolved by this study are questions concerning the relative contribution of subject characteristics, the comic book, the television and radio spots, and other coincident events in determining knowledge and behavior levels.

There are two promising approaches to untangling the causal mechanisms operating. One is to query respondents directly about their reasons for choosing, for example, to read or not read the comic book; or to ask them about the source and duration of knowledgability and behavior. A second approach would be to conduct educational sessions under conditions of experimental control, with subjects randomly or systematically assigned to treatment groups, and with the researcher determining that both subjects who might prefer to read and not to read the comic book actually both read or don't read it. Such a design would separate the effects of motivation to read from the effects of reading.

REFERENCES

Putnam GL, Yanagisako KL (1982). Skin cancer comic book: evaluation of a public educational vehicle. Community Cancer Program of Hawaii, Cancer Center of Hawaii.

Wagstaff D (1982). Skin cancer report: health awareness survey, 1980-1982. Community Cancer Program of Hawaii.

Supported in part by NCI Contract Number N01-CN-75399.

Progress in Cancer Control IV: Research in the Cancer Center, pages 145–152

POPULATION-BASED ASSESSMENT OF THE CHARACTERISTICS OF
POTENTIAL USERS OF A CANCER INFORMATION SERVICE (CIS)

Sharon R. Haymaker, M.S.N.
Laura L. Morlock, Ph.D.
David D. Celentano, Sc.D.
Donna S. Cox, M.Ed.
T. Phillip Waalkes, Ph.D., M.D.

The Johns Hopkins Oncology Center and The
Johns Hopkins School of Hygiene and Public
Health
Baltimore, Maryland 21205

The Cancer Information Service (CIS) is a component of
the Cancer Communication Network Office sponsored by the
Johns Hopkins Comprehensive Cancer Center. The office is
part of a nationwide network operating under contracts from
the National Cancer Institute. The Johns Hopkins CIS provides a toll-free telephone inquiry service within its
designated area of Maryland that supplies information
regarding cancer and cancer-related resources to the general
public, to health professionals, and to cancer patients and
their families. This communication link between the
National Cancer Program and the public is viewed as essential
because of the need to supplement existing communication
patterns between patients and providers. In addition, the
CIS provides a means of addressing the problem of public
misinformation which often surrounds the topic of cancers
and their treatment.

A persistent problem in attempting to evaluate the
effectiveness of Cancer Information Services is the difficulty in assessing selection factors that may be operating
with respect to the utilization of such services. In order
to determine the overall impact of such programs it is
necessary to attain a better understanding of how utilizers
of the service compare to the general population of nonutilizers. A household survey recently completed for the

Johns Hopkins Oncology Center provided an opportunity to begin to address these issues through an assessment of how survey respondents who expressed an interest in utilizing the Cancer Information Service differed from those individuals who indicated they had no interest in using such a service.

METHODOLOGY

The major purpose of the study was to ascertain levels of knowledge and behaviors related to cancer prevention. Telephone interviews were conducted in a random sample of 500 households located in a section of Baltimore City selected because of its relatively high rates of cancers of the lung, breast and cervix. The survey was fielded in the spring of 1981 by the Johns Hopkins Research and Development Center using trained interviewers with experience in cancer control surveys. The response rate obtained was 74.1 percent, resulting in completed interviews with 308 women and 193 men. During the interview, all respondents were read the following statement:

"The Cancer Information Service is free and they have a toll-free telephone number which you can call to get information about cancer, cancer screening, or treatment and to answer any questions or concerns you might have.

Do you think you might want to call sometime?"

Of the total sample, 92% expressed a definite preference with regard to utilization of the CIS, with 66% stating an interest in calling compared to 26% who expressed no such desire. Only 8% expressed no definite preference in either direction. The racial mix of the sample who were definite in their desire to either call or not call was 43% black, 55% white and 2% "other". The age distribution was 36% below age 41, 35% between the ages of 41 and 60, and 29% over age 60. Sixty-two percent of the sample was female. The number of years of education was twelve years or less for two-thirds of the sample with the remaining one-third attaining over twelve years. Approximately half (47%) of the respondents had a family income less than $15,000 a year. An analysis of differences between the characteristics of individuals who expressed an interest in using the CIS in comparison to those who indicated no such interest was conducted as part of ongoing evaluation activities of the CIS. The analysis specifically examined demographic characteristics, knowledge related to cancer, concern about health, and opinions concerning the adequacy of community resources.

DEMOGRAPHIC CHARACTERISTICS

Analysis of differences between the characteristics of individuals who expressed an interest in using the CIS in comparison to those who expressed no such desire indicates that potential CIS utilizers were significantly less likely to be over age 60, and twice as likely to be black (51% vs. 25%). (See Table 1) There were no significant differences between the two groups with regard to sex, marital status, income or education.

CANCER-RELATED KNOWLEDGE LEVELS

Analysis of knowledge levels related to cancer indicates that the potential utilizers of CIS, in contrast to the potential nonutilizers, were significantly more likely to know that bleeding, a change in bowel habits, or a persistent cough could serve as a warning sign of the possible presence of cancer. The two groups were not significantly different in their knowledge of other warning signs or symptoms such as the presence of a lump or having difficulty swallowing. Potential CIS utilizers were, however, significantly more likely to be able to state at least one specific way in which to decrease their likelihood of getting cancer.

CONCERN ABOUT HEALTH

In comparison to individuals not expressing an interest in calling CIS, the group of potential utilizers were less likely to describe their general health as excellent. There was no difference, however, between the two groups with regard to whether they had ever had a symptom which they believed might indicate the presence of cancer. (See Table 2) Furthermore, there was no difference noted in whether they

TABLE 1

DESIRE TO CALL CIS BY DEMOGRAPHIC CHARACTERISTICS
(Figures Percentaged by column)

Demographic Characteristics	Desire to call CIS	
	No	Yes
Age		
40 and under	29%	39%
41-60	31%	36%
Over 60	40%	25%
N	(130)	(327)
		$p < .05*$
Sex		
Male	43%	36%
Female	57%	64%
N	(129)	(325)
		$p < 0.2$
Race		
Black	25%	51%
White	74%	48%
Other	1%	1%
N	(130)	(327)
		$p < .001*$
Income		
Under $5,000	14%	12%
$5,000-$9,000	9%	18%
$10,000-$14,000	25%	16%
$15,000-$19,000	14%	13%
$20,000-$29,000	21%	25%
$30,000+	17%	16%
N	(104)	(287)
		$p < 0.2$
Education		
12 years or less	60%	66%
Over 12 years	40%	34%
N	(130)	(327)
		$p < 0.3$

*Level of significance based on Chi-Square test for independence.

TABLE 2

DESIRE TO CALL CIS BY CONCERN ABOUT HEALTH
(Figures Percentaged by Column)

Perceived Susceptibility	Desire to Call CIS	
	No	Yes
General State of Health		
Poor	3%	7%
Fair	26%	16%
Good	38%	54%
Excellent	33%	23%
N	(130)	(327)
	p<.005*	
Concern about Health in Past Month		
Very concerned	16%	18%
Somewhat concerned	46%	52%
Not at all concerned	38%	30%
N	(129)	(326)
	p<.40	
Specific Worries About Health		
None	68%	54%
Cancer	19%	29%
Other	12%	15%
All-General	1%	2%
N	(128)	(323)
	p<.10	
Concern About Getting Cancer		
Very Concerned	31%	51%
Somewhat concerned	22%	24%
Not at all concerned	47%	25%
N	(129)	(324)
	p<.001*	
Perceived Likelihood of Getting Cancer		
Very likely	40%	54%
Somewhat likely	30%	29%
Not likely	30%	17%
N	(108)	(267)
	p<.10	

*Level of significance based on Chi-Square test for independence.

had at the time seen a doctor for an evaluation of this symptom. However, the potential CIS user was significantly more concerned than the potential non-user about the possibility of getting cancer (51% vs 31%). They also specifically identified cancer as their major worry about health (29% vs. 19%) and were more likely to perceive that they had a strong probability of getting cancer (54% vs. 40%).

PERCEIVED ADEQUACY OF COMMUNITY RESOURCES

Potential utilizers in contrast to potential nonusers tended to perceive existing community resources for the care of cancer patients as inadequate (37% vs. 26%). (See Table 3) The potential users were also significantly more likely than nonusers to perceive a need for additional community resources (45% vs. 20%). When asked what resources they believed were needed, 35% stated that more services were needed for screening, 25% believed there was a need for more education and family support services, 17% saw a need for more physicians and general services, and 9% wanted more resources for home follow-up and care. An interesting finding was the significantly higher interest expressed by the potential users of the CIS in the formation of a community organization for smoking cessation. A total of 222 respondents stated that they would be interested in the formation of such an organization. This represented 73% of all respondents who expressed an opinion related to the specific question asked during the interview and 45% of the total sample.

SUMMARY

In summary, the analysis suggests that blacks are significantly more likely, and individuals over age 60 and those who perceive their health as excellent are significantly less likely to express a desire to utilize a Cancer Information Service. The group of potential CIS utilizers are also significantly more likely to identify cancer as their greatest worry relative to their own health, to be concerned about getting cancer, and to perceive a strong likelihood that they will actually get cancer in the future. They are more knowledgeable about cancer symptoms and are able to state at least one specific way to decrease the risk

TABLE 3

DESIRE TO CALL CIS BY OPINIONS ABOUT COMMUNITY RESOURCES
(Figures Percentaged by Column)

Perceptions Regarding Community Resources	Desire to Call CIS	
	No	Yes
Perceived Adequacy of Community Resources		
Very adequate	31%	19%
Adequate	43%	44%
Inadequate	26%	37%
N	(84)	(219)
	p<.10	
Perceived Need for Community Services for Care of Cancer Patients		
No	80%	55%
Yes	20%	45%
N	(86)	(207)
	p<.001*	
Interest in Formation of Community Organization for Smoking Cessation		
No	46%	20%
Yes	54%	80%
N	(78)	(225)
	p<.001*	

---

*Level of significance based on Chi-Square test for independence.

of getting cancer. The group also believes that existing community resources are inadequate and that additional resources are necessary for the care of cancer patients.

The survey results suggest that there is a substantial number of individuals who worry about getting cancer, who perceive themselves to be at high risk for this possibility, and who perceive existing community resources as inadequate. Data analysis suggests that a Cancer Information Service with sufficient visibility could help address unmet needs, particularly with respect to providing education related to cancers and their treatment. The study results also support the role of a CIS in serving as a catalyst by identifying other types of perceived needs as expressed by CIS utilizers and then communicating these concerns to other relevant community agencies and services.

This analysis was supported by a Cancer Communication Network Contract (1 CN 25576) from the National Cancer Institute to the Johns Hopkins Oncology Center.

Progress in Cancer Control IV: Research in the Cancer Center, pages 153–160
© 1983 Alan R. Liss, Inc., 150 Fifth Avenue, New York, NY 10011

APPLYING MARKETING TECHNIQUES TO PROMOTION OF THE CANCER
INFORMATION SERVICE

Russell C. Sciandra
Roswell Park Memorial Institute
Buffalo, New York   14263

Judith A. Stein
Division of Resources, Centers, and
   Community Activities
National Cancer Institute
Bethesda, Maryland   20205

The Cancer Information Service (CIS) is a network of
21 offices, most funded by the National Cancer
Institute (NCI) and based at cancer centers. CIS provides
information on cancer through toll-free telephone lines
to concerned laymen and health professionals in 27 states
and the District of Columbia. A national toll-free line
operated by a contractor in Bethesda serves other states
and provides evening backup to regional offices. Since its
inception in 1976 the network has responded to over one
million inquiries, with the rate of use rising steadily
throughout that time. In the six months between January
and June of 1982 the network recorded 112,784 calls.

Two thirds of callers are females. About one third
are cancer patients or family members. To the extent
there is a typical CIS caller she is white, between 30
and 50, has a better than average education and higher
than average income. She is calling with a specific
question about her own health or that of a family member.
We observe that certain groups, most notably blue-collar
males, minorities and healthy people over 50, call at a
lower rate than would be expected from their proportion in
the population.

Experience has shown that promotion of CIS is
important to maintaining a high level of response.

Promotion consists of national publicity for the network as a whole as well as centrally prepared advertising tailored to a specific center-based CIS. Individual offices also conduct independent promotion activities within their service areas.

Promotion efforts have included: television and radio public service announcements; print ads for newspapers and magazines; news releases for print and electronic media; brochures and posters exhibited in a wide variety of public settings; telephone directory listings; use of inter-mediaries, such as the American Cancer Society, who refer people to CIS, and a variety of other methods. While these efforts have been successful in stimulating a large number of calls, many in the network felt they could be improved.

Like many similar efforts in the health field, CIS promotion had proceeded without a coherent plan and with insufficient research. No specific long term goals were set and target audiences were often identified on the basis of program priorities rather than significant demographics. As a result, target groups frequently included those least disposed to call CIS. Publicity campaigns were short-lived and did not produce a consistent image of CIS in the public mind. Local and national campaigns often were not coordinated. Little was known about public knowledge, attitudes and practices with regard to cancer and less was used in the selection of messages and communications channels.

To rectify some of these problems a Task Force con-sisting of network representatives, the CIS project officer and specialists from the NCI Office of Cancer Communications, was assembled. The Task Force decided to apply social marketing techniques to the development of a comprehensive promotion plan.

The term "social marketing" was coined in the early 70's to describe the application of marketing concepts and techniques to the promotion of a socially beneficial cause rather than commercial products or services. In the market-place, goods or services are offered in exchange for payment. In promoting socially beneficial behaviors or ideas, marketers recognize that the individual adopting them is being asked to pay a price, not only in money, but in less tangible but equally real psychological, energy and time costs. Marketers also recognize that to different individuals and groups the perceived benefits and costs of the desired behavior will vary. Thus, health promotion is seen as an exchange process in which the offering must be responsive to consumer appetites and cost expectations in order to be accepted. A social marketer will not make the mistake (as many in the health field do) of assuming his offering is inherently desirable to everyone and that lack of interest is due to consumer ignorance of its obvious benefits.

Because it begins with the consumer, a marketing program relies on research into the wants, needs, perceptions, attitudes, habits and satisfaction levels of its audience. It then divides the audience into homogeneous groups and develops unique marketing plans for the individual target segments. This recognizes that different segments are in varying stages of readiness to accept the offering and will require varying incentives to adopt a new behavior or idea. A marketing plan may call for changes in product characteristics or at least in the way the product is presented or packaged to maximize its appeal to target segments. It is also important to recognize that various segments acquire information through diverse channels.

The Task Force has adopted several marketing principles which it followed in developing its plan. These are:

1. Audience segmentation with a separate but complementary promotion strategy for each target audience.

2. Selection, when possible, of target audiences in a readiness stage who are most likely to respond to promotion by calling CIS.

3. Selection of channels appropriate to the target groups, including mass media, health professionals and other intermediaries.

4. Use of positive, anxiety-reducing appeals delivered by sources appropriate to the target audience.

5. Clarity through use, especially in broadcast advertising, of a single message: that immediate benefit can be gained by calling CIS.

6. Locally-developed promotion campaigns which, as much as possible, complement the message and tone of the network-wide program.

In preparing its plan, the CIS Task Force examined published surveys and the existing literature, consulted an unpublished NCI consumer analysis based on focus group interviews, and reviewed its collective experience to develop a picture of the national audience. The Task Force found cancer to be the most feared of diseases. The variation in attitudes towards cancer lies in how people cope with their fear.

The Task Force divided the public into four groups useful in determining who is likely to utilize CIS and for what reasons.

One group, the "Diligent", attempt to reduce the risk of cancer by initiating behavior changes, taking early detection measures, and actively seeking cancer information. Members of this group are most typically women of middle or high socioeconomic status.

"Fatalists", on the other hand, believe little can be done to prevent or cure cancer and therefore see no reason to change their behavior. While receptive to information about cancer, Fatalists are not likely to act in response to it. They will face cancer when it comes, but until then have more important things on their minds. This group is made up of the elderly, blue collar workers, men of low socioeconomic status, blacks and Hispanics.

A third group, primarily males, fear cancer on a personal level. Pessimistic about cancer, they cope with their fear by denial. This group actively avoids information about cancer. Their fear leads to paralysis.

A final group, composed mainly of young people, is oblivious to cancer or to illness in general. They are less likely to have acquaintances with cancer and do not regard it as a threat. Typically, they know little about cancer and are not interested in learning more.

Clearly, Cancer Information Service is not for every-one. No amount of publicity will make people contact a service for information which they don't want. Historically, a large proportion of CIS callers have been high SES women from the "Diligent" group. A much lower proportion of calls have come from people representative of the latter two groups (the avoiders and unconcerned young).

Perhaps the largest and most important potential audience for CIS lies in the "Fatalist" group. Many from the focus group interviews expressed frustration and confusion over the welter of contradictory information about cancer to which they are exposed. By clarifying issues and providing perspective, CIS can help "Fatalists" identify spheres in which behavior change could make a difference. CIS is supportive of the idea that people can and should participate in their own health care and therefore is suited to a campaign which shows people that information does give them some control over the threat of cancer.

There are other characteristics of CIS which make it attractive to many people.

First, it is credible. Because CIS is sponsored by NCI, cancer research centers and, in some cases, the American Cancer Society, it is seen as authoritative and trustworthy. Secondly, because it is staffed by laypeople (often volunteers) perceived by potential callers as similar to themselves, speaking a language they can under-stand, CIS may be a more acceptable source of information than are health professionals.

Finally, the easy access and lack of monetary cost (a free telephone call) of CIS make it a convenient, attractive source of information.

The Task Force decided to accentuate these characteristics in a series of promotion campaigns aimed at specific population segments which fall into the "Fatalist" and "Diligent" groups. The specific character-istics which will be stressed in promotion will vary according to the identified needs and attitudes of the specific target group.

The groups selected are Persons Over 50 Years Old, Blacks, Smokers Who Want to Quit, and Cancer Patients and Their Families. Marketing tests for the latter three groups are being conducted by individual CIS offices. Results of their varying promotion techniques will be utilized in planning future nationwide campaigns. The Task Force is currently developing a marketing plan for the first group which will include recruitment of appropriate intermediaries, identification of the best channels for reaching this target segment and production of print and broadcast advertising.

There is abundant research showing that older Americans have a high interest in health. Confounding the picture, however, is the tendency among older people to avoid thinking about their own risk of cancer. Two focus groups of people age 60+ showed a "clear and nearly universal" desire to avoid thinking about cancer in terms of one's own health. In addition, many older people have a fatalistic attitude about cancer. This "appears to be a function of information overload," according to the focus group analysts.

The Task Force has decided that in promoting to this segment CIS will be positioned as an easily reached provider of clear, authoritative information on cancer. A pamphlet or fact sheet specifically addressing this age group is being developed which will answer common questions about cancer and discuss issues such as early detection and obtaining optimal health services. This piece of literature shall be the primary offering. Its' tone and that of all advertising will be very positive with a stress on health maintenance, not on cancer risk.

Newspapers and television will be the major publicity channels as marketing research shows this age group to be heavier readers and TV viewers than the general population. We also will involve national and local groups concerned about the health of older people, such as the National Institute for Aging.

We believe other cancer control and public information programs would benefit from similar recognition that different members of the public have different attitudes and perceptions with regard to cancer and cancer-related services and that these offerings should be positioned to meet their perceived needs and expectations. Program leaders should be certain to select information channels utilized by their target segments and to involve influential intermediaries in the planning stages of the campaigns.

In other words, outreach programs should be based, not on our preconceptions of what a monolithic public wants, but on sound research into the cancer related knowledge, attitudes and practices of a diverse populace.

Members of the CIS Publicity and Promotion Committee

James Bromley-Diaz (Director of Communications, Cancer Information Service, Comprehensive Cancer Center for the State of Florida)

Gordon Cohn (Principal Investigator/Contract Coordinator, Cancer Information Service, USC Comprehensive Cancer Center)

Bob Denniston (Chief, Information Projects Branch, Office of Cancer Communications, National Cancer Institute)

Bill Erwin (Associate Director of Public Relations, Duke University Medical Center)

Nancy McCormick-Pickett (Information Projects Branch, Office of Cancer Communications, National Cancer Institute)

Marion Morra (Communications Director, Cancer Information Service, Yale Comprehensive Cancer Center)

Russell Sciandra, Chairperson (Contract Coordinator, Cancer Information Service, Roswell Park Memorial Institute)

Judith Stein (Project Officer, Cancer Communications Network, Division of Resources, Centers, and Community Activities, National Cancer Institute)

Carlos Ugarte (Associate Director, Cancer Information Service, Comprehensive Cancer Center for the State of Florida)

Julie Woo (Communications Coordinator, Cancer Information Service, Cancer Center of Hawaii)

References

Andreason AR, (1982). Nonprofits: check your attention to customers. "Harvard Business Review", May-June.
Bloom PN, Novelli WD (1981). Problems and Challenges in social marketing. "Journal of Marketing", Spring.
Fox KFA, Kotler P (1980). The Marketing of Social Causes: the first 10 years. "Journal of Marketing", Fall.

Progress in Cancer Control IV: Research in the Cancer Center, pages 161–170
© **1983 Alan R. Liss, Inc., 150 Fifth Avenue, New York, NY 10011**

A METHODOLOGY FOR CANCER CONTROL UTILIZING CANCER
INFORMATION SERVICE DATA

Dorothy Eckert, Ph.D.

Michigan Cancer Foundation
Evaluation Department, Division of Epidemiology
110 E. Warren Avenue
Detroit, MI 48201

Introduction

The Cancer Information Service (CIS) for the state of
Michigan has been in effect in the metropolitan Detroit
area since January 16, 1982 and throughout the state since
May, 1982. It was proceeded by a Public Response Program
(PRP) in Metropolitan Detroit. The CIS is administered by
the Comprehensive Cancer Center of Metropolitan Detroit,
housed in the Michigan Cancer Foundation, which is located
in the medical complex of Detroit, Michigan. The service is
part of a network sponsored by the National Cancer Institute (NCI), encompassing 20 offices located mainly, in
regional cancer centers. It offers authoritative cancer
information to the lay-pubic, paraprofessionals and professionals on cause, prevention, early detection, diagnosis,
treatment, rehabilitation, continuing care and community
resources (Stein, Kean 1982).

Hypothesizing that an analysis of the data regularly
collected from telephone callers is a methodology that
yields: 1) Information about the public's utilization of
the system; 2) identification of those segments of the
community which may require special assistance in contact-
ing the service, and 3) measurement of the response to
existing CIS promotional strategies, a study of telephone
calls for three major cancer sites is presented.

*This study was made possible through Contract No. 1-CN-255-78.
Acknowledgement is due to Verna Lee Dennert and Judy Homberg
for abstracting the CIS data.

Materials and Methods

All incoming telephone calls to the Michigan CIS requesting information for lung, breast, and colorectal
cancers for a 5½ month period (Jan. 16-June 30, 1982) are
analyzed as to: number of calls, sex, and age of caller;
whether the information requested was for self or "other";
the relationship of the caller to the "other"; and the
kinds of information requested.

For effective cancer control the design of a technical
evaluation plan should reflect and build upon the existing
epidemiologic base (Kosecoff 1982). Incidence data (SEER
1982), therefore, for these three major cancer sites are
examined as a matrix for analyzing these CIS data (Table 1).
The SEER Metropolitan Detroit data is used because 44% of
the state's population (1980 U.S. Census) reside in
Metropolitan Detroit and because there is no extant comprehensive state tumor registry.

The examination of the SEER data for these three sites
as compared to all sites reveals that they account for 58.4%
of all incident cancers. The median ages are: white males,
67 years-of-age and white females, 65 years-of-age; black
males, 65 years-of-age, and black females, 62 years-of-age.

The three sites considered represent 48.2% of all telephone calls received for this period. When analyzed by each
county, the proportion of the number of telephone calls for
the three sites remain in the same range with the exception
of colorectal for Wayne county, which includes Detroit.
(Numbers for the remainder of the state are too small and
the service too new to be representative) (Table 2).

When colorectal cases in Wayne County are selected by
zip code from the Metropolitan Detroit SEER Program, the data
place the majority of cases in the heavily populated areas
of Detroit where older populations reside. (Study in progress)
These data, coupled with the CIS data showing fewer calls
than expected from Wayne County, serve as an indirect
measure of the lack of usage by this population. It would
bear investigation as to whether there may be other factors
at work such as: earlier detection with less morbidity,
another system that is taking care of these needs, or if
the needs are unmet.

TABLE 1

THE NUMBER AND MEDIAN AGE OF MALIGNANT PRIMARY SITE CASES
FOR LUNG AND BRONCHUS, FEMALE BREAST AND COLORECTAL CANCER
DIAGNOSED IN METROPOLITAN DETROIT 1973-77[1]

Percent of Cases Compared to All Sites[1]

	W. Males All Ages	% of All Cases	Median Age	W. Females All Ages	% of All Cases	Median Age	B. Males All Ages	% of All Cases	Median Age	B. Females All Ages	% of All Cases	Median Age
All Sites (N=63,690)	26,102	40.9	66.6	26,639	41.8	62.5	5,936	9.3	64.2	5,013	7.8	59.4
Lung and Bronchus	5,883	22.5	65.2	2,007	3.5	61.9	1,591	2.5	62.0	434	.7	59.0
Female Breast	-	-	-	7,536	11.8	59.0	-	-	-	1,269	2.0	55.9
Colon Rectosigmoid	2,568 1,379	6.2	69.8 67.5	2,628 1,033	5.7	71.2 68.1	470 159	2.4	67.9 65.3	502 180	1.1	67.1 65.0
	3,947			3,661			629			682		
TOTAL	9,830	28.7	-	13,204	21.0	-	2,220	4.9	-	2,385	3.8	-

[1]NCI Monograph 57, SEER, Incidence and Mortality Data, 1981.

NOTE: SEER data is available only for Metropolitan Detroit (Wayne, Oakland and Macomb counties.)

TABLE _2_

CANCER COMMUNICATIONS NETWORK/CANCER INFORMATION SERVICES (CIS) FOR MICHIGAN
TELEPHONE INQUIRIES FOR LUNG, BREAST AND COLORECTAL CANCER
(JANUARY 16, 1982 - JUNE 30, 1982)

Metropolitan Detroit by County Compared to Calls from the Remainder of State

	LUNG N=543		FEMALE BREAST N=523		COLORECTAL N=270	
	N	%	N	%	N	%
Macomb	71	13.1	66	12.5	21	12.4
Oakland	129	23.8	131	24.8	41	24.1
Wayne (includes Detroit)	266	49.0	268	50.8	73	42.9
Total	466	85.9	465	88.1	135	79.4
Remainder of the State	53	9.7	46	8.7	19	11.2
Out of State	-	-	1	2.2	2	1.2
Unknown	24	4.4	16	3.0	14	8.2
Total	543	100.0	528	100.0	170	100.0

The trend for fewer calls for colorectal information
in Detroit is further identified when a comparison is
made with three other network systems, University of Southern
California, Los Angeles, M.D. Anderson, Houston, Texas, and
Johns Hopkins, Baltimore, Maryland (Table 3). Historically,
the percentage of calls for these sites have been roughly
the same for all the Cancer Information of Services
(Personal communication).

Sex and Age of Callers

The frequency of calls to the CIS made by males, for
the two cancer sites shared by both sexes, is 26.8% for
lung and 21.1% for colorectal. The total number of calls
made by males for all sites is 20.8%. Female use of the
system for the three sites, accounted for 72.7% for lung,
88.8% for breast and 75.8% for colorectal. That women are
the main public for this CIS network is consistent with
other studies (Wilkinson, 1978). They represent 78.1% of
all calls made to the Michigan CIS for this period (Table 4).

TABLE 3

CANCER COMMUNICATIONS NETWORK/CANCER INFORMATION SERVICE (CIS) FOR MICHIGAN
TELEPHONE INQUIRIES FOR LUNG, BREAST AND COLORECTAL CANCER
(JANUARY 16, 1982 - JUNE 30, 1982)

A COMPARISON OF THREE CIS TEST AREAS (SEPTEMBER, 1982)

	Lung and Bronchus	Percent Based On Total N	Breast	Percent Based On Total N	Colo- Rectal	Percent Based On Total N
Michigan (CIS) (N=2571 for all sites)	543	21.1 [7.8%]*	528	20.5	170	6.6%
CIS Test Areas (N-1830 for all sites)	121	6.6	379	20.7	161	8.7

[1]These data are compiled from a summary of a pretest for a new data collection form for CIS conducted by M.D. Anderson CIS, Houston, Texas; John Hopkins University CIS, Baltimore, MD; and the University of Southern California CIS, Los Angeles.

*When adjusted for calls pertaining to information/literature as required in the new form the result is 7.8%.

TABLE 4

CANCER COMMUNICATIONS NETWORK/CANCER INFORMATION SERVICE (CIS) FOR MICHIGAN
TELEPHONE INQUIRIES FOR LUNG, BREAST AND COLORECTAL CANCER
(JANUARY 16, 1982 - JUNE 30, 1982)

BY SEX OF CALLER

	MALE		FEMALE		UNKNOWN		TOTAL	
	N	%	N	%	N	%	N	%
LUNG	146	26.8	395	72.7	2	0.3	543	100.0
BREAST	56	10.6	469	88.8	3	0.6	528	100.0
COLORECTAL	36	21.1	129	75.8	5	2.9	170	100.0
ALL SITE TELEPHONE CALLS	536	20.8	2009	78.1	26	1.0	1241	100.0

When all callers are looked at by age it is found that 81.1% are in their "middle years" (41-55), or are the "young old" 50.5% (56-65). Those requesting lung cancer information encompass a wider range from 20-55 years of age (68.3%). However, these data include more calls from an asymptomatic population than is represented in the other two sites. Lung cancer prevention (smoking) information weights this category. The majority of requests for breast cancer information come from ages 31-40 (24.1%), 41-55 (23.5%), 56-65 (25.2%) (Table 5).

TABLE 5

CANCER COMMUNICATIONS NETWORK/CANCER INFORMATION SERVICE (CIS) FOR MICHIGAN
TELEPHONE INQUIRIES FOR LUNG, BREAST AND COLORECTAL CANCER
(JANUARY 16, 1982 - JUNE 30, 1982)

BY AGE OF CALLER

	LUNG		BREAST		COLORECTAL	
	N	%	N	%	N	%
-20	22	4.0	5	4.9	3	1.7
20-30	116	21.3	81	15.3	18	10.5
31-40	125	23.0	127	24.1	24	14.1
41-55	131	24.1	177	33.5	40	23.5
56-65	78	14.3	58	11.0	43	25.2
66-75	35	6.4	27	5.1	18	10.5
75+	6	1.1	13	2.5	7	4.1
Unknown	30	5.5	40	7.6	17	10.0
Total	543	100.0	528	100.0	170	100.0

Who Calls for Whom?

For whom is the caller seeking information for these sites? The data reveal the following relationships: 33.4% of all calls are for self-information; 27% are family members. For calls for family members who are part of the nuclear family (wife, husband, mother, father, daughter or son), females (10%) call twice as often as do males (5%). Daughters (7.5%) are the most frequent callers. Not "patient related" calls represent 28%, with lung cancer (56.9%) skewing the total. When friends (5%) and volunteers are added to family inquiries the lay-patient network consists of 32% of the total calls. Health professionals (4%) add to the profile (Table 6).

TABLE 6

CANCER COMMUNICATIONS NETWORK/CANCER INFORMATION SERVICE (CIS) FOR MICHIGAN
TELEPHONE INQUIRES FOR LUNG, BREAST AND COLORECTAL CANCER
(JANUARY 16, 1982 - JUNE 30, 1982)

RELATIONSHIP OF CALLER TO PATIENT

	LUNG		BREAST		COLORECTAL		TOTAL	
	N	%	N	%	N	%	N	%
Self	39	7.2	322	61.0	54	31.8	415	33.4
Wife	33	6.1	0	0.0	24	14.1	57	4.6
Husband	13	2.4	20	3.8	7	4.1	40	3.2
Mother	0	0.0	6	1.1	2	1.2	8	0.6
Father	2	0.4	0	0.0	0	0.0	2	0.2
Daughter	44	8.1	28	5.3	21	12.4	93	7.5
Son	7	1.3	3	0.6	3	1.8	13	1.0
Sister	9	1.7	15	3.8	2	1.2	26	2.1
Brother	6	1.1	2	0.4	2	1.2	10	0.8
Family Members	50	9.2	27	5.1	7	4.1	84	6.8
Friend	25	4.6	28	5.3	7	4.1	60	4.8
Health Professional	0	0.0	49	0.3	0	0.0	40	3.9
Volunteer	0	0.0	0	0.0	1	0.6	1	0.1
Unknown	6	1.1	3	0.6	27	15.9	36	2.9
Not Patient Related	309	56.9	25	4.7	13	7.6	347	28.0
TOTAL	543	100.0	528	100.0	170	100.0	1241	100.0

People calling for information for themselves, are
asking mainly for: 1) information or literature; 2) for
doctor reference 3) patient care referral (Table 7).
Inquiries for "others" ranked in the same order followed
by Hospital or Clinic referral and referral for other
resources. Information and literature requests rank first
for others (497) and for self (174) (Table 8).

Summary

Analysis of the data disclose that 60% of the telephone
calls are from what has been called the "primary audience"
(Blumberg 1982), the patient (33%) and family and friends
(27%). The network is a resource of support to the patient
and to the patients' social support network, the family.
In giving reliable information to the person who is close

TABLE   7

CANCER COMMUNICATIONS NETWORK/CANCER INFORMATION SERVICE (CIS) FOR MICHIGAN
TELEPHONE INQUIRIES FOR LUNG, BREAST AND COLORECTAL CANCER
(JANUARY 16, 1982 - JUNE 30, 1982)

SELF-INQUIRIES FOR SELECTED CATEGORIES OF INFORMATION[1]

	LUNG		BREAST		COLORECTAL	
	N=39		N=321		N=54	
	N	%	N	%	N	%
Info/Lit	23	59.0	140	43.4	11	20.4
Symptoms	-	-	2	0.6	8	14.8
Doctor Referral	6	15.4	88	27.4	11	20.4
Hosp./Clinic Referral	3	7.7	22	6.8	13	24.1
Patient Care Referral	4	10.3	14	4.4	5	9.3
Supplies	-	-	-	-	-	-
Diet	-	-	-	-	4	7.4
Chemo/Med.	-	-	3	0.9	2	3.7
Pain	-	-	-	-	-	-
Other Resources Referral	3	7.7	52	16.1	-	-
	39	100.0	321	100.0	54	100.0

[1]May reflect multiple requests.

to the patient (Cobb & Erbe) it is bolstering the information support network, for the patient and those who have
taken the responsibility for managing the patient, either
through the acute or chronic aspects of the disease.

The data is consonant with other studies inasmuch as
we are dealing with older people (Table 5) who overwhelmingly
rely on support from relatives and/or friends rather than
formal networks of support (Branch and Jetty). While
assuming, globally, that social support for the patient will
come from family and friends (Eardley, A 1976), it may be
important to develop a contextual profile of those who are
offering social support to the patient (Satariano, Eckert
1982) and include them as a target population.

The methodology presented is a tool for developing
such a profile. While descriptive statistics are used as an

TABLE 8

CANCER COMMUNICATIONS NETWORK/CANCER INFORMATION SERVICE (CIS) FOR MICHIGAN
TELEPHONE INQUIRIES FOR LUNG, BREAST AND COLORECTAL CANCER
(JANUARY 16, 1982 - JUNE 30, 1982)

OTHER THAN SELF-INQUIRIES FOR SELECTED CATEGORIES OF INFORMATION[1]

	LUNG		BREAST		COLORECTAL	
	N	%	N	%	N	%
Info/Lit.	319	63.0	129	63.0	49	44.1
Symptoms	8	1.6	1	0.5	9	8.1
Doctor Refer.	47	9.4	31	15.1	13	11.7
Hosp. Clinc Refer.	36	7.1	6	2.9	6	5.4
Patient Care Refer.	31	6.2	14	6.8	13	11.7
Supplies	5	1.0	-	-	2	1.8
Diet	-	-	-	-	5	4.5
Chemo/Med.	5	1.0	3	1.4	10	9.0
Pain	-	-	-	-	1	0.9
Other Resource Referral	51	10.1	21	10.2	3	2.7
TOTAL	502	100.0	205	100.0	111	100.0

[1]May reflect multiple requests.

illustration, a multivariate analysis is indicated for the variety of variables needed, to help target, shape and direct CIS cancer control for each of these three high incident cancer sites (Mendelsohn 1976). Such a profile when used concomitantly with epidemiological data can be an effective tool for cancer control in a regional cancer center.

References

Blumberg BD (1982). "NCI's Coping With Cancer Information and Education Program - evaluation, planning and implementation." In Cancer Screening and Communications. New York: Alan R. Liss, p. 84.

Branch L, Jetty AM (1980). Unpublished report to the National Heart Lung and Blood Institute on the Framingham Disability Study, pp. 47-8.

Cobb S, Erbe C (1978). Social Support for the Cancer Patient. Unpublished manuscript, p. 11.

Eardley A, Davis F, Wakefield J (1976). Health Education by Chance: The unmet needs of patients in hospitals and after." In Public Education About Cancer. Ed. J. Wakefield, UICC Technical Report Series: Vol. 24, p. 65.

Freidson E (1966). Client Control and Medical Practice Am J Soc 65:374-382.

Kosecoff J, Fink A, Cullen J, Kean T, Arnold M, Swanson GM, Greenwald P (1982). Guidelines for Evaluating Cancer Control Programs. Preventive Med. 11:2 pp. 187-198.

Mendelsohn H (1976). Mass Communications and Cancer Control. In Cancer: The Behavioral Dimensions. Eds. Cullen, Fox, Isous. NY Raven Press. pp. 203-204.

Personal Communication: D Mullins, University of Southern California, Los Angeles (CIS), JA Ward, M.D. Anderson, Houston, Texas (CIS).

Satariano W, Eckert D (1982). "Social Ties and Functional Adjustment Following Mastectomy: Criteria for Research." In Progress in Cancer Control III, N.Y.: Alan R. Liss.

U.S. Dept. of Commerce, Bureau of Census, Census Population and Housing, Summary Tape 2B, Table 94, 1980.

Wilkinson GS, Mirana EA, Walsh DL, Wilson JL, Graham S (1978). Utilization of a Cancer Telephone Information Facility: A comparison of callers and non-caller controls. A J PH, 68:12 pp. 1211-13.

Progress in Cancer Control IV: Research in the Cancer Center, pages 171–182

COMMUNICATIONS STRATEGIES, CANCER INFORMATION AND BLACK
POPULATIONS: AN ANALYSIS OF LONGITUDINAL DATA

Les Butler, Gary King, and Jack E. White, M.D.

Howard University Cancer Center
2041 Georgia Avenue, N.W.
Washington, D.C. 20060

INTRODUCTION

This paper represents the analysis and discussion of
4.5 years of data from Black callers to the Cancer Information Service (CIS) at the Howard University Cancer Center. Officially known as the Cancer Communications Network (CCN), the CIS is the telephone information component of the overall program which is designed to dis-
seminate cancer information to the lay public and health
professionals. The CCN program for the Washington, D.C.
area is jointly sponsored by the Howard University Cancer
Center and the Vincent T. Lombardi Cancer Center at
Georgetown University.

This paper gives an overview of the analysis of data
collected on Blacks who called the CIS between January
1978 through June 1982. The authors discuss the inherent
difficulties in reaching Blacks (males and females) due to
the limitations in the use of mass media and sociological
factors. Also discussed are the communication strategies
which are presently employed that are beginning to prove
effective in reaching the Black population.

In addition, sociological factors which may inhibit
dissemination to Blacks are explored as well as the
positive role of the health professional in the community
outreach segment of cancer control. A programmatic model
is outlined which is currently under consideration for
implementation by this CIS office.

FINDINGS

The data presented in this paper were collected from
persons who called the CIS and identified their racial
group as Black. A total of 2,934 telephone calls were
received from members of this group over the 4.5 year
period. These callers accounted for slightly more than 30%
of the total volume of calls (9,360) received from all
Whites and Blacks. A short instrument was used (i.e., Call
Record Form) which recorded the reasons a person called and
asked a series of questions including how they learned about
CIS and certain demographic characteristics such as age,
sex, residence and race. Our discussion of these data will
be primarily limited to the cumulative period rather than
the nine bi-annual periods which comprise the 4.5 year
period. References will however be made to individual CIS
bi-annual periods. (See Figure 1.)

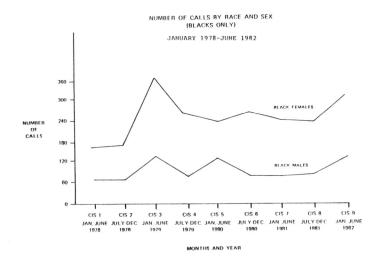

Black females account for 72% and Black males represent 28% of the total number of Blacks who have called the
CIS during the above time period. Most of the callers (57%)
came from persons who were less than 35 years old. The
25-34 year old cohort represents 35% of all Black callers.
(As expected, the overwhelming majority of calls from Blacks
were from those who resided in the District of Columbia.

This group accounts for about 67% of the total number of callers. A relatively large percentage (26%) of calls were received from Blacks who resided in Maryland and a much smaller percentage from Virginia (5%) and elsewhere (2%).)

Of the 41 different cancer sites that were used to identify the focus of a caller's inquiry, seven specific sites and one undefined cancer site predominated in terms of callers' concerns. They are lung, breast, cervix related, an undefined other category, GI tract, skin, colon-rectum and prostate. Taken together, these eight sites account for about 80% (N=1,494) of all the cancer sites the callers mentioned as their primary focus or interest. The types of questions Black callers seem most concerned with were literature requests, cancer symptoms, risk factors, detection and screening, general cancer information, and information about the CIS. Approximately two-thirds (N=1,976) of all questions were about one of these sites.

Regarding the means by which Black callers stated they learned about the CIS, about 26% indicated that television was their primary source of referral. Information about CIS received via the telephone white pages (14%) health professionals (12%), radio (11%), and an undefined "other" category and brochures and pamphlets accounted individually for 10% of the total volume of calls. The most obvious inference from these data is that TV is probably the most effective means of inducing Black audiences to call the CIS.

Cross classification analysis of the variables indicates that there were some important differences between Black male and female callers to the CIS. A clear pattern exists between Black males and females with regard to these two sites. As might be expected, 51% of the Black male callers compared to about 28% of the Black female callers focused their inquiries on lung cancer. In contrast, only 8% of Black males asked about breast cancer, whereas for Black females the number was 34%. A slightly smaller, but no less pronounced difference is apparent when one looks at the number of calls about GYN-related and prostate cancers by sex. To some degree these patterns reflect the fact that women, generally, regardless of race, are more likely to inquire about health education and information sources. It also suggests that there is little cross-over interest on the part of Black males with respect to cancer sites that are not statistically associated with their sexual status.

Another important difference between Black male and female callers to the CIS can be found in the sources of referral to the CIS. Although both a greater percentage of Black male (24%) and female callers (27%) indicated they learned about the service via television, there is a clear difference regarding the effectiveness of radio as a means of reaching either of the two groups. Seventeen percent of Black male callers compared to 8% of Black female callers reported they learned about the CIS through radio. Further evidence supporting this finding is found in the individual CIS bi-annual periods. In the one six-month CIS period in which there was an intensive radio campaign to promote the CIS to Blacks in the Washington, D.C. SMSA, the most dramatic increase occurred in calls from Black males. The percentage of calls received from this group increased 59% from the previous period.

Regarding the variable of age and the focus of a caller's inquiry, the findings reveal that most of the calls received are from those under 35 years of age who are primarily interested in information about lung and breast cancer. Younger Blacks between the ages 15-24 were for the most part, mainly interested in lung cancer information. Almost 50% of the members of this age cohort asked about this form of cancer while 37% of those between 25-34 asked questions focusing on breast cancer. These findings may suggest a perceived need among younger Blacks to seek out information on primary and secondary cancer prevention. There is a consistent decrease in the number of calls received about all cancer sites as the age of the callers increases.

An almost even percentage of Black males (22%) and females (25%) who called the CIS asked a question requesting literature about particular cancer sites or the CIS. If we confine our analysis to the five most frequently asked questions of Black callers (N=1,976), we find that about 25% of them requested cancer-related literature. This finding suggests a general misconception about Blacks and their desire to read materials about cancer. We point out that a distinction has to be made between using the print media to encourage Blacks to call

a CIS and the use of print media to inform Blacks about
cancer after they have called a CIS. It is not correct to
equate the former with the latter strategy primarily
because it is likely that those persons calling a CIS may
not have the concerns or problems of the general
population with respect to cancer. Furthermore, our
results indicate that printed advertisements are neither
particularly effective with Whites or Blacks in getting
them to call a CIS. However, additional research on this
topic is needed because of the many factors one must
consider in regards to media exposure to racial
minorities. We do, however, strongly encourage the
dissemination of appropriate and carefully selected
information about cancer to Black callers to a CIS.

COMMUNICATIONS STRATEGIES

In developing communication strategies for the
promotion of a Cancer Information Service to any audience,
we suggest the social marketing approach.

Social marketing is defined as the design, implementation and control of programs seeking to increase the
acceptability of a social idea or practice in a target
group(s). It utilizes concepts of market segmentation,
consumer research, idea configuration, communication,
facilitation, incentives and exchange theory to maximize
target group response. (Kotler 1975)

In keeping with this concept, consider the goals and
objectives of the CIS program of the Howard Unviersity
Cancer Center:

1. General Goal:

To reduce the cancer incidence, morbidity and mortality,
in the Washington, D.C., SMSA through information dissemination and education mechanisms.

2. Specific Goals:

(a) To increase and maintain the lay public's, cancer
patients' and health profesionals' "general" awareness of
cancer at a meaningful level (e.g. primary and secondary
cancer prevention), and awareness of the CIS as a resource.

Publicity and Promotion Plan Objectives:

- Establish a positive service image and awareness for the CIS within the defined service area (Washington, D.C., SMSA)

- Increase the volume of calls to the CIS by a stated percentage point.

- Target promotion to high-risk groups as defined by epidemiologic and biostatistical studies conducted by both the Howard and Georgetown Cancer Centers and the National Cancer Institute.

Based on the epidemiological studies (Parker and White, 1979), and analysis of CIS data conducted over the past 4.5 years, the CIS has for marketing and communications purposes developed three categories of audiences:

Primary Audience

Race	Sex	Age	Priority Geographic Location
White	Females	25–64	Va., Md., and D.C.
Black	Females	18–55	D.C., Md., and Va.
White	Males	25–64	Va., Md., and D.C.
Black	Males	18–55	D.C., Md., and Va.

High-Risk Audience

Black	Males	18–55	D.C., Md., and Va.
Black	Females	18–55	D.C., Md., and Va.
White	Males	25–64	Va., D.C., and Md.
White	Females	25–64	Va., d.C., and Md.

Target Group*

Black	Males	55+	D.C., Md., and Va.
Black	Females	55+	D.C., Md., and Va.
White	Females	55+	Va., D.C., and Md.
White	Males	55+	Va., D.C., and Md.

*Target audiences as defined by the Howard-Georgetown CIS are: a) groups having high-risk cancers which may be preventable, b) groups for which primary and/or secondary prevention activities can be most beneficial, and c) groups (e.g., Black, elderly and cancer patients) which have difficulty with gaining access to health care and health care information.

Media Objectives:

● Increase CIS awareness by concentrating on media and audience which will provide maximum reach of the service area.

● Select media which will provide the most efficient combination of reach, frequency and continuity within an established budget.

● Coordinate media efforts where possible with intra- and extra-institutional groups and organizations.

Media Selection:

During the 4.5 year period discussed in this paper, the use of mass media specifically targeted towards Blacks by the CIS was minimal. Promotional activities were instead aimed at the general population within the Washington, D.C. SMSA in an attempt to produce an overall increase in calls. Not until CIS Period 8 (July-December, 1981), was there a specific and aggressive effort to reach Blacks. As a result of these efforts, the volume of calls from all Blacks (318) increased 11.2% over the previous period. (See Figure 1.) In CIS Period 9 (January-June, 1982), there was a 37.4% increase (437) in calls from Blacks.

Possible explanations for the increase in calls from this group are the following:

● Focused public relations efforts towards Black oriented radio stations to play CIS public service announcements (p.s.a.).
● Increased use of intermediaries (e.g., health professionals, teachers, clegy, etc.)

● Increase in CIS staff visibility in the Washington, D.C. community.

In previous CIS periods, cancer information was not tailored to the particular cultural and social attitudes and practices of Blacks which this CIS and commercial advertisers have found to be a neccessary requirement.

The use of television and to a lesser degree radio p.s.a.'s presents challenges to the health communicator, such as: a) the inability to control the placement of messages in day parts where viewer/listenership is highest for the targeted audience(s), b) in large Metropolitan areas, the fierce competition from other cancer and cancer/health related groups for the limited amount of public service air space, c) development of a creative approach to communicate a cancer message which must first penetrate the viewer/listeners' pre-attentive processing, and d) cost of quality production.

SOCIOLOGICAL FACTORS

In addition to the pragmatic and day-to-day operational promotions of CIS to Black audiences, it is equally important that we as health educators and communi- cators be cognizant of some of the broader sociological parameters which affect how our efforts are perceived by Black communities. In this connection, we make specific reference to such factors as institutional racism, the inequity of health care delivery systems, socio-economic status, health belief systems and health care seeking behavioral patterns.

For example, health and medical institutions which have a history of racial discrimination and insensitivity to the needs of Black communities are likely to experience greater difficulty in inducing Black audiences to call their CIS. This is also likely to be the case with other health care institutions whose present track records are less than satisfactory in regards to the employment of Black professionals and staff, community outreach networks and Black patient care.

It is also important that CIS staff persons understand the limitations and problems of the health care delivery system and the impact these dynamics may have on cancer communication efforts to the poor and minority group members. A two-tier health and medical system which does not adequately address the preventive health care problems of those most in need will make it much more difficult for a CIS to serve these populations. In order for information, knowledge, and recommendations about cancer prevention and treatment to be optimally effective in reducing cancer morbidity and mortality it must be supported by a health care delivery system which is accessible, equitable and responsive to all. (Greenwald 1982)

The salience of socio-economic status (e.g., income, education and occupation) to cancer morbidity and mortality as well as to cancer prevention and education (Warnecke 1981, and Jackson 1982) has been well documented. Hence, to the extent that Blacks and other groups are continually denied the advantages of equal opportunity in employment practices, education, housing and other social spheres, cancer educators and communicators will continue to face immense and intractable difficulties in reaching these populations. This suggests the need for the CIS to be advocates of public policies related to cancer control that are non-medical determinants of increased cancer rates and education.

Lastly, since there are fewer studies of the health care beliefs about cancer and the health care seeking behavior of Blacks (Jackson 1982), we must accept the reality that there is a lot that we do not know about these areas as they relate to Blacks. This situation has implications for the assumptions, programmatic strategies and conclusions we make about this population. It is suggested that in the absence of definitive and valid data that health communicators refer to the plethora of social science literature on cultural and behavorial patterns in Black communities in designing programs.

HEALTH PROFESSIONALS IN COMMUNITY OUTREACH

In the dissemination of cancer information to Blacks, our data indicate that the health professional plays a vital role. In the context of this paper and cancer control efforts as defined by the CIS, health professionals are the following: (a) doctors, (b) nurses, (c) allied

health personnel, (d) cancer information service staff, and
(e) individuals whose responsibility it is to provide
health care, education and information in an official
capacity.

Results of our data analysis indicate that the health
professional accounted for the third largest category
through which Blacks learned of the CIS. Health
professionals as a source of referral may be relatively
more effective in inducing Black males to call than they
are with Black females. Although the cumulative findings
do not support this supposition, we cautiously suggest this
based on the data in the last year of the 4.5 year period.
During the period July 1981 to June 1982, there was a
rather sizeable increase in the number of calls from both
Black males and females. This was mainly a result of
callers who reported health professionals as their sources
of referral. Since there was no specific health
professional promotional campaign undertaken during the 4.5
years, it is not known if these callers specifically
learned of the CIS from doctors, nurses, CIS staff, etc.
However, one theory is that as the CIS has increased its
visibility in the Washington area, a positive reputation
has been achieved among health professionals and hence,
individuals were referred to the program. We also
hypothesize that health professionals and particularly
physicians have much greater leverage in persuading
patients to contact a CIS and as noted previously, our data
suggest this is especially the case with Black males.

Access to information regarding health care in general
is lower among lower socioeconomic groups and there is a
positive correlation between income and information and
access to health care. According to Gombeski and his
colleagues, (1981), "the poorly informed were more likely
than the well informed to report they have received their
health information from a physician or television, whereas
the well informed were more likely to report they received
their information from print media (i.e. newspapers,
magazines and books)." (Gombeski et al 1981.) This study
supports many of our basic contentions.

PROGRAMMATIC MODEL FOR COMMUNICATING CANCER INFORMATION

The development of a model for the dissemination of

cancer information to Blacks will possibly vary from CIS to CIS. Sociological factors must be considered as previously mentioned as well as the methods of public service programming by local television and radio stations.

During the 4.5 years discussed in this paper, the method of disseminating cancer information was in somewhat of a blanket approach. Information was generated/disseminated by the CIS pertaining to usually a general audience concerning a general topic. Data analysis has indicated that this method, though sporatically effective, does not provide for the best outcome and utilization of funds and staff resources when communicating to specific target audiences.

It is important to note that this CIS office as well as others in cancer control are still experimenting with a wide variety of communications models. The planned direction for our efforts will constantly seek to try new (new to this CIS) models. Currently under consideration is specific concentration by CIS staff in given areas of professional expertise, availability of resources and interest in focusing attention on the three main groups: a) lay public, b) cancer patients, and c) health professionals.

CONCLUSIONS

It is our hope that the beginning of our evaluation of how Blacks utilize a Cancer Information Service, will add to the common body of knowledge in this aspect of cancer control. This information should prove useful to others who have as their priority the dissemination of cancer information to Black audiences.

REFERENCES

1) Greenwald, Howard P. (1980). "Social Problems in Cancer Control." Cambridge, Mass.: Ballinger Publishing Company.

2) Gombeski WR., Jr., Moore TJ., Contant CF., Ramirez AG., Farge EJ., Jautz JA: (1981) "Health Information Sources of the Poorly Informed: Implications for Health Educators and Communicators." Health Values: Achieving High Level Wellness 5:5.

3) Jackson, Jaqueline Johnson, (1981). "Urban Black Americans" in Ethnicity and Medicine by Alan Harwood (ed). Cambridge, Mass.: Havard University Press.

4) Kotler Phillip (1975). "Marketing for Nonprofit Organizations" Prentice Hall, Inc.

5) Parker D.F., White J.E. (1979). The Distribution of Cancer Mortality in Washington, D.C.: 1971-1976. Howard University Cancer Center.

Progress in Cancer Control IV: Research in the Cancer Center, pages 183–191

CONSUMER EDUCATION MODIFIES CANCER PHOBIA - BEHAVIORAL
CHANGES CREATE A NEW HEALTH PROBLEM

Charlene T. Luciani and Jack S. Gruber, M.D.

Wright State University
School of Medicine
Dayton, Ohio 45401

In the mid 70's, reports that estrogen use was associated with the occurance of endometrial carcinoma resulted in thousands of women stopping their estrogen replacement therapy out of fear (Ziel and Finkle 1975). Mass media releases were disturbing to patients and physicians alike. There was little effort from the media to balance the benefits against the risks. The proponents of estrogen therapy were understandably cautious. Reviews of how estrogen replacement therapy was being prescribed were undertaken; it was found that by far the most prevalent regimens were to use estrogens unopposed in either a continuous or cyclic regimen.

Rust et al reported that of 75 physicians surveyed, composed of an equal number of Generalists, Internists, and Gynecologists, that 90% of them did not use progestogens with the estrogen and of the 10% who did, 87% of them were Gynecologists. None of the Internists, and only 5% of the Generalists, were opposing the estrogen with cyclic progestogens (Rust et al 1977). Ninety-five percent of the physicians believed that the benefits outweighed the risks and 63% of them believed that estrogens would prevent osteoporosis. Fifty-five percent of the physicians reported that they were going to change their prescribing policies as a result of the fears of endometrial cancer, but the proposed changes were not specified.

By the late 70's, increasing reports convinced many health care providers that depriving women of estrogen contributed to degenerative osteoporosis. Mortality and mor-

bidity was much higher for degenerative osteoporosis and
complications related to fractures than for cancer of the
endometrium (Gordan and Greenberg 1976).

The association of osteoporosis with the postmenopausal
estrogen-deficient state is not new. It was first described
by Albright in 1940 (Albright 1940). Albright observed that
40 of his 42 osteoporatic patients were women; all were
postmenopausal. Balance studies showed that they were
losing calcium and phosphate, the principal minerals of bone
(Albright 1941).

It is clear from the several publications since the development of methods for quantitation of bone mass that all
untreated castrates and postmenopausal women lose bone
(Meema et al 1965). Also, it is known that the incidence
of fractures from osteoporosis is much higher for women than
men. The rate increases shortly after menopause (Alffram
and Bauer 1962). The incidence of clinically apparent degenerative osteoporosis is 25% and 17% will have fractures,
and of those having a hip fracture, 50% will die within six
months.

The first long-term study of prevention of osteoporosis
was reported by Gordan (Gordan 1977). He reports a 25 year
study of the use of conjugated estrogens and with 0.6 mg of
conjugated estrogen, a fracture rate of 2.5 per 100 patient-
years. With 1.25 mg of conjugated estrogen, a fracture rate
of only 0.3 per 100 patient-years.

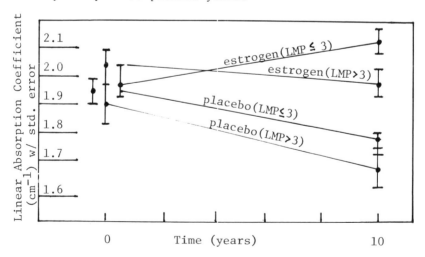

Fig. 1. Redrawn from Nachtigall's graph showing linear absorption coefficients in treated patients with LMP $\leq$ 3 years, treated patients with LMP > 3 years, control patients with LMP $\leq$ 3 years, and control patients with LMP > 3 years.

The benefits of complete sex-steroid replacement therapy in the prevention of fractures and degenerative osteoporosis are shown from a 10-year, double-blind study by Nachtigall (Nachtigall et al 1979). It was shown that daily estrogen plus cyclic progestogens prevented loss of bone mass in all patients. If started within three years of the menopause, it could even put bone back.

<u>Endometrial Carcinoma in Postmenopausal Women</u>

	Incidence of Cancer	Incidence/1000
No steroid	1/510	2/1000
Estrogens with/or without Progestogens	6/2300	2.6/1000
Estrogen only	1/212	4.7/1000
Estrogen and Progestogen	1/1240	0.8/1000

Fig. 2. R.D. Gambrell, Jr., M.D., Estrogens Progestogens and Endometrial Cancer.

The secrets of how to take sex hormones safely lie in the physiological concepts of the normal menstrual cycle. It has been known for some time that carcinoma of the endometrium was very rare in women having normal ovulatory menstrual cycles. Gambrell showed that women who have an intact uterus and are postmenopausal who took no sex steroids at all have an incidence of cancer of the uterus of approximately 2 per 1,000 (Gambrell et al 1980). The women who took estrogen, regardless of whether or not they took progestogens, have an incidence of cancer of the uterus of approximately 2.6 per 1,000. But, when it is divided into those women who took estrogen only, the incidence is 4.7 per

1,000. In those women who opposed their estrogen with progestogens, the incidence of cancer of the endometrium is
only 0.8 per 1,000, less than women who took no sex hormone
at all. The highest incidence of endometrial carcinoma in
any study using 'unopposed estrogen' is 14 per 1,000. The
addition of progestogens reduces that to less than 1 per
1,000. Keep in mind, that 986 per 1,000 won't get cancer
no matter how you replace their sex steroids.

The ovary makes estrogens every day in sufficient quan-
tities to stimulate proliferation of the endometrium. After
ovulation, the corpus luteum produces progesterone for
approximately 14 $\pm$ 2 days. A menstrual period is progesterone withdrawal of an estrogen-primed endometrium, so why
did anybody ever design a sex hormone replacement regimen
of 21 days on and 7 days off? It makes no physiological
sense (Kupperman 1976). The normal ratio or estrogen only
to estrogen opposed by progesterone is 1:1. Giving a short
course of a progestogen, five to seven days, at the end of
a cycle has been shown to prevent hyperplasia of the endometrium in most patients. Giving a progestogen for a more
physiologic time, 10 to 13 days, is even better. Present
recommendations are to oppose the estrogen in the presence
of a uterus with "Provera" (medroxyprogesterone acetate) 10
mg for 10 to 13 days (Gambrell 1981).

Now we can tell postmenopausal women and their physicians it's safe to take estrogen daily to prevent degenerative osteoporosis, but that in the presence of a uterus,
it should be opposed with a progestogen to prevent the uncommon but life-threatening cancer of the endometrium.

To inform the consumer of how they can safely take sex
hormones, an educational program, "Estrogen - Should I or
Shouldn't I?", was developed.

The Cancer Activities Office of Wright State University
School of Medicine's consumer education program design is
as follows:

      I.   Initiates Program Based On:

            A. New information
            B. Consumer request
            C. Surveys

II.   Contacts Local Unit of American Cancer Society

      A. Promotes cooperative relationship
      B. Plans program that is effective and cost efficient

III.   Press Release Provided by Cancer Activities Office - Wright State University School of Medicine

      A. American Cancer Society publicizes via:

          1. public service announcements
          2. media
          3. posters
          4. mailings
          5. service clubs and churches

IV.   Programs Held At:

      A. Schools
      B. Churches
      C. Public buildings

V.   Program Format

      A. One and one-half hour evening program
      B. Two physicians - two twenty-minute didactic presentations
      C. Forty-five minute question and answer session

*Discussion period - from our experience, the greatest learning occurs here; participants have the opportunity to express fears/concerns and receive information and reassurance.

The objectives of the program were:

1. women currently taking estrogen therapy would discuss their personal concerns with their physician;

2. women attending the program would 'multiply'

program impact through discussions of estrogen
pros and cons with family and friends;

3. women currently involved with unopposed estrogen
    therapy and exposed to the program content would
    consider the wisdom of changing their sex hor-
    mone therapy; and

4. the program attendees would experience reduced
    anxiety levels because their fears/concerns
    could be resolved.

The purpose of this program was to describe to the consumer estrogen plus progesterone hormone replacement therapy, to discuss the benefits of estrogen, as well as estrogen's supposed risks.

The educational program consisted of reviewing the normal role of estrogen and progesterone, describing the physiological changes caused by estrogen, discussing the causes
of early or normal loss of estrogen, and describing the
benefits of estrogen and progesterone therapy.

The benefits of the combined estrogen and progesterone
therapy that were emphasized are mainly the prevention or
stabilization of osteoporosis, and the reduction of endometrial carcinoma.

To study the impact of the program, a survey was carried out in two components. The participants were surveyed
immediately at the end of the program, then three months
later a survey was distributed. This was sent out as a
stamped, self-addressed, postcard-type form.

The information survey included the following questions:

1. Your age:

    _____under 30   _____30-55   _____over 55

2. Did you discuss your personal medical situation
    related to this program with your physician?

    _____Yes   _____No   _____Plan to

3. Did you obtain additional consultation as a result of attending this workshop?

   _____Yes   _____No   _____Plan to

4. Did you discuss the information received at the workshop with family, friends, etc.?

   _____Yes   _____No

5. Are you currently taking the birth-control pill?

   _____Yes   _____No

6. Have you taken or are you currently taking estrogen therapy?

   _____Yes   _____No

7. Are you taking post-menopausal estrogen therapy?

   _____Yes   _____No

8. Have you or do you plan to change your sex hormone therapy as a result of attending this workshop?

   _____Yes   _____No

9. Do you have less anxiety about sex hormone therapy as a result of attending this workshop?

   _____Yes   _____No

Eighty-three consumers attended one of two workshops. Seventy-two percent of the participants completed the immediate survey, while 82% of the participants completed the followup survey.

Program Objective 1 stated that women currently taking estrogen therapy would discuss their concerns with their physician. Fifty-seven percent of the participants indicated that they would contact their physician about their estrogen replacement therapy.

Forty percent of the participants were either taking

birth control pills or postmenopausal replacement therapy. Twenty-two percent of the women were taking postmenopausal replacement therapy. Of those women, nine had already seen their physician, and three more planned to do so. So, 80% of the attendees contacted or planned to contact their physician about their replacement therapy.

The participants were asked if they had discussed estrogen therapy with other people close to them; 99% of the participants indicated that they had done so.

As a result of the program, 44% of the participants who completed the survey said that they planned to change their sex hormone therapy regimen.

When asked whether or not the program reduced their anxiety about sex hormone replacement therapy, 91% of the participants responded to this question, and of those who responded, 84% stated that they were less anxious about sex hormone replacement therapy. Ten participants reported they were not less anxious. It may be that they were taking no sex hormone replacement therapy and found that they were facing degenerative osteoporosis.

Among 27 participants who were taking sex hormones of some type, 85% reported that they were less anxious as a result of attending the program. Fifteen women were taking postmenopausal therapy and of those, 93% were less anxious.

Our survey did not allow us to determine how many of these women didn't have a uterus and didn't need to change their therapy, or were already on estrogen plus progesterone.

Anxiety associated with the use of estrogen can be reduced through consumer education. Caution must be taken in evaluating reduction of anxiety in this program since informing women that they will develop degenerative osteoporosis if they do not take sex hormones may create a new anxiety.

Informing women that opposing the effect of estrogen with adequate progestional intake does appear to reduce their anxiety about their fear of cancer of the endometrium.

Albright F, Bloomberg E, Smith PH (1940). Post-menopausal osteoporosis. Trans Assoc Am Physicians 55:298.

Albright F, Smith PH, Richardson AM (1941). Post-menopausal osteoporosis: its clinical features. J Am Med Assoc 116: 2465.

Alffram PA, Bauer GCH (1962). Epidemiology of fracture of the forearm. J Bone Joint Surg 44-A:105-114.

Gambrell RD (1981). Preventing endometrial cancer with progestin. Contemporary Ob/Gyn 17:133.

Gambrell RD, Massey FM, Castaneda TA, Ugenas AJ, Ricci CA, Wright JM (1980). Use of the progestogen challenge test to reduce the risk of endometrial cancer. Obstet and Gynecol 55:732.

Gordan GS (1977). Postmenopausal osteoporosis: cause, prevention and treatment. Clinics in Obstet and Gynecol 4: 169.

Gordan GS, Greenberg BG (1976). Exogenous estrogens and endometrial cancer. Postgrad Med 59:66.

Kupperman HS (1976). Estrogen: why and how to use it. Female Patient 1:21.

Mack TN, Pike MC, Henderson BE, Pfeffer RI, Gerkins VR, Arthur M, Brown SE (1976). Estrogen and endometrial cancer in a retirement community. N Engl J Med 294:1262.

Meema HE, Bunker ML, Meema S (1965). Loss of compact bone due to menopause. Am J Obstet Gynecol 26:333-343.

Nachtigall LE, Nachtigall RH, Nachtigall RD, Beckman EM (1979). Estrogen replacement therapy I: a 10-year prospective study in the relationship to osteoporosis. Ob/Gyn 53:277.

Rust JA, Langley II, Hill EC, Lamb EJ (1977). Estrogens: do the risks outweigh the benefits? Am J Obstet Gynecol 128:431.

Smith SC, Ross P, Thompson DJ, Hermann WL (1975). Association of exogenous and endometrial carcinoma. N Engl J Med 293:1164.

Ziel HK, Finkle WD (1975). Increased risk of endometrial carcinoma among users of conjugated estrogen. N Engl J Med 293:1167.

We would like to acknowledge William S. Donaldson, Ed.D., from the Cancer Control Consortium of Ohio, Ohio State University, Columbus, Ohio, for his assistance in providing the statistical data for the paper.

Progress in Cancer Control IV: Research in the Cancer Center, pages 193–200
© **1983 Alan R. Liss, Inc., 150 Fifth Avenue, New York, NY 10011**

NEWSPAPER COVERAGE OF LAETRILE CLINICAL TRIALS RESULTS

Robert W. Denniston, Rose Mary Romano,
  and Holly Keck
Office of Cancer Communications
National Cancer Institute
Bethesda, Maryland 20205

Public awareness of health issues is largely dependent on the mass media. While health professionals and word-of-mouth are important sources of health information, the media provide the public with daily exposure to important issues such as health care costs, newly-identified causes of disease, successful treatments, medical personalities, and medical controversies (Dunn, 1978; Greenberg, 1979).

In a 1978 survey, the most often mentioned source of cancer information was mass media. Specifically, 82 percent of the respondents reported having heard about cancer on television, 65 percent through newspapers, 61 percent through magazines, and 42 percent through radio (American Cancer Society, 1976). Similar figures have been reported in other studies (Lieberman, 1980, National Cancer Institute, 1980).

Cancer is the chief health concern of more Americans than any other disease (American Cancer Society, 1976; Lieberman, 1980; National Cancer Institute, 1980). Consequently, public interest is high, especially when the media are seemingly filled with stories about causes, cures, "breakthroughs" and personal tragedies. But little of this is useful to the general public until the disease strikes. Then the lack of a sure cure for cancer sends some patients and their families seeking alternative therapies, especially if conventional treatments are not successful. Patients may feel they have nothing to lose by seeking unproven methods of treatment.

The results of clinical trials of new cancer treatments seldom are of public interest. Patients tend to rely on their physicians, as they should, for advice about diagnosis and treatment. But in the case of unproven methods, the dissemination of results may be important, for cancer patients are in the position literally to choose their own treatment without the counsel or expertise of a physician. Thus the proper dissemination of information about the value of unproven methods is more critical than the results of most clinical trials, where patients rely on physicians to recommend and provide therapy. An uninformed public can be expected to grab at a chance for a successful treatment, especially if other therapies have proven useless.

BACKGROUND ON LAETRILE

Laetrile (amygdalin) is a substance found naturally in the pits of apricots and some nuts. Animal tests conducted from 1957 to 1977 showed no convincing evidence that Laetrile had cancer treatment value. However, the National Cancer Institute continued to be concerned about the estimated 70,000 Americans who were leaving potentially curative treatment in pursuit of Laetrile.

Normally Laetrile would not have been tested in human cancer patients, since it failed to show any therapeutic effect against cancer in experimental animals. But due to the extraordinary public debate over Laetrile, the National Cancer Institute in 1978 initiated a formal study to determine the value of the drug against human cancer. Four medical centers participated: Memorial Sloan-Kettering Cancer Center in New York, Jonsson Comprehensive Cancer Center at UCLA, the University of Arizona at Tucson, and the Mayo Clinic in Minnesota. A total of 156 patients with advanced cancers were chosen for the study. For each patient, conventional therapies had not worked, so Laetrile represented a last alternative.

It was found that Laetrile injections and oral doses, combined with a special diet of fresh fruits, vegetables and whole grains, did not shrink the present tumors, nor prevent the cancers from seriously progressing. Laetrile was found to be ineffective. The results of the study were presented in a paper, "A Phase II Trial of Amygdalin (Laetrile) in the Treatment of Human Cancer," by Dr. Charles G. Moertel of the Mayo Clinic at a meeting of the American Society for Clinical Oncology on April 30, 1981. Dr. Moertel also announced the results of the study at a news conference at the meeting.

PURPOSE OF NEWSCLIP ANALYSIS; METHODOLOGY

The purpose of this analysis is to determine how major daily newspapers reported the news conference announcing the results of the study and the accompanying news release. The analysis extends from the period of May 1 to May 31, 1981. Articles were collected from the 72 U.S. daily newspapers with the largest circulations. The sample of articles was gathered from a commercial news clipping service. For the purposes of this study, the sample is considered exhaustive, although it is not a systematic review of all newspapers. Fifty-six newspapers carried stories about the research findings, and 84 articles were clipped and analyzed for this study. This included news stories, editorial comments and letters to the editor.

The coding instrument enabled analysis by region of publication, story origination and format, story length, balance, primary and other sources cited, and whether the opinions of pro-Laetrile groups were included. One trained coder was used for this analysis; the results were checked by two others.

RESULTS

Region of Publication   (n=84)

Region	Frequency	% of total
Northeast	29	35%
South	21	25%
North Central	19	23%
West	15	18%

Of the 84 stories included in this analysis, the greatest number came from newspapers in the Northeast; proportionately fewer appeared in the South and North Central regions, and the least appeared in the West.

Origination of the Article   (n=84)

The greatest number of stories (27) were locally originated, usually by a staff writer. The second highest number of stories (24) originated from the Associated Press. A nearly equal number came from the United Press International and the various syndicated news services. Six percent were compiled.

	Frequency	%
Story written by or for this paper (local)	27	32%
United Press International	12	14%
Associated Press	24	29%
Syndicated Services	11	13%
Compiled from wires	5	6%
Unknown	5	6%

Format of the Article   (n=84)

	Frequency	%
Hard news	57	68%
Editorial/commentary	26	31%
Feature	1	1%

About two-thirds of the stories were hard news, that is, straight, factual accounts of the press conference. Many included an in-depth discussion of the Laetrile trials and the research findings. Several began with the opening quote used by Dr. Moertel at the news conference: "Laetrile has been tested. It is not effective." The editorials, comprising one-third of the sample, included five letters to the editor. Only one story was a feature, which dealt with the personal accounts of cancer patients and their families and described patients returning from Mexican Laetrile clinics after unsuccessful treatments.

Length of the Articles   (n=84)

	Frequency	%
Short (up to 10 col. in.)	8	10%
Medium (10-40 col. in.)	74	88%
Long (over 40 col. in.)	2	2%

The length category is an indicator of the depth and completeness of coverage. Most were of medium length, using the definitions in the table, determined by the number of column inches for each story. Both of the long articles were in the hard news format.

Fairness of Coverage   (n=84)

	Frequency	%
Coverage made no judgment or was balanced	67	80%
Favorable coverage of results	14	15%
Unfavorable coverage of results	4	5%

This category assessed whether the coverage was balanced. Four out of five stories were neutral -- that is, the reporter did not make a judgment on the Laetrile study or provided a balance of both favorable and critical information about the research findings. The focus was limited to the language and tone about the research specifically. If the story gave favorable coverage, it did not question the accuracy of the study and made no mention of what Laetrile advocates thought of the research. If the story gave both favorable and unfavorable information about the study, it reported the NCI view that the findings were conclusive, and also included the opinion of Laetrile advocates who tried to refute the study.

Description of the Research Findings as Definitive (n=84)

	Frequency	%
Yes	79	94%
No	5	6%

Virtually all of the stories described the Laetrile study findings as definitive. They used quotations such as "Laetrile has been tested and it is not effective," or "Vincent DeVita said that the study findings present public evidence of Laetrile's failure as a cancer treatment," or similar comments. The five stories which did not describe the results as definitive said "Laetrile advocates insist nothing was proved by human tests in which the NCI reports the controversial substance failed and therefore should be considered worthless," or "a Government study branding Laetrile as ineffective against cancer was labeled a farce today by a user of Laetrile in Kansas."

Primary Source of Research Findings   (n=84)

	Frequency	%
Charles Moertel, M.D.	37	44%
National Cancer Institute	27	32%
Mayo Clinic	4	5%
Arthur Holleb, M.D.	2	2%
Vincent DeVita, Jr., M.D.	1	1%
American Cancer Society	1	1%
Other	12	14%

This category identified the first person or institution mentioned in the story as the primary source. Dr. Moertel, the principal investigator at the Mayo Clinic, was most often mentioned first. His statement was quoted in the lead or the second paragraph in 44% of the stories. Fourteen percent cited other primary sources, such as "researchers at four cancer centers," "Federal Government," "Food and Drug Administration," and "the American Society for Clinical Oncology."

Other Sources Cited in the Articles   (n=84)

	Frequency	%
Mayo Clinic	50	60%
Food and Drug Admin.	48	57%
National Cancer Institute	45	54%
Four cancer centers	40	48%
Vincent DeVita, Jr., M.D.	38	45%
American Cancer Society	28	33%
Charles Moertel, M.D.	19	23%

Multiple codes were possible in this category, used to analyze the depth of coverage. The more sources cited, the more complete and detailed the coverage. In most cases, the Mayo Clinic was mentioned in addition to the primary source, largely because the principal investigator, Dr. Moertel, was from the Mayo Clinc. An average of four additional sources were mentioned across all of the stories. The hard news stories mentioned or quoted an average of five additional sources of information about the study. As might be expected, the editorials contained the fewest references to additional sources, averaging only one per editorial.

Opinions of the Pro-Laetrile Groups   (n=84)

	Frequency	%
Yes	73	87%
No	11	13%

This category determined whether the opinions of those individuals and groups touting Laetrile, such as Robert Bradford and the Committee for Freedom of Choice, were included. Most of the stories made mention of the pro-Laetrile statement which was presented at the same time the study results were released. The stories either mentioned or quoted Robert Bradford, spokesperson for the Committee for Freedom of Choice, or generally referred to comments from "Laetrile advocates."

CONCLUSIONS

The data from this newsclip analysis indicate that coverage of the Laetrile study results followed traditional coverage of hard news events. Coverage was heavy, with 80 percent of the newspapers running a story based on the press conference, and many stories on page one. Almost all of the news stories used direct quotes from the press release and the news conference. The articles tended to give a balance by covering the results of the Laetrile study together with the negative response to the research results presented by the Laetrile advocates. The data showed that, for the most part, the coverage was either totally favorable or balanced. Only a few stories were negative or hostile towards the results of the study.

Editorials and letters to the editor appeared after the initial hard news stories -- at least one day later, up to several weeks after the news story appeared. With the exception of three newspapers, all of the editorials were preceded by at least one news story on the study results. Of 24 editorials, only two gave unfavorable views of the Laetrile study results. The others were either favorable in their reviews or balanced (without judgment or presenting both sides). Thus, the editorials, which represent more opinionated writing than the hard news format, tended to be supportive of the scientific research on the value of Laetrile.

The editorials and letters to the editor referred to themes of state and local issues (e.g., legislation permitting the use of Laetrile), freedom of choice or the difficulties encountered by cancer patients as they seek various therapies. None of the negative editorials or hard news stories criticized the research findings as being questionable or unscientific. Rather, the critical articles simply questioned the larger issue of whether the Government should prohibit Laetrile and thereby limit the public's freedom to choose alternative medical treatments.

Overall, the newspaper coverage examined in the study was fair, balanced, and detailed. Most of the articles were of medium length and cited the research findings as being definitive. The majority of articles were either favorable or at least balanced in their presentation. The detail and depth of the articles, in terms of the number of sources cited and viewpoints represented, also contributed to thorough coverage of the Laetrile clinical trial results.

REFERENCES

American Cancer Society. "What Californians Think, Feel, and Do About Cancer." The ACS Volunteer, Vol. 22, 1976.

Dunn W (1978). What To Tell the Public. In Proceedings of the Fourth National Cancer Communications Conference, Bethesda, Maryland: National Cancer Institute, USPHS, DHEW.

Greenberg R, Freimuth VS, Bratic E (1979). Newspaper Coverage of Cancer. In Nimmo D (ed): Communication Yearbook, New Brunswick, NJ: Transaction Books.

Lieberman Research Inc. "A Basic Study of Public Attitudes Towards Cancer and Cancer Tests." (1980) American Cancer Society: New York.

National Cancer Institute (1980). "National Survey of Public Knowledge, Attitudes and Practices Related to Breast Cancer." Bethesda, Maryland: USPHS, DHEW.

II. CANCER ETIOLOGY, PREVENTION, AND DETECTION

Progress in Cancer Control IV: Research in the Cancer Center, pages 203–215
© **1983 Alan R. Liss, Inc., 150 Fifth Avenue, New York, NY 10011**

CHARACTERISTICS OF WOMEN WITH CERVICAL INTRAEPITHELIAL DYSPLASIA

Robert Michielutte, Ph.D., Robert A. Diseker, Dr.Ph., Wayne T. Corbett, V.M.D., Dr.Ph., W. Joseph May, M.D.

Bowman Gray School of Medicine
Winston-Salem, North Carolina 27103

The consistent decline in the rate of invasive cervical cancer has been, in part, attributed to the success of screening for early detection. Greater effectiveness in the screening process would be achieved if it were possible to focus efforts on groups of women known to be at high risk for invasive cervical cancer or its precursors. An important question, however, is whether efforts to identify risk factors should be limited to carcinoma in situ and invasive cervical cancer, or also include cervical intraepithelial dysplasia.

The majority of evidence to date suggests that (1) cervical cancer is a mildly contagious, sexually transmitted disease, and (2) cervical dysplasia, carcinoma in situ, and invasive cervical cancer appear to be part of a continuum (Briggs 1979). The hypothesis of a continuum with the final stage being invasive cervical cancer has been generally supported by recent epidemiological research. Several studies have found that the risk factors for cervical dysplasia and carcinoma in situ are similar to the factors found for invasive cervical cancer (Meisels et al. 1977; Harris et al. 1980; Sweetnam et al. 1981). It is important to note that the results are not entirely consistent, and some studies have found that dysplasia is epidemiologically different from carcinoma in situ and invasive cervical cancer (Thomas 1973; Thomas and Anderson 1974; Terris et al., 1980).

The inconsistent results with respect to dysplasia appear to be partly due to differences in the methodology employed in the various studies, particularly with respect to a lack of multivariate analysis of risk factors or deficiencies in such analysis, and partly due to differences in the definition of dysplasia. Many studies have examined all dysplasia together (mild and severe), and Terris et al. (1980) have suggested that dysplasia may include a mixture of diagnoses of which only some, the more severe dysplasias, are part of the continuum leading to cervical cancer. Thus, it may be that mild dysplasias would differ epidemiologically from cervical cancer while the more severe dysplasias would show a similar pattern. At present, then, it appears to be most profitable to focus on identifying groups of women at high risk for severe dysplasia, in addition to carcinoma in situ and invasive cervical cancer.

The two risk factors consistently identified as being important predictors of all cervical neoplasia are age at first coitus and number of sex partners (Briggs 1979). Women with an early age at first coitus and who have had multiple partners are at higher risk. Other variables less consistently identified as high risk factors include low socioeconomic status, early marriage, multiple marriages, early age at first pregnancy, and high parity (Briggs 1979; Harris et al. 1980; Lambert et al. 1980). Multivariate analyses of several implicated factors are rare, but the recent work of Harris et al. (1980) suggests that experience with multiple sex partners may be the most important factor, and many other presumably important high risk factors are covariables rather than being of direct importance. The predominant importance of multiple sex partners is also supported by anthropological evidence (Spriggs 1981).

Of particular interest is recent research suggesting that cigarette smoking and the use of oral contraceptives may be risk factors in the development of dysplasia, carcinoma in situ, and invasive cervical cancer (Harris 1980; Briggs 1979). However, the research results dealing with oral contraceptives have been contradictory and highly controversial, and comparative evidence on cigarette smoking is still quite limited.

The present report describes the results of a study of factors associated with severe cervical dysplasia in a homogeneous sample of women attending a county family planning clinic. Several previously identified risk factors, including use of oral contraceptives and smoking behavior, are considered together with a set of variables which summarize the womens' prior medical history.

METHODS AND MATERIALS

The sample of cases consists of woman attending the Forsyth County, North Carolina Family Planning Clinic who were found to have severe dysplasia (Stage III or higher on a five stage classification scheme) between January 1, 1980 and June 30, 1981. A total of 199 cases with dysplasia were identified during this time period, and background information was available for 195 women. A stratified random sample of 195 controls was selected from the records of other women in the clinic who were free of dysplasia (severe or mild) during this time period. Selection of controls was stratified by age and race in order to obtain a similar distribution of cases and controls for these variables. This procedure removed the confounding effects of age and race in assessing other risk factors, and assured a sufficient sample size to make comparisons within age-race groups.

Information on cases and controls was obtained by reviewing clinic records for age, race, marital status, educational attainment, medical history, sexual activity, age of coital onset, contraceptive use, number of pregnancies, number of live children, and number of abortions/miscarriages. In order to obtain the correct temporal ordering of risk factors, background information on the women was obtained for the most recent update of the clinic record prior to the Pap smear which identified each woman as having severe dysplasia or being normal. Although clinic records are usually updated at each visit, complete information was not available for all women on all variables of interest.

The Forsyth County Family Planning Clinic serves a primarily low-income nonwhite population. Racial composition of the sample, cases and controls, reflects the character of the clinic and is approximately 70 percent black and 30 percent white. Mean age of the women is 21 years and less than 15 percent are over 25 years of age. Educational attainment is somewhat misleading since many of the women are still in school. However, among the women age 21 and over, approximately half had not completed high school, and about 10 percent have had some schooling beyond high school.

Initial analyses of the data are presented as percentage differences between cases and controls, with the chi-square test being used to assess the statistical significance of differences between the two groups. It is recognized that neither the cases nor the controls represent simple random samples, and the tests of statistical significance are employed to assess the probability of cases and controls ordering themselves in the manner observed for each potential risk factor within our sample, without reference to a larger population. Multiple discriminant analysis is used to examine the relative importance of risk factors and to determine the value of significant risk factors in correctly identifying women as having dysplasia or being normal. The criterion for statistical significance is $p \leq .05$, two-tailed test.

RESULTS

The preliminary analysis of all variables revealed no significant differences between cases and controls with respect to educational attainment, number of pregnancies, number of living children, number of abortions/ miscarriages, current sexual activity (virtually all the women were sexually active), and age at coital onset. Controls for age and race did not alter these findings.

Since age at coital onset has been found to be one of the most important risk factors for cervical neoplasia in previous studies, additional analyses were conducted to determine if its effect was being suppressed by other factors. Age at coital onset was entered in all subsequent multivariate analyses, but in no instance did it emerge as a significant factor.

Marital status, contraceptive use, and several items in the women's medical history were found to significantly differentiate between cases and controls.

Marital status can be viewed as a crude indicator of experience with multiple sex partners, particularly in a

young population such as the one attending the family
planning clinic. Early marriage reduces the probability of
multiple sex partners. Approximately 22 percent of the
women in the total sample were married during the study
period, but almost twice the percentage of controls were
married as compared to the cases with dysplasia (Table 1).
Never married women, and the few (N = 28) who were
separated or divorced all showed the same pattern of
increased risk for cervical dysplasia, and marital status
has been treated as a dichotomy of married, spouse present
vs other. It should be noted that the observed effect of
being married as a factor in reduced risk of dysplasia is
probably diluted somewhat due to the fact that some women
in the "other" category will have been living monogamously
with a man during the study period and are misclassified.
Thus, the estimate of marital status as a risk factor is
likely to be conservative.

Contraceptive use differs for cases and controls, but
in a manner different from the relationship reported in
recent research. While other studies have suggested a
possible increased risk from the use of oral
contraceptives, the results shown in Table 1 indicate that
women using no contraceptives are at highest risk. Over 18
percent of the cases were using no contraceptive prior to
the identification of dysplasia as compared to

TABLE 1

Marital Status, Contraceptive Use, and Cervical Dysplasia

	Cases	Controls	
Percent Married	16.0(187)*	28.0(189)	$\chi^2 = 7.87$, p = .005
Percent not using contraceptives	18.2(192)	3.2(189)	$\chi^2 = 23.14$, p <. 001

* Total sample size on which percent is based in
parentheses.

approximately three percent of the controls. Since almost all of the women in our sample who practice contraception use oral contraceptives, the data suggest that sexual activity together with no contraceptive use is associated with increased risk of dysplasia and, conversely, use of oral contraceptives is associated with a reduced risk.

The relationships between selected health problem categories dealing with the womens' medical history and cervical dysplasia are shown in Table 2. Eight of the fifteen categories show significant differences between the cases and controls. For each of the eight categories, a larger proportion of women with dysplasia have a health problem of some type. Thus prior health problems, or problem behavior in the use of cigarettes/alcohol/drugs, appear to be significant risk factors for cervical dysplasia.

It is important to point out that several of the problem categories included as part of the clinic medical history were not analyzed separately. The categories defined as symptoms of pregnancy, phlebitis-varicose veins, embolism-CVA, cardiac disease, breast mass-discharge-cancer, liver disease-hepatitis, and pelvic tumor-fibroid-cancer all had too few women (a total of 10 or less for cases and controls combined) to permit a separate statistical analysis of each problem category.

Further analyses of the problem categories reported in Table 2 were conducted in an attempt to determine the relative importance of each one. Multiple discriminant analyses which also controlled for marital status and contraceptive use revealed that four health problem categories continue to significantly discriminate between the cases and controls; 1) use of cigarettes/alcohol/drugs, 2) visual problems, 3) asthma or allergies and 4) use of medications. However, a clear interpretation of the results is not possible due to the fact that many of the health variables are highly intercorrelated. The problem of multicollinearity suggests that simultaneous analysis of the separate health problem categories is not appropriate for our sample, although the analysis was of some use in that it demonstrated the consistently strong direct relationship between the use of cigarettes/alcohol/drugs and dysplasia.

TABLE 2

Medical History and Cervical Dysplasia

Problem	Cases	Controls	Level of Significance
Sample Size	195	195	
Dysmenorrhea	27.9	30.3	NS
Menorrhagia, Inter-menstrual bleeding	17.3	6.2	p < .001
Amenhorrhea	12.5	3.1	p < .001
Medications (e.g. anti-coagulants)	9.4	1.0	p < .001
Seizures, Nervousness, Depression	10.4	2.1	p < .001
Visual Problems	18.4	2.1	p < .001
Asthma, Allergies	22.2	7.8	p < .001
Anemia, Sickle Cell	11.9	7.8	NS
Migraine Headaches	16.4	7.8	p = .009
Kidney, Gallbladder Disease	8.8	6.7	NS
Vaginitis, Other Infection	21.9	15.6	NS
Cigarettes, Alcohol, Drugs	60.0	16.3	p < .001
Diabetes, or Family History of	24.9	19.4	NS
Hypertension, or Family History of	31.1	37.4	NS
Breast Cancer, or Family History of	7.5	6.4	NS

Since a large number of the health problem categories were related to the occurrence of dysplasia, it was decided that an alternative approach would be to conceptualize a women's cumulative health history as a risk factor in dysplasia. In order to examine cumulative health history, a health history score was computed from the 15 problem categories in Table 2 and the seven categories which could not be separately analyzed. One point was assigned for every category in which a health problem was reported. The maximum possible score is 22, and the actual scores ranged from 0 to 11 for both cases and controls. The distribution of scores is shown in Table 3.

TABLE 3

Health History Score and Cervical Dysplasia

Score	Percent	
	Cases	Controls
0 - 1	27.7	50.8
2 - 3	37.9	34.9
4 - 5	18.5	13.3
6 - 11	15.9	1.0
Total	100.0	100.0
Sample Size	195	195

$\chi^2 = 40.59$, p < .001

A comparison of cases and controls with respect to the health history score reveals that cumulative health history is clearly a significant risk factor for dysplasia among women in this sample. Over half the controls have the lowest possible scores of 0 or 1, while only about one quarter of the cases scored this low. At the upper end of the score, slightly less than 16 percent of the cases have scores between 6-11 as compared to one percent of the controls. Briefly stated, the more health problems a women has experienced in the past, the greater the risk of cervical dysplasia.

Multivariate Analysis of Risk Factors

In order to determine the relative importance of marital status, contraceptive use, and health history as risk factors for dysplasia, a set of multiple discriminant analyses were performed on the total sample, and also by race and age. Race was found to have little effect on the relationships whether alone or in combination with age. The three risk factors significantly discriminated between cases and controls in the same way for both whites and nonwhites.

In contrast, the risk factors differ in their effects by age of the women (Table 4). All three factors discriminate significantly between cases and controls regardless of age, but in younger women (under 21) the standardized discriminant function coefficients indicate that marital status is the most important risk factor, followed by the health history score. Contraceptive use shows the weakest relationship with dysplasia for the younger women.

The health history score is by far the most important risk factor among older women (21+). Contraceptive use is second in importance, with the weakest effect attributed to marital status.

The use of marital status, health history, and contraceptive use to predict the occurrence of dysplasia resulted in more accurate classification for older women. Sixty-seven percent were correctly classified as cases or controls for women 21 and over, as compared to approximately 59 percent for the younger women. The difference between the two age groups is largely due to the strong influence of the health history score among the older women.

CONCLUSION

The present investigation has identified marital status, contraceptive use, and a woman's history of health

TABLE 4

Multiple Discriminant Analysis

Variable	Standardized Discriminant Function Coefficients		
	Total Sample	Women Age 20 or Younger	Women Age 21 or Older
Health History	.717	.550	.807
Marital Status	.374	.659	.177
Contraceptive Use	-.406	-.437	-.346
Percent Correctly Classified as Dysplasia or Normal	63.6%	58.6%	67.0%
N	368	162	206

problems as significant risk factors for severe cervical dysplasia. Women in our sample who are unmarried, use no method of contraception, and who have a history of many health problems are at higher risk for cervical dysplasia.

In light of the fact that virtually all the women in the sample were sexually active at the time of the study, and almost all began sexual activity at an early age, marital status has been conceptualized as a crude indicator of experience with multiple sex partners. In this context, the observed relationship with dysplasia supports the results of earlier research which has found number of sex partners to be one of the most important risk factors for all cervical neoplasias. This interpretation of marital status is further supported by the result of the multiple discriminant analyses. Marital status is the most important risk factor for younger women, and the least important for older women. This is the pattern that would be expected since being married would have a much more direct effect in limiting the total number of sex partners for young women, while it may or may not have had this effect for older women who have had a larger period of potential sexual activity. Duration and number of marriages would be more important factors for older women; variables which unfortunately were not available on the clinic records.

The result with respect to the relationship between dysplasia and one category of health problems, cigarettes/alcohol/drugs, also provides some support for the results obtained in earlier research. Harris et al. (1980) found a strong relationship between cigarette smoking and carcinoma in situ and dysplasia even after controlling for other risk factors. A similar relationship was found in the present study. Although our measure of smoking is relatively crude, including alcohol and drug use as well, the persistence of this relationship with dysplasia suggests it is worth pursuing further.

In contrast to the results obtained with respect to marital status and cigarette/alcohol/drug use, the observed relationship between contraceptive use and dysplasia appears to contradict some recent research. Our data suggest that sexually active women who use no contraceptive are at higher risk for dyplasia, while women who use oral contraceptives are at lower risk. Previous research such as that of Harris et al. (1980) suggests that use of oral contraceptives carries an increased risk of dysplasia. Although it is only possible to speculate on reasons for the contradictory findings, it may be that the effects of oral contraceptive use may be dependent on duration of use. In a young population of the type dealt with in the present study, the effects of such use may require more time to be noticeable. At this point in time, both sexual activity and lack of contraceptive use may be indicators of an overall lifestyle that predisposes to dysplasia among young women.

The results dealing with the relationship between age at first coitus and dysplasia is also in opposition to most earlier research and requires some elaboration. Age at first coitus has previously been found to be one of the most important risk factors for cervical neoplasia, though no relationship was found in the present study. After a comprehensive review of epidemiological studies in cervical cancer, Rotkin (1973) concluded that only early intercourse before the age of 17 years was important in its effect as a risk factor. In the present sample, 62.6 percent of the women had engaged in intercourse by age 16 and over 80 percent had done so by age 17. Thus, the lack of an observed relationship between age at first coitus and dysplasia in the present study may be due to a lack of variation around the critical age of 17 years. In effect, age at first coitus, may be almost a constant in our sample in terms of its effect on dysplasia.

The final variable identified as a risk factor for cervical dysplasia, a woman's prior health history, may provide an added dimension to the understanding of risk factors affecting cervical dysplasia. The data obtained for the present study are crude and analysis is limited by lack of a direct measure of number of sex partners, but our results suggest that health history is a potentially powerful risk factor that exerts an independent effect on dysplasia. However, there are at least three alternative hypotheses worth pursuing with more appropriate data which may explain how health history affects the chances of contracting cervical dysplasia.

The first hypothesis simply suggests that prior health history exerts an independent effect in addition to such factors as number of sex partners and age of first coitus. Women with a history of prior health problems may have a deficient immune system which increases their chances of getting dysplasia even if they have had only one sex partner or have a late age at first coitus.

The second hypothesis would define prior history of health problems as another component of a lifestyle which includes early age at first coitus, multiple sex partners, poor nutrition, sporadic or no use of contraceptives, many pregnancies, etc. If in fact, multiple sex partners and age at first coitus are the predominant factors, the relationship between health history and dysplasia may be spurious and would disappear when controlling for these factors.

The third hypothesis would suggest an interaction effect. It may be that the influence of a woman's health history on dysplasia is mediated by such variables as the number of sex partners and age at first coitus. A history of health problems may be strongly related to dysplasia among women who have had multiple sex partners. In this case women with many health problems would be particularly susceptible to exposure to the initiating factor through sexual contact and would be at increased risk of dysplasia. On the other hand, if a women has not had multiple sex partners, a history of health problems would have little or no relationship to dysplasia. Briefly stated, the relationship between health history and dysplasia would be dependent on prior sexual experience.

REFERENCES

Briggs RM (1979). Dysplasia and early neoplasia of the uterine cervix. Obstet Gynecol Survey 34:70.

Harris RWC, Britton LA, Cowdell RH, et al. (1980). Characteristics of women with dysplasia or carcinoma in situ of the cervix uteri. Br J Cancer 42:359.

Lambert B, Morisset R, Bielmann P (1980). An etiologic survey of clinical factors in cervical intraepithelial neoplasia. J Rep Med 24:26.

Meisels A, Begin R, Schneider V (1977). Dysplasias of uterine cervix. Cancer 40:3076.

Rotkin I (1973). A comparison review of key epidemiological studies in cervical cancer related to current searches for transmissible agents. Cancer Res 33:1353.

Spriggs AI (1981). Natural history of cervical dysplasia. Clinics Obstet Gynecol 8:65.

Sweetnam P, Evans DMD, Hibbard BM, Jones JM (1981). The Cardiff cervical cytological study. J Epidemiol Comm Health 35:83.

Terris M, Wilson F, Nelson JH (1980). Comparative epidemiology of invasive carcinoma of the cervix, carcinoma in situ, and cervical dysplasia. Am J Epidemiol 112:253.

Thomas DB (1973). An epidemiologic study of carcionoma in situ and squameous dysplasia of the uterine cervix. Am J Epidemiol 98:10.

Thomas DB, Anderson RI (1974). An epidemiologic study and serologic comparison of uterine carcinoma in situ and squamous dysplasia. Am J Epidemiol 100:113.

Progress in Cancer Control IV: Research in the Cancer Center, pages 217–235
© 1983 Alan R. Liss, Inc., 150 Fifth Avenue, New York, NY 10011

The Acquired Immune Deficiency Syndrome

Peter W.A. Mansell, M.D., Guy R. Newell, M.D.,
Evan M. Hersh, M.D.
Departments of Cancer Prevention and Clinical
Immunology, UTSCC M. D. Anderson Hospital and
Tumor Institute, Houston, Texas

In early 1981 an outbreak of pneumocystis carinii pneumonia (PCP) was reported on the west coast of the USA in young male homosexuals.[1-3] Since there has emerged an epidemic of opportunistic infections consisting largely of PCP but also of other diseases associated with malignancy, particularly Kaposi's sarcoma (KS). The epidemic has now risen to over 900 reported cases of opportunistic infections with or without malignancy from America and foreign countries.

Although the malignant disease most often associated with the syndrome is KS, there have also been cases reported of lymphoma[4,5] and extensive squamous cell cancer.[6] One of the unanswered questions obviously is why should the predominant neoplasm be KS? KS, first described in 1872[7], is usually seen in this country in elderly men of Jewish or Mediterranean extraction, the incidence is approximately 0.05/100,000.

Kaposi's sarcoma has a striking predominance in males, less than 10% of all cases occurring in females.[8] Skin on any part of the body may be affected and almost every internal structure can be involved, most common is the gastrointestinal tract.[9,10] Cases have been described in almost every part of the world but particularly from the countries surrounding the Mediterranean and from Eastern Europe. Several early authors concluded that there was a preponderance in Jews.[11,12] It is also found to be common in Northern Italy and in one series of 356 cases, 111 were Italian and 45

Jews.(13) More recent series report a high incidence in
Jews.(14,15) The disease is also common in Western Africa
making up 10% of all malignancies in Zaire.(8) In French
Equatorial Africa, it constitutes as much as 16.8% of all
sarcomas(16) and 4.6% of all tumors seen in
Malawi.(17,18)

The age distribution differs by race. The commonest
age in Caucasians is in the 6th and 7th decades(13)
whereas in Africa the incidence is highest in the fourth
and fifth decades.(16,19,20) In two published series
Caucasian females accounted for only 6% and 9.6% of cases
respectively.(21,22) In Africa the female incidence of
KS is similarly low.

In Africa the disease is rapidly progressive often
involving lymph nodes, a common form of presentation is in
the gastrointestinal tract. The disease now being seen in
the USA is more like the African disease in its
presentation and natural history than that commonly seen
in this country. Of interest, in this regard, is the
recently reported outbreak of Kaposi's sarcoma among young
Haitian since the Haitian people derive from freed slaves
originating on the west coast of Africa.(23)

Pneumocystis pneumonia (PCP) has been the most often
reported opportunistic infection in this epidemic(1-3,24)
although other infectious diseases have been
seen.(2,25-27) Little is known of the epidemiology and
immunology of PCP infection. (28,29) Pneumocystis carinii
may be passed by human contact(30,31) and a proportion of
unaffected individuals have antibodies against this
organism.(31,32) The association of PCP and
cytomegalovirus seen in the recent outbreak also occurs in
post-transplantation patients in whom PCP is relatively
common.(33) Cytomegalovirus is known to be
immunosuppressive(34) and infection with the virus may
thus provide the background against which PCP can become
established. (33,35) Malnutrition may also be related
to this present outbreak.(28,35)

There is a strong association between immune
depression and this epidemic and a variety of
abnormalities have been described by ourselves and
others.(2,3,26,36-40) Also reported have been the presence
of radiosensitive suppressor cells(41); elevated thymosin

α_1[39] and lysozyme[41] levels. It seems clear that the immunological defect, whatever its cause, is progressive and long lasting, patients with overt infection or neoplasm being more depressed than ambulatory patients with the prodrome. Apparently healthy subjects without clinical abnormality may be immunologically suppressed to an unexpected degree.

Other related factors are the use of recreational drugs, in particular the use of nitrites which are known to be mutagenic and at least potentially carcinogenic[42-44] and immunosuppressive both in vitro and in vivo.[44,45] The effects of other commonly used drugs are presently unknown although marijuana has been shown to be an immunosuppressant. [46] Both in our own study and others, drug taking, particularly nitrite inhalation, is extremely common, 80-90%, in the homosexual community.[47,48] A case control study conducted by the CDC uncovered a number of factors which were more common in cases than in controls specifically a history of syphilis, hepatitis, treatment with Flagyl, high number of sexual partners, sexual experiences in bath houses and "fisting".[48,49]

Of great interest are the recent studies of major histocompatibility antigens in both classical and epidemic KS[36,51] which demonstrate an increased frequency of HLA DR5 and BW35. These findings suggest possible predisposing immunogenetic host factors. HLA DR5 has also been found to be increased in patients with scleroderma,[52] rheumatoid arthritis, [53] renal cell carcinoma,[54] and mycosis fungoides.[55]

It has been proposed that chronic antigenic stimulation with sperm may be a factor in producing immune suppression: experimental evidence in a small series of individuals supports this.[56] Mice injected intravenously with allogeneic sperm also become immunosuppressed. [57,58]

Kaposi's sarcoma appears to be a tumor which is related to the host immune system. It has been reported in patients with systemic lupus during immunosuppressive therapy and in patients with plasma cell dyscrasia, thymoma, polymyositis and temporal arteritis.[59-65] Also in renal transplant recipients following steroid therapy.(66-68) There have been reports of the high incidence of second primary malignancies in KS.(69,70) Immune suppression as measured by hypersensitivity to DNCB and blastogenic responses is seen in KS patients.(71-75)

Although the causes of AIDS are unknown one of the most likely factors is a transmissable agent. This theory is based on a cluster of cases found on the West Coast,(76) the apparently centrifugal spread of the disease from New York and reports from other countries coming after the initial reports from this country(38,49,50) some of which point to the fact that affected individuals in Europe and elsewhere had visited New York shortly before they became ill. Recent reports of cases of PCP in persons with Haemophilia A(77) also raise the suspicion of a transmissable agent. The suggestion has been made in light of the incidence of disease recently reported in Haitians(23) that the "agent" may have originated in the Caribbean. In this regard the discovery of the human lymphocyte transforming virus (HLTV) is certainly of interest since it has been identified in the Caribbean Basin. (78)

Of much more obvious interest is cytomegalovirus (CMV), known to be associated with the Kaposi's sarcoma since the early 1970s.(79-83) Cytomegalovirus is immuno-suppressive (34,84) and capable of transforming human cells in tissue culture(85),is excreted in urine, semen and other body fluids and is carried by up to 90% of the male homosexual population.(86) When semen and CMV are given together intravenously to experimental animals together profound immunosuppression results.(87) Although CMV is an ubiquitous pathogen it seldom causes serious disease except in immunosuppressed hosts.(88-90)

Other members of the DNA herpes group of viruses which are at least putatively, if not actually, oncogenic in man are the Epstein-Barr virus (EBV) and Herpes II.(91-95) High levels of anti-EBV antibody are found in many AIDS patients and in the CDC case control study(49) this was one of the characteristics which differentiated cases from controls. There are many parallels between EBV and CMV. EBV probably causes Burkitt's lymphoma rather than infectious mononucleosis because of immunosuppression perhaps caused by endemic malaria. CMV may act similarly although the immune suppression is possibly due to facts such as previous infections, drugs, nutrition and allogeneic sperm. Burkitt's lymphoma although rare in the country has recently been reported in male homosexuals in the West Coast.(5) Thus in the usual situations CMV may cause a mononucleosis which in its more florid form is recognized as the AIDS "prodrome" but when the stage is set in susceptible individuals, possibly predetermined by some hereditable trait, the full blown malignancy is seen. The immunological defect is probably due to a large number of known or suspected factors or to some agent as yet undiscovered and may have even wider consequences.(96)

The therapy of PCP and other opportunistic infections is standard although it should be very aggressive in this situation as the mortality is extremely high. A number of therapeutic options exist for KS particularly in regard to the use of cytotoxic agents. The most successful combination hitherto has been Adriamycin, Velban, and Bleomycin while the best single agent appears to be VP16.(97,98) Unfortunately, the results have been of short duration with a large number of relapses within four to six months and an unacceptably large number of infectious complications. Interferon on the other hand seems to offer certain advantages particularly in respect to the lack of adverse side effects both in this institution (99) and at Memorial Sloan Kettering Institute.(100) Studies are now underway evaluating partially pure leukocyte interferon in low doses.(99)

As for prevention, the most obvious method would be elucidation of the cause of the syndrome but, since immune suppression appears to be the central common denominator, a number of agents which are immune restoratives and have already been tested in immunologically deficient cancer patients, namely thymic hormone, cimetidine, Azimexon, Isoprinosine, and Indomethacin amongst others(101-105) and many others should be considered. We already have experience with these agents and protocols for AIDS patients are being considered. Since the epidemic seems to be gaining momentum rather than fading(106, 107) the need for active intervention in the near future is all the more pressing.

The Department of Cancer Prevention at The University of Texas M. D. Anderson Hospital began a Preventive Medicine Clinic to serve as the clinical basis for the

Kaposi's Sarcoma and Opportunistic Infection Program in
Houston and has seen 150 subjects in the period beginning
January 1982. To date 116 patients have been seen who
were referred by their private physicians either with a
diagnosis of Kaposi's sarcoma or opportunistic infection
or because of factors such as lymphadenopathy, fever,
weight loss, or previous history of infection suggesting
high risk for development of AID or subsequent
complications. Each individual was given a complete
physical examination and subjected to a screen of
hematological, biochemical, immunological and virological
tests designed to determine the existence and extent of
any immunological or other abnormality. At the same time
a prospective serum bank has been begun and approximately
500 serum samples have been stored at -20°C in order to
have the capability to answer the question as to whether
any change has occurred in levels of, for instance,
anti-viral titers in pre-and post-diagnosis serum should
any of the cohort become sick in the future. Both the
clinic patients and the prospective cohort will be part of
an epidemiological long term study. An extremely
extensive lifestyle and previous medical history
questionnaire was also completed not only by the 150 cases
seen in the Preventive Medicine Clinic but also those
individuals who's serum is stored in the serum bank. A
preliminary analysis of the first 62 questionnaires from
the group seen in the Preventive Medicine Clinic reveal
that 30% had had previous urethritis, 30% had had
persistent diarrhea at least once lasting for more than 2
weeks, 50% had had swollen lymph nodes at one time in the
recent past. Only 5% reported regular use of skin
ointments containing steroids, 50% were nonsmokers and
approximately 20% were frequent or heavy drinkers. So far
as drug use is concerned, 35% used marijuana and nitrites
more than once a week and 15% amphetamines. Social habits
revealed that 90% went to cruise bars and 60% to dance
bars while 40% frequented baths and bookstores, 30%
thought that they were underweight, 60% of this group were
engaged in sexual relations with someone of the same sex
at least 3 times per week and 40% had sexual relationships
with 3 or more different individuals weekly. Forty
percent gave a history of syphilis and 60% a history of
hepatitis, 25% had had herpetic infections and 30%
intestinal infections requiring treatment. Eighty five
percent were either active or passive in anal intercourse
while 30% were active and 15% passive in the homosexual

activity known as fisting. The results of these lifestyle questionnaires are currently being correlated with clinical and immunological parameters and some preliminary correlations have been performed.

Preliminary results have shown that certain of the immunologic tests show a tendency to be associated significantly with selected questionnaire items, namely reported elevating thymosin α_1 and lysozyme levels associated with sexual practices and reported drug uses. Skin tests which are 60 to 90% negative for those tested, however, have not generally shown significant associations when tested univariately with the individual questionnaire items.

The immunological characteristics of the group show a variety of abnormalities Of the first 33 patients studied, only 7% compared to 46% controls reacted to dermatophytin in the delayed hypersensitivity skin test, 26 versus 71% to varidase, 30 versus 60% to mumps. However, 52% of patients had a skin test reaction to candida compared to 82% of the controls. There was a slight decrease in total T cells and a marked deficiency of OKT_4+ (T helper) cells with a small but significant rise in the number of OKT_8+ (T suppressor) cells thus giving an inverted helper/ suppressor cell ratio of 0.85 in patients compared to 1.92 in controls. Lymphocyte blastogenic responses to phytohemagglutinin (PHA) were slightly reduced but responses to Concanavalin-A (Con-A) and pokeweek mitogen (PWM) were markedly reduced compared to controls. Natural killer (NK) cell activity and antibody dependent cell mediated cytotoxicity (ADCC) were both esentially normal in patients as compared to controls, however, monocyte adherence was markedly reduced in the patient group. Two striking serological findings relating to cell mediated immunity were found. Thymosin α_1 levels which might have been expected to be reduced in view of the depressed T cell numbers, inverted H/S ratios and other signs of depressed cell mediated immunity were in contrast, markedly elevated thus perhaps suggesting an end organ deficit. In view of the low level of adherent peripheral blood monocytes it might have also been expected that lysozyme levels would be low. On the contrary, however, they were significantly elevated above normal perhaps indicating a sequestering of macrophages in tissues (39,40, 108).

In an attempt to detect the presence of active suppressor cells rather than simply enumerating OKT_8+ cells, co-cultivation experiments were performed and radiosensitive suppressor cells were found in 12 out of the first 21 individuals tested which were capable of reducing the response of a normal individual's peripheral blood lymphocytes to mitogens (41).

Since the suggestion has been made that chronic exposure to allogeneic semen may be a factor in producing the immune deficit, a study to investigate this has been completed at this institute Asymptomatic, monogomous homosexual male couples whose role vis a vis of sexual activities was clearly defined were studied. A significantly enhanced mixed lymphocyte reaction was detected in one of three couples between responding lymphocytes from an exclusive sperm recipient and stimulating mononuclear cells from his sperm donor partner when compared to the MLC reaction stimulated by cells from a universal, unrelated donor. Specific anti-sperm antibodies were detected in the serum of another sperm recipient homosexual against target sperm from his partner and effector suppressor T cell ratios (Te/Ts) were significantly reduced in two exclusively sperm recipient homosexuals but not in their exclusively sperm donor partners. Both partners of a third homosexual couple who had an alternating role in regard to their sexual practice also displayed a reduced Te/Ts ratio. In the asymptomatic monogomous sperm recipients the Te/Ts ratio reduction was not associated with a significant reduction in the local GVH reduction. However, these two parameters were linearly correlated in a group of 13 symptomatic, non-monogomous homosexuals who were tested by both parameters. Seminal plasma did not exert an immunosuppressive effect on the local GVH reaction following incubation with a partner's mononuclear cells in vitro (56).

In view of the interest in the possible role of the nitrites (poppers) as etiological agents in acquired immune deficiency, a study was conducted at this institute to determine the effect of isobutyl nitrite in vitro on several parameters of lymphocyte function. Concentrations of isobutyl nitrite dissolved in ethyl alcohol from 0.001 to 1.0% were added to in vitro leukocyte cultures. At 1% concentration the agent lysed leukocytes and reduced

viability from 95% to 21% in 24 hours. At a concentration
of 0.5% or below, cell count and viability were unaffected
but the agents inhibited in vitro lymphocyte blastogenic
responses to PHA, PWM and Con-A. It also inhibited NK
cell activity, lymphocyte mediated ADCC and monocyte
mediated ADCC and also reduced in vitro monocyte adherence
and transformation to macrophages. The inhibitary effects
were greater than 90% at the 0.5% concentration but still
detectable at 0.01%. The agent inhibited the
incorporation of leucine, uridine and thymidine
approximately equally in lymphocyte cultures and the
effects were not reversable after 24 hours exposure to the
agent. Thymidine incorporation into both myeloid and
solid tumor cell lines was also inhibited by the same
concentrations of isobutyl nitrite which inhibited
leukocyte functions. Also the the induction of alpha beta
interferon by polyriboinosinic-polyribocytidylic acid in
mouse embryo fibroblasts was inhibited by pre-treatment of
the cells by isobutyl nitrite. These data suggest that
isobutyl nitrite has non-specific cytotoxic activity for
various cells in vitro and could have immunosuppressive
effects on tissues exposed in vivo to high contrations
during its recreational use. The results relating to the
reduction in production of alpha beta interferon also
suggest that isobutyl nitrite is a possible carcinogen
(44).

A study was made of the histopathological features of
lymph nodes removed from 11 of the early patients all of
whom presented with lymphadenopathy of more than 3 months
duration accompanied in the majority of cases by fever and
weight loss. One patient showed lymphoid depleted nodes
with absent germinal centers and a prominent vascular
skeleton. The remainder showed reactive follicular and
sinusoidal hyperplasia, the marginal sinuses being packed
with monomorphic round sinuosidal cells associated with
neutrophils. In one of these cases, however, granulomas
were also seen particularly in the subcapsular sinuses.
The only patient who did not have an inverted
helper/suppressor cell ratio in this group was the one
who's lymph nodes showed the granulomatous reaction in
addition to reactive follicular hyperplasia (109).

So far as the therapy of Kaposi's sarcoma is
concerned, it was decided, on the basis of reported
results, to use Interferon as the primary treatment

modality for patients with Kaposi's sarcoma. This
institute has pioneered the clinical investigation of
interferon in a variety of different tumors and has shown
tumor regression in a number including Kaposi's sarcoma.
To date no serious side effects have been seen except
for the usual one of fever, lassitude and headache. One
patient's markedly abnormal liver function tests for
chronic active hepatitis have returned to normal, no
serious opportunistic infections have been seen in the
treated group. The immunological monitoring of treated
patients is currently being analyzed. Studies are
underway to evaluate low doses of partially purified
leukocyte interferon in these patients.

In preliminary tests of immunorestorative agents in
vitro the agent Azimexon when added to peripheral blood
lymphocytes, caused a reduction in the suppressor cell
population both in normal patients and in patients with
acquired immune deficiency with a corresponding change in
the H/S ratio in normal patients from 1.8 to 2.5 and in
patients with acquired immune deficiency from 0.65 to
1.37. There is also a correlation between the improvement
in the H/S cell ratio and an improvement in the graft
versus host assay (110). Azimexon is one of a number of
agents which are potential candidates for in vivo trials
of immune restoration, others include isoprinosine,
Interferon, thymic hormones, Cimetidine, and ludocin.

Literature Cited

1. Centers for Disease Control. Kaposi's Sarcoma and
    Pneumocystis Pneumonia in Homosexual Men -New York
    and California. Morbid and Mortal Weekly 30:305-307,
    1981.
2. Gottlieb MS, Schroff R, Schanker HM, Weisman JD, Fan
    PT, Wold RA, and Saxon A. Pneumocystis Carinii
    Pneumonia and Mucosal Candidiasis in Previously
    Healthy Homosexual Men. Evidence of a New Acquired
    Cellular Immunodeficiency. N Engl J Med
    305(24):1425-1430, 1981.
3. Masur H, Michelis MA, Greene JB, Onorate I, Vande
    Stouwe RA, Holzman RS, Wormser G, Brettman L, Lange
    M, Murray HW, and Cunningham-Rundles S. An Outbreak
    of Community-Acquired Pneumocystis Carinii Pneumonia.
    Initial Manifestation of Cellular Immune Dysfunction.
    N Engl J Med 305(24):1431-1438, 1981.

4. Centers for Disease Control. Diffuse, Undifferentiated Non-Hodgkins Lymphoma Among Homosexual Males-United States. Morbid and Mortal Weekly 31:277-284, 1982.
5. Zeigler J, Miner RC, Rosenbaum E, Lennette ET, Shillitoe E, Casavant C, Drew WL, Mintz L, Gershaw J, Greenspan J, Beckstead J, and Yammamoto K. Outbreak of Burkitts-like Lymphoma in Homosexual Men. Lancet ii:631-633, 1982.
6. Conant MA, Volberding P, Fletcher V, Lozada FI, and Silverman S. Squamous Cell Carcinoma in Sexual Partner of Kaposi Sarcoma Patient. Lancet i:286, 1982.
7. Kaposi M. Idiopathisches Multiples Pigmentsarkom der Haut. Arch Dermatol Syphiol, 4:265-273, 1872.
8. Lothe F. Kaposi's Sarcoma in Ugandan Africans. Acta Path Microbiol Scand Supp 161, 1963.
9. Philippson L. Weber das Sarcoma Idiopathicum Cutis Kaposi. Ein Beitrag Zur Sarcomlehre. Virchows Arch 167:58-81, 1902.
10. MacKee GM, Cipollaro AC. Idiopathic Multiple Hemorrhagic Sarcoma (Kaposi). Am J Cancer 26:1-28, 1936.
11. Bernhardt R. Weitere Mitheilungen uber Sarcoma Idiopathicum Multiplex Pigmentosum Cutis. Arch f Derm u Syph 62:237-262, 1902.
12. Mierzecki H. Sarcoma Idiopathicum Multiplex Kaposi. Arch f Derm u Syph 165:577-584, 1932.
13. Dorffel J. Histogenesis of Multiple Idiopathic Hemorrhagic Sarcoma of Kaposi. Arch Derm Syph 26:608-634, 1932.
14. McCarthy WD, Pack GT. Malignant Blood Vessel Tumors. A Report of 56 Cases of Angiosarcoma and Kaposi's Sarcoma. SG&O 91:465-482, 1950.
15. DiGiovanna JJ, and Safai B. Kaposi's Sarcoma. Retrospective Study of 90 Cases with Particular Emphasis on the Familial Occurrence, Ethnic Background and Prevalence of Other Diseases. Amer J Med 71:779-783, 1981.
16. Pellisser A. La Maladie de Kaposi en Afrique Noire (Angio-reticulo-endothelio-fibro-sarcomatose). A Propos de 18 Cases. Bull Soc Path exot 46:832-839, 1953.
17. O'Connell KM. Kaposi's Sarcoma: Histopathologic Study of 159 Cases from Malawi. J Clin Path 30:687-695, 1977.

18. Oettle AG. Geographical and Racial Differences in the Frequency of Kaposi's Sarcoma as Evidence of Environmental or Genetic Causes. Acta Unio Int Contra Cancrum 18:330-363, 1962.
19. Kaminer B, Murray JF. Sarcoma Idiopathicum Multiplex Haemorrhagicum of Kaposi With Special Reference to its Incidence in the South African Negro and Two Case Reports. S Afr J Clin Sec 1:1-25, 1950.
20. Thijs A. L'Angiosarcomatose de Kaposi au Congo belge et Ruanda Urundi. Ann Soc belge Med-Trop 37:295-308, 1957.
21. Choisser RM, Ramsey EM. Angioreticuloendothelioma (Kaposi's disease) of the Heart. Amer J Path 15:155-177, 1939.
22. Bluefarb SM. Kaposi's Sarcoma. Charles C. Thomas, Springfield, IL. 1957.
23. Centers for Disease Control. Opportunistic Infections and Kaposi's Sarcoma Among Haitians in the United States. Morbid and Mortal Weekly 31:353-354, 360-361, 1982.
24. Follansbee SE, Busch DF, Wofsy CB, Coleman DL, Gullet J, Aurigemma GP, Ross T, Madley WK, Drew WL. An Outbreak of Pneumocystis Carinii Pneumonia in Homosexual Men. Ann Int Med 96:705-713, 1982.
25. Siegal FP, Lopez C, Hammer GS, et al. Severe Acquired Immunodeficiency in Male Homosexuals, Manifested by Chronic Perianal Ulcerative Herpes Simplex Lesion. N Engl J Med 305:1439-1444, 1981.
26. Sexual Transmission of Enteric Pathogens. Editorial. Lancet ii:1328-1329,1981.
27. Fainstein V, Bolivar R, Mavligit G, Rios A, Luna M. Disseminated Infection Due to Mycobacterium Avium-intercellulare in a Homosexual Man with Kaposi's Sarcoma. J Infect Dis 145:586, 1982.
28. Symposium on Pneumocystis Carinii Infection. NCI Monograph 43, 1976.
29. Walzer PD, Perk DP, Krogstad DJ, Rawson PG, Schultz MG. Pneumocystis Carinii Pneumonia in the United States, Epidemiologic, Diagnostic and Clinical Features. Ann Int Med 80:83-93, 1974.
30. Singer CC, Armstrong D, Rosen PP. Schottenfeld D. Pneumocystis Carinii Pneumonia: A Cluster of Eleven Cases. Ann Int Med 82: 772-778, 1975.
31. Williams DM, Kriela JA, Remington JS. Pulmonary Infection in the Compromised Host. Am Rev Resp Dis 114:359-394, 593-627, 1976.

32. Hughes WT. Pneumocystis Pneumonia. N Engl J Med 297, 1381-1383, 1977.
33. Rubin RH, Cosimi AB, Tolkoff-Rubini ME, Russell PS. Infectious Disease Syndromes Attributable to Cytomegalovirus and Their Significance Among Renal Transplant Recipients. Transplantation 24:458-464, 1977.
34. Carney WP, Hirsch MS. Mechanisms of Immunosuppression in Cytomegalovirus Mononucleosis: II. Virus-monocyte Interactions. J Infect Dis 144:47-54, 1981.
35. Hughes WT, Price RA, Sisko F, Havron WS, Kafatos AG, Schonland M, Smythe PM. Protein Calorie Malnutrition: A Host Determinant for Pneumocystis Carinii Infection. Am J Dis Child 128:44-53, 1974.
36. Friedman-Kien AE, Laubenstein LJ, Rubinstein P, Buimovici-Klein E, Marmor M, Stahl R, Spigland I, Kim, KS, Zolla-Pazner S. Disseminated Kaposi's Sarcoma in Homosexual Men. Ann Int Med 96:693-704, 1982.
37. Fauci AS. The Syndrome of Kaposi's Sarcoma and Opportunistic Infections: An Epidemiologically Restricted Disorder of Immunoregulation. Ann Int Med 96:777-779, 1982.
38. Gerstoft J, Malchow-Moller A, Bygbjerg I, Dickmeiss E, Enk C, Halberg P, Haahr S, Jacobsen M, Jensen K, Mejer J, Neilsen JO, Thomsen HK, Sondergaard J, Lorenzen I. Severe Acquired Immunodeficiency in European Homosexual Men. Brit Med J 285:17-19, 1982.
39. Reuben JM, Hersh EM, Mansell PWA, Newell GR, Rios A, Rossen R, Goldstein AL, McClure JE. Immunological Characterization of Homosexual Males. Cancer Research (in press)
40. Hersh EM, Mansell, PWA. Acquired Immune Deficiency Syndrome: A New Clinical Entity. Clinical Immunology Newsletter (in press)
41. Hersh EM, Mansell PWA, Reuben JM, Frank J, Rios A, LaPushin R, Newell GR. Suppressor Cell Activity Among the Peripheral Blood Leukocytes of Selected Homosexual Subjects. Cancer Research (submitted)
42. Coulston F, Dunne JF. The Potential Carcinogenicity of Nitrosable Drugs. WHO Symposium, Geneva, June 1978. Ablex Publishing Corporation, Norwood, NJ, pp 1-16, 1980.

43. Jorgensen KA, Lawesson SO. Amyl Nitrite and Kaposi's Sarcoma in Homosexual Men. N Engl J Med 307:893-894, 1982.
44. Hersh EM, Reuben JM, Bogerd H, Bielski M, Mansell PWA, Rios A, Newell GR, Sonnenfeld G. Effect of the Recreational Agent Isobutyl Nitrite on Human Peripheral Blood Leukocytes and on In Vitro Interferon Production. Cancer Research (in press)
45. Goedert JJ, Wallen WC, Mann DL, Strong DM, Neuland CY, Greene MH, Murray C, Fraumeni JF, Blattner WA. Amyl Nitrite May Alter T Lymphocytes in Homosexual Men. Lancet 412-416, 1982.
46. Nahas GG, Suciu-Focee N, Armand JP, Morishima A. Inhibition of Cellular Mediated Immunity in Marijuana Smokers. Science 183:419-420, 1974.
47. Goode E, Troiden RR. Amyl Nitrite Use Among Homosexual Men. Am J Psych 136:1067-1069, 1979.
48. Vandenbroucke JP, Hofman A. Amyl Nitrite Use by Homosexuals. Lancet i:503, 1982.
49. Special Report: Epidemiologic Aspects of the Current Outbreak of Kaposi's Sarcoma and Opportunistic Infections. N Engl J Med 306:248-252, 1982.
50. Curran, J. Personal communication.
51. Pollack MS. Unpublished results.
52. Gladman DD, Keystone EC, Baron M, Lee P, Cane D, Mervert H. Increased frequency of HLA-DR5 in Scleroderma. Arthritis Rheum 24:854-856, 1981.
53. Tosato G, Steinberg A, Blaese M. Defective EBV-Specific Suppressor T-Cell Function in Rheumatoid Arthritis. N Engl J Med 305:1238-1243, 1981.
54. DeWolf WC, Lange PH, Shepherd R, Martin-Alosco S, Yunis EJ. Association of HLA and Renal Cell Carcinoma. Human Immunology 1:41-44, 1981.
55. Safai B, Pollack M, Myskowski P, Dupont B. Increased Frequency of HLA-DR5 in Mycosis Funoides and Kaposi's Sarcoma. Fed Proc 41:414, 1982.
56. Mavligit GM, Talpaz M, Hsia FT, Wong WL, Lichtiger B, Mansell PWA, Mumford DM. Chronic, Sperm-Induced Allo-Antigenic Stimulation: A New Hypothesis for Immune Dysregulation in Homosexual Males. N Engl J Med (in press).
57. Hurtenbach U, Shearer GM. Germ Cell Induced Immune Suppression in Mice. Effect of Incubation of Syngeneic Spermatozoa on Cell-Mediated Immune Responses. J Exp Med 155:1719-1729, 1982.

58. Anderson D, Tarter T. Immunosuppressive Effects of Mouse Seminal Plasma Components In Vivo and In Vitro. J Immunol 128:535-539, 1982.

59. Klein M, Pereira F, Kantor I. Kaposi's Sarcoma Complicating Systemic Lupus Erythematous Treated with Immunosuppression. Arch Dermatol 110:602-605, 1974.

60. Leung F, Fam A, Osoba D. Kaposi's Sarcoma Complicating Corticosteroid Therapy for Temporal Arteritis. Amer J Med 71:320-322, 1981.

61. Kapadin S, Krauise J. Kaposi's Sarcoma After Long-Term Alkylating Agent Therapy for Multiple Myeloma. Southern Med J 70:1011-1013, 1977.

62. Mazzaferri E, Penn G. Kaposi's Sarcoma Associated with Multiple Myeloma Arch Intern Med 122:521-525, 1968.

63. Dentzig P. Kaposi's Sarcoma and Polymyositis. Arch Dermatol 110:605-607, 1974.

64. Law I. Kaposi's Sarcoma and Plasma Cell Dyscrasia. JAMA 229:1329-1331, 1974.

65. Ettinger D, Humphrey R, Skinner M. Kaposi's Sarcoma Associated with Multiple Myeloma. Johns Hopkins Med J 137:88-90, 1975.

66. Myers B, Kessler E, Lepi J, Pick A, Rosenfeld J, Tikvah P. Kaposi's Sarcoma in Kidney Transplant Recipients. Arch Intern Med 133:307-311, 1974.

67. Harwood A, Osoba D, Hofstader S, Goldstein M, Cardella C, Holecek M, Kunynetz R, Giammarca R. Kaposi's Sarcoma in Recipients of Renal Transplants. Am J Med 67:759-765, 1979.

68. Hardy M, Goldfarb P, Levein S, Dattner A, Muggia F, Levitt S, Weinstein R. De Novo Kaposi's Sarcoma. CA 38:144-148, 1976.

69. Moertel C. Multiple Primary Malignant Neoplasms, Their Incidence and Significance. In: Recent Results in Cancer Research. Springer-Verlag, New York, 7:34-47, 1966.

70. Safai B, Mike V, Giraldo G, Beth E, Good R. Association of Kaposi's Sarcoma with Second Primary Malignancies. CA 45:1472-1479, 1980.

71. Master S, Taylor J, Kyalwazi S, Ziegler J. Immunological Studies in Kaposi's Sarcoma in Uganda. Br Med J 1:660-662, 1970.

72. Taylor J, Junge U, Wolfe L, Deinhardt F, Kyalwazi S. Lymphocyte Transformation in Patients with Kaposi's Sarcoma. Int J Cancer 8:468-474, 1971.

73. Taylor J. Lymphocyte Transformation in Kaposi's Sarcoma. Lancet i:883-884, 1973.
74. Taylor J and Ziegler J. Delayed Cutaneous Hypersensitivity Reactions in Patients with Kaposi's Sarcoma. Br J Cancer 30:312-318, 1974.
75. Safai F, Cunningham-Rundles S, Matsuoka L, Dupont B, Good RA. Cell Mediated Immune Reaction in Kaposi's Sarcoma. Clin Research 28:9-81, 1980.
76. Centers for Disease Control. A Cluster of Kaposi's Sarcoma and Pneumocystis carinii Pneumonia among Homosexual Male Residents of Los Angeles and Orange Counties, California. Morbid and Mortal Weekly 31:305-307, 1982. 77. Centers for Disease Control. Pneumocystis Carinii Pneumonia Among Persons with Hemophilia A. Morbid and Mortal Weekly 31:365-367, 1982.
78. Posner LE, Robert-Guroff M, Kalyanaraman VS, Poiesz BJ, Ruscetti FW, Fossieck B, Bunn PA, Minna JD, Gallo RC. Natural Antibodies to the Human T Cell Lymphoma Virus in Patients with Cutaneous T Cell Lymphomas. J Exp Med 154(2):333-346, 1981.
79. Giraldo G, Beth E, Haguenau F. Herpes-type Virus Particles in Tissue Culture of Kaposi's Sarcoma from Different Geographic Regions. J Natl Cancer Inst 49:1509-1526, 1972.
80. Giraldo G, Beth E, Kaurilsky F, Henle W, Henle G, Mike V, Haurax J, Anderson M, Ghardi M, Kyalwazi S, Puissant A. Antibody Patterns to Herpes Viruses in Kaposi's Sarcoma: Serological Association of European Kaposi's Sarcoma with Cytomegalovirus. Int J Cancer 15:839-848, 1975.
81. Giraldo G, Beth E, Henle W, Henle G, Mike V, Safai B, Haurax J, McHardy J, De The G. Antibody Patterns to Herpes Viruses in Kaposi's Sarcoma. II. Serological Associations of American Kaposi's Sarcoma with Cytomegalovirus. Int J Cancer 22:126-131, 1978.
82. Giraldo G, Beth E, Huang E. Kaposi's Sarcoma and its Relationship to Cytomegalovirus. III. CMV, DNA and CMV Early Antigens in Kaposi's Sarcoma. Int J Cancer 26:23-29, 1980.
83. Boldogh I, Beth E, Huang ES, Kyalwazi SK, Giraldo G. Kaposi's Sarcoma. IV. Detection of CMV DAN, CMV RNA and CMNA in Tumor Biopsies. Int J Cancer 28(4):469-474, 1981.

84. Rinaldo CR, Carney WP, Richter BS, Black PH, Hirsch MS. Mechanisms of Immunosuppression in Cytomegaloviral Mononucleosis. J Infect Dis 141:488-495, 1980.
85. Geder L, Laychock AM, Gorodecki J. Alterations in Biological Properties of Different Lines of Cytomegalovirus-Transformed Human Embryo Lung Cells Following In Vitro Cultivation. IARC Sci Publ 24:591-601, 1978.
86. Drew WL, Mintz L, Miner RC, Sands M, Ketterer B. Prevalence of Cytomegalovirus Infection in Homosexual Men. J Infect Dis 143(2):188-192, 1981. 87. Shearer GM. Personal communication.
88. Rubin RH, Cosimi B, Tolkoff-Rubin, NE, Russell PA, Hirsch MS. Infectious Disease Syndromes Attributable to Cytomegalovirus and Their Significance Among Renal Transplant Recipients. Transplantation 24(6):458-464, 1977.
89. From the National Institutes of Health. Summary of a Workshop on Cytomegalovirus Infections during Organ Transplantation. J Infect Dis 139(6):728-734, 1979.
90. Feletti C, Musiani M, Bonomini V. Early Diagnosis of Cytomegalovirus Infection in Renal Transplantation. Proc Eur Dial Transplant Assoc 17:473-477, 1980.
91. Epstein MA, Achong BG, Barr YM. Virus Particles in Cultured Lymphoblasts from Burkitt's Lymphoma. Lancet i:702-703, 1964.
92. Henle G, Henle W, Diehl V. Relation of Burkitt's Tumor Associated Herpes Type Virus to Infectious Mononucleosis. Proc Nat Acad Sci 59:94-101, 1968.
93. Henle G, Henle W, Clifford P, Diehl V, Kafwiko GW, Kirya BG, Klein G, Morrow RH, Monube GMR, Pike P, Tijkel PM, Ziegler JL. Antibodies and Epstein Barr Virus in Burkitt's Lymphomas and Control Groups. JNCI 43:1147-1157, 1969.
94. Henle W, Henle G, Ho HC, Burtin P, Cachin Y, Clifford P, de Schryver A, de The G, Diehl V, Klein G. Antibodies to Epstein Barr Virus and Nasopharyngeal Carcinoma, Other Head and Neck Neoplasms and Control Groups. JNCI 44:225-231, 1970.

95. Nahmias AJ, Naib ZM, Josey WE. Genital Herpes and Cervical Cancer, Can a Causal Relation Be Proven? Proceedings Synp Oncogenesis and Herpes Type Viruses. Ed. de The G and Biggs PM. Cambridge University Press, 1972.

96. Morris, L, Distenfeld A, Amorosi E, Karpatkin S. Autoimmune Thrombocytopenic Purpura in Homosexual Men. Ann Int Med 96:714-717, 1982.

97. Hymes K, Green J, Marcus A, William D, Cheung T, Prose N, Ballard H, Laubenstein L. Kaposi's Sarcoma in Homosexual Men -A Report of Eight Cases. Lancet 598-600, 1981.

98. Laubenstein L, Hymes K, Krigel R. Phase II Trial of VP-16213 in Disseminated Kaposi's Sarcoma. Proc Am Soc Clin Oncol 1:175, 1982.

99. Gutterman, J.U. Personal communication. (also see Appendix I)

100. Krown S. Personal communication.

101. Low TLK, Thurman GB, Chinçarini C, McClure JE, Marshall GD, Hu SK, Goldstein A. Current Status of Thymosin Research: Evidence for the Existence of a Family of Thymic Factors that Control T-Cell Maturation. Ann NY Acad Sci 332:33-48, 1979.

102. Low TLK, Thurman GB, McAdoo M, McClure J, Rossio JL, Naylor PH, Goldstein AL. The Chemistry and Biology of Thymosin. Isolation, Characterization, and Biological Activities of Thymosin alpha 1 and Polypeptide Beta$_1$ from Calf Thymus. J Biol Chem 254(3):981-986, 1979.

103. Bicker U. BM 06.002. A New Immunostimulating Compound. In: Immune Modulation and Control of Neoplasia by Adjuvant Therapy. MA Chirigos, Ed. Raven Press, New York, 389-401, 1978.

104. Wybran J, Govaerts A, Appelboom T. Inosiplex, a Stimulating Agent for Normal Human T Cells. J Immunol 121:1184-1187, 1978.

105. Goodwin JS. Prostaglandin E and Cancer Growth: Potential for Immunotherapy with Prostaglandin Synthetase Inhibitors. In: Augmenting Agents in Cancer Therapy. EM Hersh, Ed. Raven Press, In Press, 1981.

106. Guinan ME, Auerbach DM, Curran JW, Goodrich JT, Jaffe HW, Haverkos HW, Thomas PA, KSOI Task Force of the Centers for Disease Control in Atlanta, GA. Epidemic Kaposi's Sarcoma and Serious Opportunistic Infections. A Comparison of Heterosexual and Homosexual Cases. 22nd Interscience Conference on Antimicrobiological Agents and Chemotherapy, 1982.

107. Masur H, Michelis MA, Wormser GP, Lewin S, Gold J, Tapper ML, Giron J, Lerner CW, Armstrong D, Setia U, Sender JA, Siebken RS, Nichols P, Arlen Z, Maayan S, Ernst JA, Siegal FP, Cunningham-Rundles S. Opportunistic Infection in Previously Healthy Women. Initial Manifestations of a Community-Acquired Cellular Immunodeficiency. Ann Internal Med 97:533-539, 1982.

108. Hersh EM, Reuben JM, Rios A, Mansell PWA, Newell GR, McClure JE, Goldstein, AL. Elevated serum Thymosin α, levels associated with evidence of immune dysregulation in male homosexuals with a history of infective diseases or Kaposi's sarcoma. NEJM 308. 45-46. 1983.

109. Guarda LA, Butler JJ, Mansell P, Hersh EM, Reuben J, Newell GR. Lymphadenopathy in Homosexual Men: Morbid Anatomy with Clinical and Immunologic Correlations. Amer J Clin Path. (in press)

110. Patt YZ, Keating MJ, Mansell PWA, Reuben JM, Hersh EM. The granulopoietic effect of Azimexon in smouldering leukemia and Acquired Immune Deficiency Syndrome in homosexuals. Cancer Research (submitted).

Progress in Cancer Control IV: Research in the Cancer Center, pages 237–247
© **1983 Alan R. Liss, Inc., 150 Fifth Avenue, New York, NY 10011**

CANCER CONTROL: X-RAY INDUCED C3HBA TUMOR REGRESSION AND
PREVENTION OF ITS REGROWTH BY β-CAROTENE OR VITAMIN A.

Eli Seifter, Ph.D.[1,2], Jacques Padawer, Ph.D.[3],
Giuseppi Rettura, Ph.D.[1], Paul Goodwin, Ph.D.[4],
and Stanley M. Levenson, Ph.D.[1]

Department of Surgery[1], Biochemistry[2], Anatomy[3],
and Radiology[4], Albert Einstein College of
Medicine, Yeshiva University, New York, N.Y.
10461.

One approach to Cancer Control involves the use of
combined therapies to reduce tumor mass and decrease tumor
regrowth to a degree permitting a normal life span with
minimal physical signs of tumor disease. The research
discussed herein addresses the problem of how, in an animal
cancer system, the remission state may be achieved and
maintained.

Supplemental vitamin A inhibits growth of several
transplantable tumors, e.g., C3HBA and BW10232 (Rettura et
al. 1975, 1980) and increases the anti-tumor effects of
limited local tumor excision and cyclophosphamide therapy
(Rettura et al. 1978, 1982b; Seifter et al. 1981a). We had
shown previously that supplemental vitamin A abrogates some
toxic responses to chemicals and treatments used in cancer
therapy. For example, vitamin A reduces some of the
systemic reactions (stress) associated with surgical
procedures and improves wound healing and survival in
experimentally-wounded animals subjected to some cancer
chemotherapeutic agents (Freiman et al. 1970; Seifter et al.
1975, 1981b; Stratford et al. 1980). Supplemental vitamin A
may therefore permit increased amounts of therapeutic agents
to be tolerated or may increase the efficacy of the
therapeutic modalities employed.

Because β-carotene is the major dietary source of

1

vitamin A and is less toxic than supplemental vitamin A, we
have been studying the tumor preventive and therapeutic
actions of supplemental β-carotene (Dorogokuplya et al.
1973; Seifter et al. 1982a). Supplemental β-carotene, like
supplemental vitamin A, also has antitumor action against
certain viral, chemical, and transplantable tumors (Seifter
et al. 1982b; Rettura et al. 1982a). Also, we have found
that supplemental vitamin A and β-carotene each diminishes
the toxicity due to local X-irradiation or whole body ^{60}Co
or ^{137}Cs X-radiation (Seifter et al. 1981c, 1982c; Shen et
al. 1983). Because both vitamin A and β-carotene have
salutary effects on tumor-bearing or irradiated mice, we
studied the effects of these two compounds on tumor-bearing
mice subjected to local X-irradiation.

MATERIALS AND METHODS

Animals, Housing, Diets

     Five-week-old male CBA/J mice (Jackson Laboratories,
Bar Harbor, ME.) were distributed randomly, in groups of 6,
in plastic shoe box-type cages. Ground Purina Laboratory
Chow (Δ5001, Ralston Purina Co., St. Louis, MO.) was used
for the basal or control chow (CR). It contains 15,000 IU
vitamin A and 6.4 mg β-carotene/Kg diet (total = 18,000
units vit A/Kg diet), considerably more than the National
Research Council's recommended dietary allowance of vitamin
A, which averages 6,000 IU/Kg diet, for normal growth. The
basal control diet is therefore not deficient in vitamin A.
We prepared two experimental diets from the basal diet. One
was made by addition of vitamin A palmitate (150,000 IU/Kg
diet); the other was made by addition of 90 mg β-carotene/Kg
diet.

Tumors, Inoculation

     Adenocarcinoma C3HBA was passed into male CBA/J mice in
which the tumor grows well, metastasizes, and kills (Rettura
et al. 1982). Inocula were prepared from solid CBA tumors
1.4 cm in diameter, as previously described (Rettura et al.
1982). Mice were inoculated with 2×10^5 tumor cells
subcutaneously in the outer aspect of the right thigh.

Tumor Measurements

Tumor size was evaluated by methods previously
described (Rettura et al. 1982a). In experiment 1, the
average of the diameters was 6.2 mm on the day experimental
treatments were begun; in experiment 2, the corresponding
value was 5.6 mm. After treatments were begun, measurements
were made several times weekly.

Radiation

Mice were anesthetized lightly with sodium
pentobarbital (1 mg/20 g body weight, i.p.) and were then
irradiated with a Picker-Vanguard 280 KVp X-ray therapy
unit, half value layer (HVL) = 0.5 mm copper. The unit was
calibrated to deliver 450 Roentgens /minute and was timed to
deliver a single dose of 30 Gy (3000 rads) to the hind leg
bearing the tumor. The rest of the body, including the
other hind limb, was shielded by a 2 mm thick lead shield.

Experimental Plan

Two similarly-designed experiments, separated by a nine
week interval, were carried out; the first was started in
Nov. 1980, the second in Jan. 1981. Five week-old male
CBA/J mice were acclimatized to our laboratory for one week
and then inoculated with $2x10^5$ C3HBA tumor cells. On the
13th post-inoculation day for each experiment, when tumors
had a mean diameter of 6.2 mm in experiment no. 1 and 5.6 mm
in experiment no. 2, mice in each experiment were
distributed randomly into 3 groups of 10 each and housed
5/cage. These 3 groups received no radiation. Group no. 1
was continued on the control chow, while groups no. 2 and
no. 3 were started on the chow supplemented with vitamin A
or β-carotene, respectively. Thirty-six additional
tumor-bearing mice were subjected to local tumor irradiation
as described. Following this, they were divided randomly
into 3 groups of 12 mice each, housed 6/cage. Group no. 4
was continued on the control chow for the post-radiation
period. Mice of groups no. 5 and no. 6 were given the
vitamin A or β-carotene supplemented chow starting a few
hours after irradiation.

One year after radiation in Experiment 1, the diet of
some of the surviving mice was altered. Five of the eleven
mice from group no. 5 were continued on that same vitamin
A-supplemented diet, whereas 6 mice were switched back to

the control chow. Similarly, five mice from group 6 were continued on their β-carotene-supplemented diet, and the remaining 5 animals were switched back to the control ration. In the second experiment, similar dietary changes were made 13 1/2 months after irradiation and the start of the supplemental diets. In both experiments, survival studies were continued for 24 months after the day of radiation therapy, at which time survivors were killed and studied.

Statistical Analyses

Tumor size and latent period for tumor reappearance were analyzed by Student's "t" test, and survival time by ANOVA. Where warranted by the F ratio , the data were further examined by the Newman-Keuls test to establish allowable comparisons and their P values. Tumor incidence (frequency of tumor recurrence) was evaluated by a Chi Square method.

RESULTS

Chemotherapeutic Effects of Supplemental Vitamin A, β-carotene, or Local X-irradiation Used Singly.

a) Tumor Growth. As shown in Table 1, supplemental vitamin A and β-carotene each slowed tumor growth and there were no significant differences in the effects of vitamin A and β-carotene. By contrast, local radiation, by itself, caused tumor regression. In experiment 1, local irradiation caused partial tumor regression in all mice, but tumor growth resumed after a few weeks. Similarly, in experiment 2, local radiation caused partial regression in 11 of 12 mice and temporary "complete" regression on one (Table 2).

b) Survival. Mice receiving neither dietary supplementation nor radiation survived an average of 41.2 days in experiment 1 and 43.3 days in experiment 2 Supplemental vitamin A and β-carotene increased survival time to an average of 60.2 days and 61.2 days, respectively, in experiment 1, and 64.2 days and 63.3 days, respectively, in experiment 2 (p<0.001 in each case). Local radiation increased survival time even longer, to 84.4 days (p<0.001) in experiment 1 and 99.1 days (p<0.001) in experiment 2.

c) Tumor Regression. All mice receiving both radiation and supplemental vitamin A (24/24) showed complete tumor regression. However, in two cases (one in each experiment), the regression was temporary and a tumor reappeared after several months, followed by deaths of both hosts within several months. The remaining animals (22/24) survived without palpable tumor during the first year. Irradiated mice receiving supplemental β-carotene responded in a similar way (Table 2). In experiment 1, there were two deaths in β-carotene supplemented mice during the first year. In one of these mice, tumor recurred 45 days after initial regression and death followed 75 days later. The other death was accidental and not tumor related.

Table 1

Influence of Supplemental Vitamin A (VA), β-carotene (BC), and Radiation on C3HBA Tumor Size (mm)

Experiment 1

Group	Days post-radiation and post-treatment					
	0	4	8	11	14	18
No Rx	6.2	10.1	14.4	16.8	18.0	20.4
X-Ray	6.2	5.5	5.2	4.8	4.0	4.0
No Rx + VA	6.2	9.4	10.1	11.4	13.7	15.8
X-Ray + VA	6.2	4.3	2.6	0.5	0.2	0.0
No Rx + BC	6.2	9.5	7.8	8.5	10.0	12.7
X-Ray + BC	6.2	4.3	2.4	0.9	0.2	0

Experiment 2

Group	Days post-radiation and post-treatment							
	0	3	5	7	10	12	14	18
No Rx	5.6	7.4	8.9	10.0	11.7	12.8	13.9	15.4
X-Ray	5.6	5.3	4.9	4.0	3.3	3.1	2.8	3.2
No Rx + VA	5.6	6.4	7.5	8.4	9.2	10.0	10.7	13.1
X-Ray + VA	5.6	4.5	2.4	1.5	0.3	0	0	0
No Rx + BC	5.6	6.7	7.5	8.3	9.1	10.0	10.7	12.9
X-Ray + BC	5.6	4.3	2.6	1.7	0.5	0	0	0

In experiment 2, tumor recurred in one of 12 mice treated with β-carotene radiation 108 days after regression, and death occurred 64 days later.

Effects of Combined Therapy (24 Month Follow Up)

a) Supplemental Vitamin A. In experiment 1, vitamin A supplements were continued for five mice beyond the first year. Supplements were discontinued for the other six mice, and these animals were returned to the control chow one year after they had been irradiated. Of the five continued on supplemental vitamin A, none redeveloped tumors; however, three died with no evidence of tumor at autopsy by gross examination and two survived without evidence of tumor. Of the six mice switched back to the control chow, 5 redeveloped tumors and died. Tumors redeveloped 431+12 days after radiation and vitamin A supplementation and 66+3 days after the vitamin A supplement was discontinued. Deaths occurred 71+5 days after tumor recurrence. One mouse died of non-tumor cause 547 days after radiation.

b) Supplemental β-carotene (Table 2). Of the five mice continued on supplemental β-carotene in experiment 1, none redeveloped tumors. However, on mouse died of nontumor cause 664 days (lifespan for this strain of mice = 600-750 days) after the start of β-carotene supplementation and radiation, while the other 4 mice survived through the second year without evidence of tumor. Of the five mice switched back to the control chow, two redeveloped tumors 133 and 275 days, respectively, after the β-carotene supplementation was discontinued, and they died about 52 days later. Three mice died of nontumor causes 240, 277, and 291 days after stopping the β-carotene supplement.

c) Supplemental vitamin A. These results are from the experiment started by tumor inoculation on Jan. 16, 1981, followed by irradiation and initiation of feeding of experimental diets on Jan. 30, 1981. Discontinuance of dietary supplements (for appropriate groups) was carried out on March 15, 1982. Surviving mice were killed in January-- 2, years after the inoculation day. Of the five mice maintained on supplemental vitamin A throughout the experiment, none redeveloped tumors; however, 3 died of nontumor causes and 2 survived through the 22nd month without evidence of tumor. Of the six vitamin A mice switched back to the control chow (58 weeks after radiation), 3 redeveloped tumors and died, one died of

Table 2

Effect of Supplemental Vitamin A, β-Carotene, and 30Gy
on Local Radiation on Survival Time of
CBA/J Mice with C3HBA Tumors

Group	1	2	3	4	5	6
supplemt	-	Vit A[d]	β-Car	-	Vit A	β-Car
X-Ray	-	-	-	+	+	+
No. Mice, Compl. Tumor Regression:						
Exp 1	0	0	0	0	12	12
Exp 2	0	0	0	0	12	12
No. Mice Surviv. 1yr:						
Exp 1	0	0	0	0	11	11
Exp 2	0	0	0	0	11	11
Mean Surv'l of Nonsurviv. Mice, days:						
Exp 1	41.2±2.5[b]	60.2±3.0	61.2±2.1	84.4±5.4	142	136
Exp 2	43.3±0.8	63.3±1.8	64.2±1.9	99.1±5.9	182	199

P values[c], Gp:	1 vs 2	1 vs 3	1 vs 4	2 vs 3	2 vs 4
Exp 1	<.001	<.001	<.001	NS[d]	<.001
Exp 2	<.001	<.001	<.001	NS	<.001

[a]Vit A= vitamin A; β-car= β-carotene.
[b]Mean ± Standard Error of the Mean.
[c]By Analysis of Variance and Neuman-Keuls Test.
[d]Not statistically significant.

nontumor causes, and 2 survived. Tumor recurrence occurred
39, 59, and 69 days following dietary changes, and their
deaths occurred 39, 59 and 135 days after the dietary
change.

d) Supplemental β-carotene. Of the six β-carotene mice continued on their supplements, none redeveloped tumors; however, one died of nontumor causes 195 days after the dietary change while 5 mice survived without evidence of tumor. Of the five β-carotene-supplemented mice switched back to the control chow, none redeveloped tumor. However, 3 survived while 2 died of nontumor causes; deaths occurred 152 and 153 days following the dietary change.

DISCUSSION

The present studies confirm earlier reports of the additive antitumor therapeutic actions of radiation and supplemental dietary vitamin A in mice with C3HBA tumors (Brandes, Anton 1966; Brandes et al. 1967; Tannock, Marshall 1972) and, in contrast to the previously cited works, show that this added therapeutic effect can be accomplished in a remarkable way without inducing toxicity even when the supplemental vitamin A is fed for a very extended period of time. Moreover, under these conditions, protection against tumor regrowth persists for several months after supplementation is discontinued. We think that incorporating vitamin A into the diet (analogous in humans to giving a vitamin A supplement at mealtime) is more efficacious and less toxic than is intraperitoneal injection, the route most frequently employed by others. Additionally, the present studies demonstrate that supplemental dietary β-carotene, a vitamin A precursor, contributes additively to the anti-tumor action of X-irradiation in a manner similar to that of vitamin A, and exerts dramatic protective action against tumor regrowth even after feeding of the β-carotene is discontinued. This finding may be of major importance in the prevention and treatment of tumors in humans.

Radiation Dosage

Previously, we confirmed (Zaravinos 1980) Fisher's finding (Fisher et al. 1978) that 30 Gy causes partial regression of C3HBA tumors. We employed 30 Gy in the present study to determine if supplemental vitamin A and β-carotene would further enhance radiation-induced tumor regression. In these experiments we have not used β-carotene or vitamin A supplements as primary agents to obtain tumor regression; rather, we have used these compounds to (a) slow C3HBA tumor growth (Rettura et al. 1982a; Seifter et al. 1982b); (b) ameliorate X-radiation toxicity (Seifter et al. 1981c); (c) prevent the thymic involution, adrenal enlargement, and weight loss caused by C3HBA tumor growth. We are aware that single-dose local radiation is not used clinically for tumor therapy; however, we have employed it in these experiments to test our hypothesis that supplemental vitamin A and β-carotene would each add to the therapeutic effectiveness of radiotherapy. The results of our experiments show this to be the case.

General role for Vitamin A and β-Carotene in Tumor Therapy.

In addition to inhibiting tumor growth moderately and ameliorating radiation toxicity, supplemental Vitamin A and β-carotene have an additional and important action in tumor-bearing animals. Like many other tumors, C3HBA induces some responses in the host that mitigate against survival and also enhance further tumor growth. The progressive and often accelerating course of many tumor diseases is associated with immune depression and with alterations in metabolism of nontumor host tissues. Because of these events, the host ability to contain or limit the growth of even a small tumor burden is diminished, and tumor growth progresses. Catabolic responses similar to those described by Selye as stress (Selye 1936) and by Cuthbertson as metabolic response to injury (Cuthbertson 1930) derive, in part, from intensified pituitary-adrenal medullary and cortical activities that ultimately subserve tumor growth by thymolytic and lympholytic activities and by stimulating host proteolysis and gluconeogenesis. A major finding of previous work from this laboratory is the observation that supplemental vitamin A or β-carotene inhibit some of the most negative aspects of tumor-induced metabolism such as weight loss, adrenal hemorrhage, thymic involution and lymphopenia and the associated immune depression, and bleeding associated with thrombocytopenia.

The moderation of tumor-induced stress responses and enhancement of host resistance to tumors are important properties of supplemental vitamin A or β-carotene; these properties suggest that vitamin A and/or β-carotene may have general application in tumor therapy.

REFERENCES

Brandes D, Anton E (1966). The role of lysosomes in cellular lytic processes. III. Electron, histochemical changes in mammary tumor after treatment with cytoxan and vitamin A. Lab Invest 15: 987.

Brandes D, Sloan KW, Bloedorn F (1967). The effect of X-irradiation on lysosomes of mouse mammary gland carcinomas. Cancer Res 27: 731.

Cuthbertson DP (1930). The disturbance of metabolism produced by bony and non-bony injury with notes on certain abnormal conditions of bone. Biochem J 24: 1244.

Dorogokuplya AG, Troitskaya EG, Adilgireeva LK, Postolnikov SF, Chekrygina ZP (1973). Effect of carotene on the development of induced tumors. Zdavooknr Kaz 10: 32.

Fisher B, Gebhardt MC, Saffer EA (1978). Further observations on the inhibition of tumor growth by corynerbacterium parvum with cyclophosphamide. VIII. Effect of tumor radiation prior to therapy. Internat J Rad Oncol Biol Phys 4: 975.

Freiman M, Seifter E, Connerton C, Levenson SM (1970). Vitamin A deficiency and surgical stress. Surg Forum 21: 81.

Rettura G, Barbul A, Levenson SM, Seifter E (1978). Tumor excision and vitamin A supplementation increase survival of mice with C3H breast adenocarcinoma. Surg Forum 29: 170.

Rettura G, Schittek A, Hardy M, Levenson SM, Demetriou A, Seifter E (1975). Brief communication: Anti-tumor action of vitamin A in mice inoculated with adenocarcinoma cells. J Natl Cancer Inst 54: 1489.

Rettura G, Levenson SM, Seifter E (1982b). Improvement of cyclophosphamide therapeutic activity by supplemental vitamin A (VA) or beta carotene (BC). Proc 13th Internat Cancer Congr, Sept 8-15, Seattle WA. Abstr no 181.

Rettura G, Stratford F, Levenson SM, Seifter E (1982a). Prophylactic and therapeutic actions of supplemental beta carotene in mice inoculated with C3HBA adenocarcinoma cells; lack of therapeutic action of supplemental ascorbic acid. J Natl Cancer Inst 69: 73.

Rettura G, Wolfe ES, Seifter E (1980). Inhibition of WB10232 breast cancer growth by supplemental vitamin A. Fed Proc 39: 1117.

Seifter E, Crowley L, Rettura G, Nakao K, Gruber C, Kan D, Levenson SM (1975). Influence of vitamin A on wound healing in rats with femoral fracture. Ann Surg 181: 836.

Seifter E, Rettura G, Levenson SM (1981a). Decreased resistance of C3H/HeHa mice to C3HBA tumor transplants: increased resistance due to supplemental vitamin A. J Natl Cancer Inst 67: 467.

Seifter E, Rettura G, Levenson SM (1982a). β-Carotene and vitamin A palmitate protect against 7,12-dimethylbenz-(α)-anthracene (DMBA) carcinogenesis. First Conference on Radioprotectors α Anticarcinogens, June 21-24, Gaithersburg MD. Abstr no 8.

Seifter E, Rettura G, Padawer J, Levenson SM (1982b). Moloney sarcoma virus tumors in CBA/J mice: Chemopreventive and chemotherapeutic action of supplemental β-carotene. J Natl Cancer Inst 68: 835.

Seifter E, Rettura G, Padawer J, Stratford F, Goodwin P, Levenson SM (1982c). Supplemental vitamin A and β-carotene reduce morbidity and mortality in mice subjected to partial or whole body irradiation. First Conf Radioprotectors Anticarcinogens, June 21-24, Gaithersburg, MD, Abstr no 44.

Seifter E, Rettura G, Padawer J, Stratford F, Kambosos D, Levenson SM (1981b). Impaired wound healing in streptozotocin diabetes: Prevention by supplemental vitamin A. Ann Surg 194: 42.

Seifter E, Rettura G, Stratford F, Yee C, Weinzweig J, Jacobson NL, Levenson SM (1981). Vitamin A inhibits some aspects of systemic disease due to local X-radiation. J Parent Enter Nutr 5: 288.

Selye H (1936). Thymus and adrenals in the response of the organism to injuries and intoxications. Br J Exp Pathol 17: 234.

Shen RN, Mendecki J, Rettura G, Seifter E (1983). Partial prevention of radiation toxicity by supplemental vitamin A (VA) and β-carotene (BC). Fed Proc (in press).

Stratford F, Seifter E, Rettura G, Levenson SM (1980). Impaired wound healing due to cyclophosphamide: Alleviation by supplemental vitamin A. Surg Forum 31: 224.

Tannock IF, Suit HD, Marshall N (1972). Vitamin A and the radiation response of experimental tumors: An immune-mediated effect. J Natl Cancer Inst 48: 731.

Zaravinos T, Vogl S, Rettura G, Seifter E (1980). Intermittent combined radiation (RT) and chemotherapy (CT) in a murine mammary cancer. Suboptimal RT plus CT improves local tumor control with acceptable toxicity. 16th Ann Mtng Amer Soc Clin Oncol, San Diego, CA, May 26-27.

Progress in Cancer Control IV: Research in the Cancer Center, pages 249–259

A METHOD FOR ESTIMATING THE POTENTIAL EFFECTS OF PRIMARY AND SECONDARY PREVENTION ACTIVITIES IN HIGH RISK POPULATIONS

John P. Enterline, M.S.[1,2], Ellen B. Gold, Ph.D.[2]

The Johns Hopkins University Oncology Center[1] and Department of Epidemiology[2], Baltimore, MD 21205

INTRODUCTION

In recent years there has been increased interest in developing quantitative approaches for planning and evaluating cancer control activities for both community-based and national populations. Specifically, in an era of restricted resources, health planners and others wish to know which intervention activities can be expected to be most effective in meeting the needs of defined populations. In the present paper an approach is presented which can assist in quantifying the potential efficacy which might be expected for specific cancer control activities in defined populations. The approach is presented using the example of black–white differences in overall cancer mortality, incidence and survival. The basis of this approach is the examination of differences in cancer mortality between populations, with an emphasis on estimating the effects that specific primary and secondary prevention activities might be expected to produce in reducing a mortality differential between a population of interest and an appropriate comparison population. This is accomplished by a partitioning of the mortality differential into three components: (1) that portion amenable to primary prevention, (2) that portion amenable to secondary prevention and (3) that portion which is more difficult to control due to multifactorial causes. Such a quantified approach to determining the potential for specific cancer control activities can assist health planners at both the national and local levels in designing programs which have the most probable opportunity for success. The approach presented here is not a pure mathematical model in the strict sense of the term; however, for the purpose of simplicity it will be referred to in this paper as a "model".

METHODS

The model is based on the assertion that mortality rates in a population can be viewed as a function of two factors, the incidence and survival rates in that population. When an individual dies from a chronic disease, the disease usually is present for some time prior to death. The time interval from the occurrence of a disease to death from that disease is referred to as the survival time. This relationship of incidence and survival to mortality can be generalized to a population as long as secular trends in survival remain relatively constant and, thus, the relationship between incidence and mortality are fairly stable over time. With the exception of a few types of cancer, (e.g., acute lymphocytic leukemia, Hodgkin's lymphoma) such a generalized approach should be appropriate.

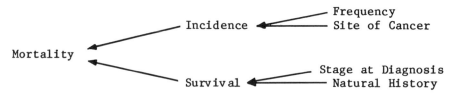

The effects of incidence and survival on the cancer death rates in a population can be further divided into two categories each. The effect that incidence has on mortality can be viewed as being composed of the absolute frequency of the occurrence of cancer and the distribution of occurrence of the different types of cancer. For example, if a population has a higher than average incidence rate of cancer but has an average distribution of cancer sites, that population will have a higher than average mortality rate. Also, if a population has an average incidence rate of cancer but a greater than average proportion of cancers with a poor prognosis (e.g., lung cancer) this will also lead to a greater than average mortality rate.

The effect that survival has on mortality rates in a population can be divided into that portion of survival which is due to the stage of disease at diagnosis, and that portion that is due to the survival within stage (i.e., survival due to factors other than stage at diagnosis). In general, the earlier stage at which a cancer is detected, the better the prognosis. However, even for persons detected at the early stages of cancers with relatively better prognoses (e.g., breast cancer), survival rates are lower than in a general population (Axtell, 1976).

The basic tenets of the above approach can be used to quantify factors responsible for differences in cancer mortality between two populations in terms of differences in (1) the incidence of cancer, (2) the distribution of the types of cancer that are occurring, (3) the distribution of the stages at which cancer is detected and (4) survival within stage. Such partitioning of factors can be helpful in plannning and evaluating population-based cancer control activities from a quantitative perspective.

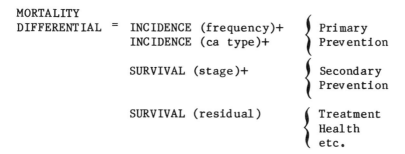

```
MORTALITY
DIFFERENTIAL  =  INCIDENCE (frequency)+     ⎧ Primary
                 INCIDENCE (ca type)+       ⎨ Prevention
                                            ⎩

                 SURVIVAL (stage)+          ⎧ Secondary
                                            ⎨ Prevention
                                            ⎩

                 SURVIVAL (residual)        ⎧ Treatment
                                            ⎨ Health
                                            ⎩ etc.
```

If a population is at a particularly high risk of dying from cancer, planners should first determine which cancer control activities might be most effective in that particular population, integrating into the overall health plan both available resources and available effective methods for primary and secondary prevention. The component of the mortality differential which is theoretically amenable to primary prevention activities is the portion due to differences in incidence rates controlling for, or within, specific cancer sites. The component of the mortality differential theoretically amenable to secondary prevention is the survival difference resulting from differences in stage of disease at diagnosis between populations. The remaining within-stage survival component of mortality differentials could result from a variety of factors including differences in overall health, nutrition, treatment, access to health care, immune systems, genetics, etc. This is an extremely difficult component of cancer mortality to control, given the intervention techniques which are currently available. However, this may be one of the most interesting areas of study from the sociologic, epidemiologic and basic science perspectives.

An example of the application of the model is presented using age-adjusted mortality, incidence and relative survival rates for cancer in blacks and whites from the Surveillance, Epidemiology, and End Results (SEER) Program of the National Cancer Institute (Axtell, 1976, Young 1978). The effects of differences between these populations in age distributions and in mortality from other causes have been minimized by using adjusted rates.   The SEER cancer registration system covers approximately ten percent of the U.S. population.   In this application of the model it has been assumed that (1) mortality, incidence and survival data are complete and accurate and (2) staging of disease is accurate.   However, the minimal assumption of the model is that the biases or inaccuracies of these elements are similar between the populations under study and consistent over time.   It should be noted that the model is best suited to a cancer-site-specific examination of mortality differentials. While it is beyond the scope of this paper to go through the calculations of a site-specific application of the model, selected results of such an application are presented.

APPLICATION OF MODEL

Notable differences in cancer mortality rates have been reported for the black and white populations in the United States (White, Enterline, 1980).   In Table 1, both age-adjusted mortality and incidence rates are presented as black-

Table 1.   BLACK-WHITE AGE-ADJUSTED RELATIVE RISKS OF MORTALITY AND INCIDENCE*: SEER PROGRAM, 1973-1976

Black/White Relative Risk for:

$$\text{MORTALITY} : \quad \frac{215.3}{165.6} = 1.30$$

$$\text{INCIDENCE} : \quad \frac{347.3}{318.9} = 1.09$$

---

*Rates per 100,000 population adjusted to the 1970 U.S. population (Young, 1978)

to-white relative risks. The black population of the SEER program has age-adjusted risks of cancer mortality and incidence of 1.30 and 1.09, respectively, relative to the white population. This translates into a 30% excess risk of mortality and a 9% excess risk of occurrence of cancer among blacks relative to whites. If the excess risks for both mortality and incidence were similar, other factors (i.e, distribution of types of cancer, stage of disease, survival within stage) would not be thought to account for the mortality differential. However, the data provided below (1.1) indicate that the majority (70%) of the total cancer mortality differential is not due to the difference in the incidence of cancer but to the other components. The first line of data provides the differential calculations and the second line of data provides the components of mortality differentials when the total mortality differential is viewed as the whole or 100% (i.e., 9% ÷ 30% = .3 or 30% of the whole).

(1.1)

MORTALITY DIFFERENCE	=	INCIDENCE DIFFERENCE	+	CA TYPE & DIFFERENCE	SURVIVAL DIFFERENCE
30%	=	9%	+	(30%	− 9%)
100%	=	30%	+	70%	

To understand the portion that survival differences between blacks and whites contribute to the mortality differential, the relative risk of the incidence can be directly adjusted for differences in distributions of cancer sites between whites and blacks (1.2). When such an adjustment is made to the incidence differential, the differences in both the incidence and the types of cancers that occur in blacks compared to whites are found to account for 19.5% of the 30% total mortality differential, or setting the total mortality differential at 100%, 65% is due to differences in the incidence and distribution of cancer sites. The remaining 35% of the difference in mortality is due to differences in survival.

(1.2)

MORTALITY DIFFERENCE =	SITE ADJUSTED INCIDENCE DIFFERENCE	+	SURVIVAL DIFFERENCE
30% =	19.5%	+	(30% − 19.5%)
100% =	65%	+	35%

From the two above partitions (1.1 and 1.2) of the data, the following partition (1.3) can be derived by subtraction.

(1.3)

MORTALITY DIFFERENCE	=	INCIDENCE DIFFERENCE	+	CA SITE DIFFERENCE	+	SURVIVAL DIFFERENCE
30%	=	9%	+	10.5%	+	10.5%
100%	=	30%	+	35%	+	35%

Thus, the difference in incidence accounts for 30% of the mortality difference (i.e., blacks have a greater risk of occurrence of cancer) and differences in the distribution of the types of cancers accounts for 35% of the mortality difference (i.e., blacks are at a greater risk of having the types of cancer that have a poor prognosis).

The remaining 35% of the mortality differential, which is due to black-white survival differences (i.e., blacks survive for shorter periods of time than whites), has two components: (1) survival differences resulting from differences in stage of disease at diagnosis and (2) survival differences due to factors other than differences in stage.

Table 2.   RACIAL DIFFERENCES IN FIVE-YEAR RELATIVE SURVIVAL RATES FOR ALL CANCERS BY STAGE: BIOMETRY BRANCH, NCI, 1965-1969

RACE	ALL STAGES	LOCALIZED	REGIONAL	DISTANT
White	39%	68%	38%	10%
Black	30%	62%	32%	8%
Difference	9%	6%	6%	2%

In Table 2 five-year relative survival rates are presented by race and stage of disease (SEER). The difference in survival for all stages between blacks and whites was 9%, but the survival difference within stage ranged from 2% to 6%.

Two facts thus emerge: (1) within each stage of disease, blacks have a poorer survival than do whites, and (2) for the "all stages" differential to be greater than any of the "within stage" differentials, the distribution of the stage of cancer among blacks must be such that blacks have a greater proportion of cancer cases in later (e.g., more "distant") stage categories than whites.

The specific contributions of differences in distributions by stage and within-stage survival to the survival component of the cancer mortality differential between blacks and whites can be examined by adjusting overall black survival rates to the distribution by stage in the white population. When such an adjustment is made (1.4), the five-year relative survival rate among blacks improves from 30.0% to 34.5% for all stages, an absolute improvement of 4.5%, (i.e., differences in stage at diagnosis account for one-half of the total 9% difference in survival). Thus, differences in distribution of cancer cases by stage at diagnosis account for 50% of the total survival difference (1.3) between blacks and whites (i.e., .5 x 35% = 17.5%), and

(1.4)

SURVIVAL DIFFERENTIAL	=	DUE TO STAGE AT DIAGNOSIS	+	DUE TO OTHER FACTORS
[39% - 30%]	=	[34.5% - 30.0%]	+	[39.0% - 34.5%]
9%	=	4.5%	+	4.5%
100%	=	50%	+	50%

differences within-stage survival account for the remaining 50% (i.e., .5 x 35% = 17.5%). It should noted that this portion of the model is based on the assumption that blacks and whites have cancers with comparable prognoses. In fact, as was shown earlier, the types of cancers occurring among blacks have a poorer prognosis than those that occur among whites. If the survival differences were not only adjusted for differences in distribution by stage but also for differences in distribution by cancer site, it is probable that a greater proportion of the survival differential would be due to within-stage survival differences rather than differences in distribution by stage. However, this adjustment would not be likely to exert a large effect on the results of the present application, and if the model were applied on a site-specific basis, the adjustment for differences in distribution by site would not be necessary.

When all partitioned components of the mortality differential are entered into the model (1.5), the following observations are made concerning the differences in cancer mortality in blacks relative to whites: (1) 30.0% of the mortality differential is due to the higher incidence of cancers occurring among blacks; (2) 35.0% of the mortality differential is due to the greater proportion of more aggressive types of cancer among blacks; (3) 17.5% is due to the later stage of disease at diagnosis among blacks; and (4) 17.5% of the differential is due to poorer survival within stage among blacks.

(1.5)

MORTALITY DIFF.	=	INCIDENCE DIFF.	+	CANCER TYPE DIFF.	+	SURVIVAL DIFF. DUE TO STAGE AT D_x	+	WITHIN STAGE SURV. DIFF.
30.0%	=	9.0%	+	10.5%	+	5.25%	+	5.25%
100.0%	=	30.0%	+	35.0%	+	17.5%	+	17.5%

PRIMARY PREVENTION   SECONDARY PREVENTION   HEALTH R_x Etc.

Thus, 65.0% of the differential in cancer mortality between whites and blacks is theoretically amenable to primary prevention activities, 17.5% is theoretically amenable to secondary prevention activities and 17.5% will require other, more difficult, activities to control.

The theoretical effect of the above values in reducing cancer mortality rates among black Americans is presented in Table 3. In 1978, there were 44,953 deaths from cancer among rblacks in the United States (NCHS). When age-specific cancer mortality rates for the white population in 1978 were multiplied by the age-specific numbers of blacks in the U.S. population for that year, the expected number of cancer deaths was found to be 37,972. Thus, an excess of 6,981 (16%) cancer deaths occurred among blacks, using white age-specific rates as a standard. This excess occurrence of death is markedly less than the 30% excess risk for cancer mortality noted in the model, due to the younger age distribution among blacks compared to whites.

Table 3. THEORETICAL* EFFECT OF PRIMARY AND SECONDARY PREVENTION IN REDUCING CANCER MORTALITY AMONG BLACK AMERICANS: 1978

Total Cancer Deaths Among Blacks.......	44,953	(100%)
Excess Cancer Deaths Among Blacks Relative to Whites	6,981	(16%)
Theoretical Reduction in Deaths Among Blacks Through Primary Prevention	4,537	(10%)
Theoretical Reduction in Deaths Among Blacks Through Secondary Prevention	1,222	(3%)
Excess Deaths Not Affected Through Either Primary or Secondary Prevention	1,222	(3%)

*Is not totally feasible given available cancer prevention techniques and knowledge

Applying the findings from the application of the model concerning black-white differences in cancer mortality to this excess number of deaths, primary and secondary prevention activities theoretically could annually prevent 4,537 and 1,222 deaths, respectively. An additional 1,222 of the excess deaths theoretically were due to racial differences in the within-stage survival rates. It should be noted that to have been effective in reducing death rates in 1978, primary prevention activities would have had to take place probably starting in the early 1950s, due to the long latency period for most cancers. Thus, these findings provide no direct indication of the current exposures affecting risks in the population unless black-white differences in exposures have remained constant over time. The reduction in deaths through secondary prevention activities provides a better estimate of what effect preventive activities instituted in the population today could be expected to produce.

One problem in these theoretical estimates is that, for many types of cancers, no well-defined cause or method of effectively detecting and treating the cancer at an early stage is known. Thus, the model is logically best applied on a site-specific basis for those cancers which have potential for primary and/or secondary prevention. Such an application was made on four cancer sites (Table 4).

Table 4. PERCENT REDUCTION OF EXCESS CANCER DEATHS* AMONG BLACKS FOR SELECTED SITES WITH VIABLE** PRIMARY AND SECONDARY PREVENTIVE MEASURES: 1978

CANCER SITE	PRIMARY PREVENTION	SECONDARY PREVENTION
Lung	9%	--
Breast	--	11%
Cervix	--	18%
Colon	--	7%

*Using U.S. white rates as a standard
**Dashes (—) represent no known effective primary or secondary prevention

For lung cancer, primary prevention could theoretically reduce mortality rates among blacks by 9%. For breast, cervix, and colon cancers, secondary prevention could theoretically reduce mortality rates by 11%, 18%, and 7%, respectively. These estimates assume that in lung cancer the excess incidence is due to a preventable cause, or that in the other sites presented, the tumors have the same aggressiveness and potentially could be diagnosed at the same stage in blacks and whites, given a comparable periodicity of screening and/or recognition of warning signs.

SUMMARY

There is an increasing need to plan and assess cancer control programs based on quantitative data. In this paper a model is presented to help planners design cancer control programs to meet the needs of defined high-risk populations. This model can be applied to demographically defined segments of the U.S. population, to geographically defined populations, and to demographic subpopulations within geographically defined areas. It is intended to allow planners to assess the cancer control needs of high risk populations in terms of lowering cancer risks using available primary and secondary prevention techniques. This model represents only one of many quantitative factors that should be integrated into planning cancer control activities.

REFERENCES

Axtell LM, Asire AJ, Myers MH (eds) (1976). " Cancer Patient Survival: Report Number Five." U.S. Department of Health, Education and Welfare, DHEW No. (NIH) 77-992.
National Center for Health Statistics (NCHS). Unpublished data.
Surveillance, Epidemiology, and End Results Program (SEER). Unpublished data.
White JE, Enterline JP (1980). Cancer in Nonwhite Americans. Current Problems in Cancer, 4(9) 6-34.
Young JL, Asire AJ, Pollack ES (eds) (1978). "SEER Program: Cancer Incidence and Mortality in the United States -- 1973-1976." U.S. Department of Health, Education and Welfare, DHEW No. (NIH) 78-1837.

(This paper was supported in part by NIH Grant #CA-06973. The authors gratefully acknowledge the assistance of Rae Kopher in the preparation of this manuscript.

Progress in Cancer Control IV: Research in the Cancer Center, pages 261–270
© 1983 Alan R. Liss, Inc., 150 Fifth Avenue, New York, NY 10011

OHIO'S MORTALITY-BASED SYSTEM FOR IDENTIFICATION OF CANCER
INTERVENTION PROGRAM SITES

William S. Donaldson, Ed.D.

Comprehensive Cancer Center
Ohio State University
Columbus, Ohio 43210

INTRODUCTION

For this discussion Cancer Control is defined as consisting of two major early-detection elements: 1) the
potential for correct diagnosis of a patient with the disease,
and 2) the potential for insuring that this patient is
presented to a physician in a timely manner (Stage 1 or 2).
It is not necessary that a widely-accepted definition of
Cancer Control precede planning of intervention strategies
of the type being discussed.

Ohio's procedure for identification of geographic sites
and subsequent development of Cancer Intervention Program
Designs (CIPD) is predicated on the maxim that patient education, proper attitudes toward site-specific screening and the
need to seek prompt medical attention--if so counseled,
awareness of early-warning signals, signs and symptoms, all
contribute to the potential for timely patient presentation.
The intent is to optimize impact of existing medical expertise
and technology. Intervention programming does not include
professional education at this time.

It has been Ohio's experience that, varying from county
to county, there are numerous geographic sites (counties)
within the state which have "cancer problems" far greater
than do other counties, and these target areas should be
responsive to development and implementation of cost-
effective, productive CIPDs. Recognizing known limitations
of cancer mortality data, particularly those clarified by
Percy, Stanek and Gloeckler (1981), it is worthwhile to use

cancer mortality data for identification purposes. The
advantages far outweigh the limitations.

Several factors must be considered if a proposed intervention program is to be effective and contribute significantly
to the reduction of incidence, morbidity and mortality due to
the disease: (1) geo-political boundaries which circumscribe
manageable areas; (2) local personalities which must be
involved to insure a successful program design and its implementation; (3) local resources which should be drawn into the
program and how these resources should be acquired without
reliance on funds from outside the area. Specifically, the
intent of the CIPD approach to be described is to minimize
dependence upon federal funding and to maximize use of local
expertise, energy and financial resources to prioritize,
design, implement, and evaluate local-level cancer intervention programming. CIPD development is depicted in Figure 1.

Local level is defined as the county level of
administration in Ohio. Counties were selected as target
units for these programs because Ohio's cancer mortality
data is readily aggregated in terms of county-of-residence.
And, it is believed that people residing within counties, at
least within counties defined as being rural, are readily
involved as volunteers, that they have knowledge of population
segments within their area which might escape definition if a
larger administrative area was chosen, that in many instances
these same volunteers are the people who have direct access
to local financial and other resources that could not be
captured by people from outside the immediate area, and that
they—the volunteers—rapidly acquire an "ownership" of the
intervention program that cannot be duplicated by outside
personalities.

Two major uses of county-level data have been made
possible by development of the Cancer Mortality Reporting
System, designed under the aegis of the Cancer Control
Consortium of Ohio (CCCO) and the Ohio State University
Comprehensive Cancer Center (OSUCCC). Although easily
separated into two categories, they are interrelated and have
obvious implications for CIPD development:

(1) Cancer Control activities defined as procedures
leading to direct screening of at-high-risk patients
within an area known to be above average mortality
with respect to a certain cancer site; and

Cancer Control — Cancer Intervention Program Design (CIPD)

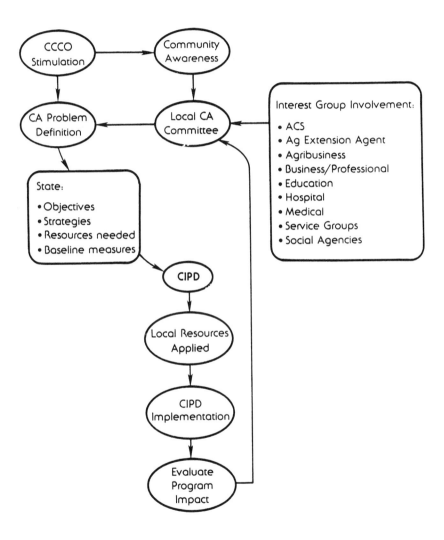

Figure 1. A Procedure for CIPD Development

(2) Epidemiological studies which investigate the cause(s) why this particular area is exceptionally high in mortality.

The first activity addresses the problem and the second assesses the cause of the problem.

There are at least six major factors to consider in determination of where a cancer intervention program should be initiated: selection of geographic site; determination of the extent of community interest, the possibility for increasing that interest, and for capitalizing on any health prevention/risk reduction programs in the area; prioritization of cancer sites to be addressed; identification of appropriate target age-groups; total mortality count for this cancer site; rank-in-state and rate. These six factors should be used to evaluate the relative importance of potential CIPDs.

The problem is both interesting and difficult. How does one best infiltrate the local setting with CIPD strategies which will reduce incidence, morbidity and mortality due to cancer? What must be done to develop local initiative/ownership to attract resources (people, dollars, facilities, etc.) vital to the success of the CIPD procedure? Moreover, it is important to forget the notion of "comparison," and to focus all available resources on intervention program planning to resolve priority needs within the defined geographic area. In short, the intent is to apply locally-available resources where they will produce the most good, relying on the principle of participatory management to create leadership to sustain the effort within the larger framework of the Consortium (Mintzberg, 1979).

OHIO'S CCCO NETWORK

During the interval 1979-1983, OSUCCC developed a statewide network of cancer control professionals and laypersons interested in applying their collective talents toward the goal of reducing incidence, morbidity and mortality in the state due to the disease. A small, central staff is housed at the university to coordinate ten Regional Councils, a Board of Trustees and an Executive Committee. Funds were not included in this contract for direct support of local-level planning and program activity, although two sub-contracts have served as prototypes for extending outreach strategies statewide.

The network established as the Consortium (88 counties grouped into 10 Regional Councils) will be extremely beneficial for establishing local-level Cancer Committees. We are now actively involved in CIPD development in one south-central county of Ohio, Highland; data used for orientation of the Cancer Committee at the Greenfield Area Medical Center will be described later in this paper.

Ohio State also has taken steps to use the same mortality data base for defining appropriate, feasible epidemiological studies to accompany the CIPD process. A Field Investigation Team with quality expertise will analyze these problems. A statewide cancer incidence reporting system now being planned will improve network members' capacity for self-analysis of local cancer problems, and will improve the Team's responsiveness to the information needs of local Cancer Committees.

THE LOCAL (COUNTY) CANCER COMMITTEE

OSUCCC has worked with the Greenfield Area Medical Center (GAMC) for approximately one year on matters directly related to Consortium goals. During this time we established strong ties with the Health Promotion/Risk Reduction Project (HP/RRP) at GAMC, an ongoing, federally-funded effort in Highland County (Daugherty, 1982). The CIPD process was used to develop a Cancer Committee at GAMC.

During this procedure, administrative strategies were incorporated to capitalize on the various types of volunteer expertise and resource connections possible in Highland County:

(1) Create ties with hospitals, local leaders and extant health education programs where possible;

(2) Identify population segments to be reached with the CIPD;

(3) Design penetration strategies appropriate to each population segment identified; and

(4) Secure planning information unique to the county, easily understood, showing minimal "comparison" displays, which motivates Cancer Committee personnel

to examine (much more closely than ever before) their own cancer problem(s).

The Cancer Committee has visibility within specific population segments of the study area, and provides unusual and unique insights into strategy development for reaching respective population segments. The role of the HP/RRP Director in this regard should not be underestimated. This person holds a position of great visibility in the area and is able to attract volunteer participation from many sources which would be unavailable by traditional study-area methods. It is clear that structuring a cancer committee at a different location should be preceded by identification of a person of similar stature in that area, the equivalent of the HP/RRP Director. This group was charged with full responsibility for CIPD development, the foundation of which was obtained from analysis of the Highland County Cancer Mortality Report.

CCCO'S CANCER MORTALITY REPORT (CMR)

Simultaneously with the emergence of the Highland County Cancer Committee, the Evaluation Coordinator of the parent Outreach Project at OSUCCC developed a county-specific Mortality Reporting System (MRS). Building on a previous system developed by the Evaluation Coordinator, the MRS uses disk-file information from the previous systems, combines it with population information from 1940, 1960, 1980, and two projections for the year 2000, to create a set of detailed, computer-printed reports (charts, tables, graphs) for the Cancer Committee. This report is divided into five sections, each of which has relevance to intervention program planning.

Summary data/ranks - three pages which describe local cancer problems in terms of 1970-1980 cancer mortality X cancer sites, including the number of deaths, crude rate, age-adjusted rate, rank in state, confidence limits, and coefficients of variation. Second, *population trends* - a series of displays showing variations across nine standard age-groups. A graph is presented showing how, within age-groups, populations are changing within the county across the sixty-year interval being reported. This section concludes with a table and graph to illustrate how "at-risk" and "not-at-risk" are changing through the years; these displays nurture an appreciation for what to expect in the year 2000.

Third, *at-risk ratios* - the Cancer Committee is asked to
consider a series of graphs which display mortality rates,
defined as total mortality divided by age-group population
(to provide standard values for comparison purposes). One
use of these graphs is to identify the age-group within the
county at which this particular cancer site becomes a problem
in terms of rapidly-accelerating mortality. The Committee
then can consider the latent period leading up to the mortality and can define an age-group for which a CIPD would be
appropriate. The graph for the site in question was prepared
using the population being considered (total, male, female).
When appropriate, this graph is followed by a second graph
called a "triple plot." Triple plots are appropriate where
cancer sites are not sex related; i.e., breast, prostate,
ovary, and uterus are sex-specific and do not offer triple-
plot opportunity.

Fourth, *contiguous-county display* - people being what
they are, we frequently are asked "How does my county compare
to other counties in the area?" Our response has been that
comparisons are not our main emphasis, but we have retreated
somewhat from this position and now provide a "Contiguous
County Profile" showing the base county and all counties
contiguous to it, across the number of cancer sites which are
appropriate to the population being studied (12 total population; 11 female population; 9 male population). These
profiles often do reveal gross differences among contiguous
counties.

Fifth, *attainable target death rate (ATDR)* - a table
which demonstrates to the Committee the reduction in mortality
that would be possible if the county could reach what is
termed attainable rate. After considerable study of Woolsey's
(1981) approach to definition of "Attainable Target Death
Rate," we have prepared this table modifying his approach
somewhat. Attainable rate here is defined as the lowest
non-zero crude rate observed in the State of Ohio over the
1970-1980 period, appropriate to the population being studied.
This information influences Committee decision-making and
warrants efforts toward more advanced methodology. The next
release of the CMR system will contain a sophisticated
approach toward definition of attainable target death rate.
OSUCCC makes this product available to any Ohio county
willing to convene a Cancer Committee and cooperate with CCCO
to initiate CIPDs.

THE GREENFIELD PROJECT AND CIPD DEVELOPMENT

Highland County demographics are not appreciably different from other rural, agribusiness counties in the state.
Prevailing health problems are related to life-styles and
chronic disease, thus indicating a low level of awareness and
practice of health promotive life-styles. These problems
highlight concerns about the future of health care in rural
areas. Accessibility to family physicians and the incidence
of chronic disease are both critical concerns.

To improve this situation Greenfield Area Medical Center
developed a program to promote healthful life-styles and the
use of prevention services: the Health Promotion Center
(HPC). Under this sponsorship, programs are conducted in
patient and consumer education utilizing the Health Belief
Model (Green, et al., 1980), focusing on wellness, early
detection and screening programs. The "Life-Time Health
Monitoring Program" (Breslow and Somers, 1977) is utilized
toward these ends. The "Health Hazards Appraisal" (Colburn,
1973) is administered to all patients at GAMC.

Community education is designed to emphasize four types
of programs: nutrition education; improvement in fitness
levels; stress management; and, reduction of abusive behavior.
In addition, education regarding the appropriate use of health
services is integrated into this component.

It is believed that attention paid to improving health
status will lower health care cost by emphasizing health-
promotive life-styles. The project was designated in 1979
by the Office of the Assistant Secretary of Health (DHEW) as
one of 18 nationally significant demonstration programs in
health promotion. The setting for this health promotion
project was well chosen. Highland County has extremely high
rates on five major cancer sites.

In this context, development of the Highland County CIPD
was predicated on information related to six fundamental considerations: number of mortalities per cancer site; above-
average rates; effective screening technique availability;
identifiable populations; known latency periods; and
identifiable age-groups for screening. These considerations
must be evaluated when attempting CIPD's at the county level,
for lack of an effective screening procedure precludes

attempts to construct a CIPD for, say, ovarian cancer. In addition, Highland County offers abundant opportunity for epidemiological study.

Extensive studies are planned to isolate cancer mortality within specific locations, and to extend the procedure into two of the contiguous counties, Fayette and Ross, by convening Cancer Committees in those counties to perform CIPD functions. There are major health-education/early-detection activities which--if well structured and housed within strategies appropriate to particular population segments--have great potential for reducing cancer mortality not only in Highland County but in any Ohio county willing to make the necessary commitment.

IN THE FUTURE

Highland County offered an unprecedented opportunity to test CIPD potential. Within four to six months, intervention programs will be developed and implemented as appropriate to particular segments of the Highland County population. Since Fayette and Ross Counties have no recognized counterpart to the Health Promotion Center in Greenfield, and since these people have not been involved until recently in discussions with the Cancer Committee in Greenfield, it will take somewhat longer to get CIPDs implemented in the two counties contiguous to Highland. Nevertheless, within six to eight months programs will be underway in those counties.

The need for immediate financial resources can be minimized through this procedure. Business and social service agencies can be asked to contribute needed funds with a high expectation that they will respond positively. It is not difficult to secure the participation of leaders who can "get things done," and who are willing to be identified with CIPD efforts.

What about transferring the Greenfield experience to other counties across the state? Our preliminary investigation of cancer mortality data revealed numerous instances where cancer problems are acute. A recent survey conducted among people on the Consortium's mailing list revealed that *very few respondents identified any cancer problems in their home counties*. Either respondents to this survey did not think they had any special problem or they do not recognize

cancer problems as and where they exist (Donaldson, 1982).
In coming months the CIPD procedure will be transferred to
at least four or five other counties in Ohio. These counties
will be identified by staff assessment of Cancer Mortality
Reports generated for these counties; those with the most
significant problems will be contacted first. Both CIPD
procedure and the Cancer Mortality Report system could be
transferred to sites outside Ohio.

CIPD development hinges (to no small extent) on
impressing local residents with the reduction in deaths that
is possible, given the willingness of volunteers and the
cooperation of their targets (response). In this regard, it is
imperative that we provide them with optimum ATDR computations
and that we add sophistication to the system used to generate
these values as rapidly as possible. Changing residents'
attitudes is easier to effect when positive results are
perceived.

REFERENCES

Breslow L, Somers AR (1977). The life-time health-monitoring
     program. NEJM 296:601-608.
Colburn HN (1973). Health hazards appraisal--a possible tool
     in health protection and promotion. Canadian J of Public
     Health 64:490.
Daugherty S (1982). Greenfield, OH community health promo-
     tion program. Greenfield Area Medical Center (Project
     Summary).
Donaldson W (1982). Evaluation report: CCCO's linking
     objective. Columbus: OSUCCC.
Green LW, Kreuter MW, Deeds SG, Partridge KB (1980). "Health
     Education Planning." Palo Alto, CA: Mayfield Publishing
     Co., pp. 72-74.
Mintzberg H (1979). "The Structuring of Organizations."
     Englewood Cliffs, NJ: Prentice-Hall, pp. 148-215.
Percy C, Stanek E, Gloeckler L (1981). Accuracy of cancer
     death certificates and its effect on cancer mortality
     statistics. AJPH 71:242-250.
Woolsey TD (May 1981). Toward an index of preventable
     mortality. Vital and Health Statistics. DHHS, Series 2-
     Number 85.

Progress in Cancer Control IV: Research in the Cancer Center, pages 271–281
© 1983 Alan R. Liss, Inc., 150 Fifth Avenue, New York, NY 10011

SOME ISSUES CONCERNING COMMUNITY BASED
CHRONIC DISEASE CONTROL PROGRAMS

Emil Berkanovic, Barry Gerber,
Helene Brown and Lester Breslow

School of Public Health
University of California, Los Angeles
Los Angeles, California 90024

Community Cancer Control/Los Angeles (CCC/LA) recently
completed a contract as one of six Community Based Cancer
Control Programs (CBCCP's) funded by the National Cancer
Institute (NCI) for the purpose of demonstrating the impact
of coordination on cancer control in the community. The
cost of the CCC/LA program over the five year lifespan of
this demonstration project was approximately $5.6 million.
A nearly equal amount was contributed locally in the form of
"in kind" services and funds. These funds were expended on
a wide range of programs aimed at the prevention, detection,
pre-treatment evaluation, diagnosis, treatment,
rehabilitation and continuing care phases of breast cancer,
cervical cancer and lung cancer. Each of these programs has
been evaluated and the results have been reported to the NCI
(Berkanovic, Gerber and Wright, 1982). The purpose of this
paper is to discuss several issues concerning community
based chronic disease control programs that have emerged
from the experience gained in conducting CCC/LA.

The CBCCP's, along with several other community based health
demonstration projects, have built a base of knowledge for
planning such programs. Out of this experience, seven
issues have been identified for consideration in planning
the next cycle of community based demonstrations. Examining
these issues may contribute to improving the effectiveness
and efficiency of future programs. The issues discussed
herein include 1) use of media; 2) amount of intervention

required to be effective; 3) lead time required to establish
programs; 4) length of time required to impact problems
effectively; 5) cumulative effects of similar programs; 6)
impact of eligibility criteria on programs; and 7) limits of
past experience in planning future programs. After
addressing these issues, the discussion examines possible
structures and processes for future community based
programming. The paper concludes by exploring the need for
a future round of community based programming.

ISSUES FOR CONSIDERATION IN THE NEXT ROUND OF COMMUNITY BASED CHRONIC DISEASE PROGRAMS

1. Use of Media

The media played a complex role in CCC/LA's programs. One
finding from the study of these programs which supports
those of other media oriented programs is that the media
activities required to recruit people to educational or
screening programs are different from those required to help
individuals change specific behaviors (Kar, 1975). It is
also clear that the media affect different groups in the
community differently and vary in their impact depending on
the context within which they are operating. For example,
both the mix and the intensity of media activity required to
persuade people to attend an educational program will vary
depending on the extent to which the sponsor of the program
is already viewed as credible by those being persuaded
(Zimbaro and Ebbesen, 1970). Further, the amount and
content of media activities required to persuade a
population will vary depending on what other persuasive
activities are occuring at the same time. For example, a
media campaign coupled with personal contacts through
community outreach will differ in both amount and content
from a media campaign alone (Weiss, 1969; Rogers, 1973;
Pool, 1973).

Five steps are necessary to persuade someone to take action.
First, an individual's attention must be obtained. Second,
he must understand the persuasive message. Third, he must
believe that the message is true. Fourth, he must be
motivated to do as the message asks. Fifth, he must develop
behavioral skills necessary to the action desired (McGuire,
1969). The achievement of each of these steps requires

different media activities. For example, because community baseline data collected by CCC/LA indicated that a large number of smokers already believed that they should quit, CCC/LA helped organize a television series on how to quit. The programs in this series were quite different in content from those aimed at motivating people to want to quit.

Future community based demonstrations should test those media activities that appear from prior experience to be most promising with respect to the step in the persuasion process at which they are aimed. Such tests will provide considerable information on how to use the media efficiently.

2. The Amount of Intervention Required to be Effective

A second issue concerns the amount of intervention required to accomplish certain objectives. For example, research indicates that smoking occurs as a developmental process that accelerates with each year during adolescence (Lanere, et al., 1972; HEW, 1979). Because several anti-smoking interventions have achieved varying levels of success for varying periods of time, a test of alternative strategies, for reducing the number of individuals who become smokers throughout the teen years would now be most appropriate. By testing these strategies, it would be possible to determine the levels of reinforcement and, therefore, the costs required to prevent smoking among various subgroups of adolescents.

A comparison of two of CCC/LA's smoking cessation programs illustrates the importance of this issue to program costs. Although the percentage of smokers who remained quit for 6 months was greater in a face to face program than in a televised program, the cost per smoker who quit was substantially (100 times) less for the televised program. Future community based programs could examine, therefore, both the percentage of smokers by type who are likely to respond to the less costly media approaches and the optimum media activity levels for maximizing cessation.

Similar questions arise with respect to any efforts to teach new behaviors. For example, although the CCC/LA evaluation ascertained the percentage of women trained in breast self examination (BSE) who were still doing BSE one year after

training, the program was not designed to test either the
amount of programmatic effort required to achieve that
percentage or the amount of additional effort required to
increase it. Because there now exist a variety of
techniques for recruiting and training people in a wide
range of health behaviors, the next cycle of community based
demonstrations could attempt to sort out not only which are
the most effective, but which are the most efficient. For
example, as noted above, persuasive campaigns can be done
through the media alone or through combined media-community
outreach programs. It remains to be determined, however,
what the most efficient combinations of media and outreach
are in specific subgroups and in relation to specific
activities about which persuasion is attempted. Because per
contact costs are generally lower for media than for
outreach activities, such studies would have important
implications for the costs of community programs.

3. Lead Time Required to Establish Programs

Programs in the community take time to become established.
Hence, there is likely to be a lag between completion of
plans and the full development of the administrative
structure needed to implement those plans. Time is also
needed to establish the credibility of new programs in the
community. Pre-implementation planning for CCC/LA's Breast
Examination Training Centers required one and one half
years. Detailed operational plans for each of the Centers
could not be developed until pre-implementation plans had
been completed, approved locally and by NCI, and the money
to operate the Centers was guaranteed. Without that
guarantee, most administrators were unwilling to expend the
resources required to do operational planning. For some
Centers, a year was required to complete such operational
plans. In addition, at least another year passed after
these centers opened before they reached relatively high
levels of operation. Soon after these levels were reached,
the scheduled wind-down of the contracts supporting the
Centers began. As a consequence, these programs were
actually fully implemented for considerably less time than
had been originally planned.

It is, therefore, worthwhile to consider the lead time
required to establish programs of various types. Further,
the differences between startup costs and costs once these

programs are fully operational need to be examined. By
examining these issues, more informed decisions can be made
regarding both the length of time required to adequately
test the interventions involved and the level of activity at
which these programmatic costs can be justified.

4. The Length of Time Required to Impact Problems Effectively

Another issue is the period over which projects are
scheduled to run. That period should be appropriate to the
magnitude of the problem which a project is intended to
address. CCC/LA's school based anti-smoking program
illustrates this point. It is clear that becoming a smoker
is a developmental process that accelerates rapidly during
the high school years (Lanere, 1972; HEW, 1979). It is also
clear that the factors influencing a person to become a
smoker continue throughout that developmental process (HEW,
1979). Because of contractual limitations, CCC/LA's schools
program was planned for four years beginning in the fifth
grade. Although the evaluation found the program to be
successful during the period it was funded, a great deal
more could have been learned had the program been funded to
continue through the 12th grade.

Complex processes govern both the amount of money that is
allocated for any particular purpose and the length of time
for which that money is allocated. Nonetheless, more could
be accomplished with the limited funding that is available
for community based programs if it were possible to spend
that money with greater flexibility. In the school anti-
smoking program, the students exposed to the program would
have been better served and the knowledge gained about such
programs would be greater it had continued throughout the
period during which these students were at the highest risk
of becoming smokers. By adjusting other programs within
CCC/LA's contract, this program could have been funded for
an appropriate length of time within the constraints of
available funds.

5. Cumulative Effects

Another issue concerns the cumulative effect of programs.
Even when the evaluation suggests that a particular program
had limited specific impact, there may be a reason to

continue to support its activities. For example, health messages of many types are frequent in the media in urban areas. Although one additional media campaign may show little specific impact under these circumstances, the frequency with which certain health behaviors are practiced might be appreciably less in the absence of any media activities at all. The history of cigarette smoking in the United States since the Surgeon General's Report provides evidence in this regard. For example, Warner (1977) presented data indicating that the percentage of cigarette smokers is less than would have been expected in the absence of extensive anti-smoking activities in the media. His data also showed that short term fluctuations in the number of cigarettes consumed per person in the United States are correlated with fluctuations in media activities aimed at smoking.

Two factors should be examined in deciding whether to continue media campaigns that appear to be unsuccsessful. First, research is needed regarding the optimal mix and intensity of media activities aimed at modifying health behavior. Such information would permit the design of campaigns that maximize the efficiency with which money spent on the media is used. Second, responsibility for maintaining appropriate levels of media activities needs to be clearly allocated among those concerned with modifying various health behaviors. Without explicit allocation of this responsibility, it is likely that some media activities which are important in "keeping the pressure on" will not occur.

6. Eligibility Criteria

The impact of eligibility criteria on recruitment to screening and training programs is another issue. In an attempt to educate and screen women at high risk, CCC/LA established eligibility criteria for both its breast and cervical cancer detection programs. The breast cancer program focused on women over 45 years of age; the cervical cancer program on Hispanic and Black women in certain high risk geographical areas.

The eligibility criteria, however, might actually have worked against the goal of teaching breast self examination. At present, there is little evidence regarding the ages at which women are most likely to be successfully trained and motivated to practice BSE.

In the case of screening, many women who did not meet the criteria participated in the two programs. There were few differences between eligibles and ineligibles in the frequency with which abnormalities were found in either of these programs. Because many women attended in groups in which not all women were eligible, eligibility criteria often impeded the recruitment process. Although CCC/LA served all women who came to these programs, announcing eligibility criteria might have resulted in some eligible women not participating because they thought their ineligible friends would not be served. These concerns indicate the importance of examining how the use of eligibility criteria impacts on the accomplishment of objectives in community based programs.

7. The Limits of Experience

A final issue is the extent to which experience in planning and implementing specific programs is valid in contexts other than the one in which it was originally gained. CCC/LA sponsored two cervical cancer education and detection programs for minority women. One of these programs was conducted by an organization that had prior experience in recruiting minority women for pap screening. In attempting to apply this experience, however, the other program encountered a number of difficulties. Although the experience of the first group may have been valid for a specific population at a specific time, the attempt to apply it to a different population was not completely successful. However, evaluation included direct comparisons of the two programs, the problems inherent in applying applying the experience of one program to design another became clear.

Because there is a limited empirical base from which to draw data for community programming, those who plan and implement such programs must depend on their experience and on the experience of others. Yet some of this experience could be tested empirically. Both of the cervical cancer programs mentioned above timed their recruitment according to the impressions of the most experienced outreach workers in the on-going program. This resulted in less recruitment than might have occured otherwise in the other program. Thus,

the recruitment strategy that was based on experience should
have been pilot tested empirically before being fully
implemented.

PLANNING AND MONITORING THE NEXT CYCLE OF
COMMUNITY BASED PROGRAMS AT THE NATIONAL LEVEL

Because demonstration projects require evaluation, they
should be viewed in the same light as any other form of
research. As such, it would be more appropriate to fund
them as grants rather than contracts. Grants permit the
flexibility required to assure the most valid test of the
research hypothesis. In community based programs, because
the research is focused on complex organizations and
activities, there is greater danger of inappropriate
monitoring than in laboratory research. Indeed, because
most of the problems of laboratory research admit to
straightforward technical solutions, the likelihood of
controversy regarding the adequacy with which they are being
done is less than in the case of community based programs in
which problems are more likely to be solved by professional
judgements (Kaplan, 1964). For this reason, the grant
system, in which controversy is resolved prior to the
beginning of the project, seems a more appropriate means of
funding community based demonstrations than the contract.

Special steps also should be taken to assure that only those
individuals with appropriate training and experience are
assigned to staff and to study sections that review and
monitor community based demonstrations. Those submitting
proposals should be assured their proposals are reviewed by
qualified peers and that project officers are technically
qualified to perform the monitoring function.

Community based programs might be designed and monitored
more efficiently, if the funding and personnel assigned to
them were pooled. Community based programs have two
features in common that are independent of the disease at
which they are aimed. First, they require staff with a
range of skills that are quite different from those required
either in the laboratory or in clinical research. Among
others, these skills include community organization,
techniques for changing behavior, administration and
management, and evaluation of social programs. Second, the
behavior change techniques used by various community based

programs are basically the same. For example, the same
skills used to change smoking behavior are also the skills
used to change eating habits or to encourage compliance with
treatment regimens (Bandura, 1969).

Because these skills differ from those required for basic or
clinical research and because these skills are the same
regardless of the behavior being changed, it may be
inefficient for the individual institutes within the
National Institutes of Health to develop, sponsor and
monitor its own community based demonstrations. It is
unlikely that most individual institutes will have the
resources needed to hire and maintain staff with the range
of competencies required to develop and monitor
sophisticated community based programs. As a consequence,
individuals might be asked to design and monitor activities
in the community for which they lack both training and
experience. Even if each institute hired staff with the
skills needed to design and monitor community based
programs, the costs of such programs would prevent most
individual institutes from sponsoring enough programs to
keep these staff fully employed.

In some instances, considerable economies could be gained by
carefully designed community based programs that test
approaches to chronic disease control jointly for two or
more institutes. This would work most readily in areas
where more than one institute addresses the same behavior.
Smoking and diet are two examples. Efficient community
based programs might be designed to test change strategies
aimed at different behaviors that are relevant for different
diseases. Indeed, because programs in the community
frequently result in changes in the organization and
delivery of health services, the efficiency of such programs
might be enhanced if they included research relating to the
health care delivery system.

Given these considerations, the scarce dollars available
for chronic disease control in the community might be spent
more efficiently if community based demonstration programs
were sponsored by a single agency. Although implementation
of this suggestion would mean reduced funds for the
individual institutes, it would also mean a reduction in the
activities across which their budgets would have to be
stretched. It is also possible that more stable funding for
community based programming would result if this suggestion

were implemented. On the other hand, a single agency might come to represent and fund only a narrow range of the legitimate approaches to community based programming that existed at any given time. This danger could be minimized if staff and study sections were required to encompass a representitive base of theory and practice.

WHY COMMUNITY BASED DEMONSTRATION PROJECTS SHOULD BE FUNDED

Community based demonstration projects facilitate the accumulation of knowledge base for testing behavior change strategies. Without a commitment to accumulating knowledge about behavior change strategies in the community, subsequent chronic disease programs are unable to do more than "reinvent the wheel." Although the behavioral sciences are still quite primitive, the evaluations of several recent demonstrations indicate that a knowledge for community based programming is developing. The only laboratory within which it can be developed, however, is the community.

In addition to developing knowledge for chronic disease control, there are three values that can be achieved by demonstration projects. First, a demonstration project calls attention to a problem. It may play an important role in helping to "keep the pressure on" a population with respect to that problem. Second, successful demonstrations may serve as the basis for new programs in the future. Even if a project is not continued after demonstration funding ends, if the results of the demonstration have been properly disseminated, new programs that might not have been thought of may be stimulated elsewhere. Third, demonstration projects in which the results have been properly disseminated inform other organizations and agencies regarding the adequacy of alternatives they may be contemplating. Considerable waste of resources might be averted thereby.

REFERENCES

Bandura, A.(1969). "Principles of Behavior Modification." New York: Holt, Rinehart and Winston.

Berkanovic, E., B. Gerber and W. Wright (1982). "Contractor's Final Report; Community Cancer Control/Los Angeles: NCI Contract Number NO1-CN-75400." Los Angeles: Community Cancer Control.

HEW: Department of Health, Education and Welfare (1979). Smoking in children and adolescents. In "Smoking and Health." Washington D.C.: U.S. Public Health Service, Chapter 17.

Kar, S.B. (1975). "Communication Research in Family Planning." New York: UNESCO.

Kaplan, A. (1964). "The Conduct of Inquiry." Chandler.

Lanere, R.R. (1972). Smoking behavior in a teenage population. American Journal of Public Health, 62:807-813.

McGuire, W.J. (1969). The nature of attitudes and attitude change. In Lindzey, G. and E. Aronson, (eds), "Handbook of Social Psychology." (2nd ed., Vol. 3) New York: Addison-Wesley, pp. 136-314.

Pool, I.S. (1973). Communication systems. In I.S. Pool, et al. (eds) "Handbook of Communications." New York: Rand McNally, pp. 3-26.

Rogers, E.M. (1973). "Communications Strategies for Family Planning." Glencoe: Free Press.

Warner, K.E. (1977). The effects of the anti-smoking campaign on cigarette consumption. American Journal of Public Health, 67:645-650.

Weiss, W. (1969). Effects of mass media of communications. In Lindzey, G. and E Aronson, (eds): "Handbook of Social Psychology" (2nd ed., Vol. 5). New York: Addison-Wesley, pp. 77-195.

Zimbaro, P. and E.B. Ebbesen (1970). "Influencing Attitudes and Changing Behavior." New York: Addison-Wesley.

Progress in Cancer Control IV: Research in the Cancer Center, pages 283–292
© **1983 Alan R. Liss, Inc., 150 Fifth Avenue, New York, NY 10011**

COMMUNITY CANCER CONTROL OF LOS ANGELES (CCC/LA):
BREAST EXAMINATION TRAINING (BET) CENTERS

Claudia Lee, Administrator

Memorial Hospital Cancer Center
2801 Atlantic, P.O. Box 1428
Long Beach, CA 90801-1428

In the United States, breast cancer is a health problem
of almost epidemic proportion with one out of eleven women
expected to develop the disease sometime during her life-
time. During 1982, there were 112,900 newly diagnosed
breast cancers and 37,300 deaths from the disease.
(American Cancer Society, 1982).

There are essentially three approaches to the control
of breast cancer: prevention, cure, and early diagnosis.
Medical science has to date, however, neither identified
preventable causative factors nor discovered an effective
cure for all stages of breast cancer. It is necessary,
therefore, to rely on a low risk, cost effective method
of early detection, such as breast self examination (BSE),
which is capable of detecting breast cancer when it is
still localized and most responsive to treatment.

The Health Insurance Plan (HIP) of Greater New York
was a randomized controlled trial, involving 31,000 women,
designed to examine breast cancer detection techniques
in terms of usefulness and survival. The 1963 HIP study
demonstrated conclusively that: (1) early diagnosis decreases
mortality from breast cancer for women over 50 (Shapiro
1977; Shapiro, Strax, Venet et al 1972); (2) physical
examination independent from mammography contributes to
earlier diagnosis (Eddy 1980; Shwartz 1978; Shapiro 1977;
Bailar 1976); and (3) physical examination is particularly
important for the 40-49 year age group (Venet 1979; Venet,
Strax, Venet et al 1971). It follows logically, therefore,
 that breast self examination should be an integral component

of health education and screening programs.

Within this framework of proven educational methods
for early detection of breast cancer, the National Cancer
Institute (NCI), through Community Cancer Control of
Los Angeles (CCC/LA), funded five hospital-based Breast
Examination Training (BET) Centers in Los Angeles. The
hospitals provided matching funds and the program was
free to the community. The purpose of the BET Centers
was educational: to teach high risk women the appropriate
technique of BSE with the anticipation that the individual/
private instruction would result in improved technique
and increased confidence, thereby leading to regular
and appropriate BSE practice. The purpose of the BET
Centers was not screening; however, it was during the
course of individual BSE training that abnormalities
were detected. At the conclusion of the demonstration
program (12/81), the five Centers had collectively operated
a total of 154 months, individually trained 25,147 women
in BSE, referred 2,161 symptomatic women to physicians,
and detected 48 breast cancers.

The educational program consisted of two components:
a small group didactic/discussion session followed by
a private practice/feedback session. The program was
offered onsite at the Center as well as offsite at the
workplace, churches, senior centers, etc. Over 800 offsite
programs were provided by the five Centers. Throughout
the program, there was a strong emphasis on wellness
and the importance of women taking responsibility for
their own health.

The group session consisted of client profile and
knowledge/behavior questionnaires, a short NCI film,
and a discussion of related issues: (1) anatomy and physiology of the breast, (2) breast diseases, both benign
and malignant, (3) symptoms of breast cancer, (4) risk
factors for breast cancer, (5) treatment options, (6)
reconstruction, and (7) recent California legislation
regarding informed consent and third party reimbursement
for reconstruction. The small group session concluded
with BSE instruction using diagrams, table top silicone
breast models, and nurse demonstration. Teaching BSE
technique was obviously an important segment of the program
as it is well documented that 90% of breast lumps are
found by women themselves (Leis 1967; Haagenson 1958).

Most lumps are found accidentally, however, when they are so large that detection is almost inevitable. The BSE instruction stressed strongly the importance of women becoming familiar with their own breast texture so that with accurate/regular BSE practice, they would be able to purposefully detect small changes much earlier. It is known that there is a higher degree of acceptance and compliance by women who learn BSE by using their own hands on their own breasts (Strax 1979). In order to provide that personal learning environment and to increase the likelihood of learning transference from the classroom model to her breasts, the group session was followed by a private session where the client practiced on her own breasts what she had learned in the classroom.

This individual session between the nurse and woman was a critical step in learning the technique. When the woman practiced on her own breasts, she received immediate feedback from the nurse about the correctness of her technique and about the idiosyncratic nature of her own breasts. Feelings of confidence and competence are both important variables in determining whether a woman will continue practicing BSE after originally learning the technique (Stillman 1977; Gallup Poll 1980; Hobbs 1971); therefore, there was an intensive effort to reinforce the skill. The nurse also performed a complete breast physical on the woman so that the woman was comfortable that she had not missed anything abnormal and that she was feeling the same thing in her breasts that the nurse felt. If an abnormality was detected at this point, the woman was referred to her own physician or selected a physician from the Center's referral list. During this private session, the nurse also had the opportunity to answer personal questions, provide emotional support, and allay unnecessary fears.

The followup evaluation consisted of a random telephone interview of 2,500 women a minimum of one year post BSE instruction. The interview was a series of tracked open ended questions designed to determine the frequency and adequacy of BSE practice and technique. This self report from the five Centers indicates 75% continued to practice BSE (Table I) with 70% reporting at least monthly practice (Table II). This conclusion must be tempered by the fact that the best single predictor of long term practice was whether the woman stated she was already practicing

BSE at the time of instruction. This indicates the training may have served more as reinforcement of behavior for some women rather than initiation of behavior. The correctness of the technique varied from Center to Center (Tables III, IV, V). Additional variables described below must be noted when interpreting the followup data.

TABLE I

TELEPHONE FOLLOWUP

FREQUENCY OF WOMEN REPORTING BSE PRACTICE

(PERCENTAGE OF TOTAL WOMEN)

	HOSPITAL A	HOSPITAL B	HOSPITAL C	HOSPITAL D	HOSPITAL E
PRACTICING BSE	74%	81%	80%	85%	74%
N=	710	668	526	298	292

TABLE II

TELEPHONE FOLLOWUP

BSE FREQUENCY

(PERCENTAGE OF WOMEN PRACTICING BSE)

	HOSPITAL A	HOSPITAL B	HOSPITAL C	HOSPITAL D	HOSPITAL E
MORE OFTEN THAN MONTHLY	19	22	24	13	12
MONTHLY	50	53	52	57	65
EVERY 2-3 MONTHS	18	10	10	18	14
WHEN I THINK OF IT	10	12	11	10	7
OTHER/NO ANSWER	3	3	4	1	2
N =	529	539	422	253	215

TABLE III

TELEPHONE FOLLOWUP

BSE TECHNIQUE

(PERCENTAGE OF WOMEN DOING BSE-

MULTIPLE RESPONSES POSSIBLE)

PARTS OF BSE:	HOSPITAL A	HOSPITAL B	HOSPITAL C	HOSPITAL D	HOSPITAL E
USES FINGERS	36	32	34	53	29
USES 4 FINGERS	12	30	35	12	24
MOVES HAND CLOCKWISE	38	50	42	38	52
USES FLAT PART OF FINGERS	22	13	10	24	18
MOVES FINGERS IN CIRCLE	34	39	46	54	24
SQUEEZES NIPPLE	2	5	7	7	6
N=	520	524	406	251	210
MEAN # RESPONSE	1.4	1.7	1.7	1.9	1.5

The five Centers (Table VI) varied greatly in terms of the ethnic, economic, and social composition of the populations served. The evaluation results, therefore, need to be presented Center by Center, not in aggregate, and could be interpreted as a series of five independent tests of the BET Center concept in five diverse communities. In addition, the sponsoring hospitals ranged in size from a 307 bed community hospital to an 848 bed teaching hospital and the total operation time varied from 40 months at the first hospital Center to 19 months at the last.

Several variables were submitted to a chi-square test to look at differences between the women included in the followup study and the women available but not included. Significant differences were found for age, income, race, marital status, and location of training. Women included in the followup study were two to five years older than

TABLE IV

TELEPHONE FOLLOWUP

BSE MANUAL CHECKS

(PERCENTAGE OF WOMEN DOING BSE –

MULTIPLE RESPONSE POSSIBLE)

CHECKS FOR:	HOSPITAL A	HOSPITAL B	HOSPITAL C	HOSPITAL D	HOSPITAL E
LUMP	92	94	90	94	96
CHANGE IN SIZE/ CONSISTENCY	38	26	30	50	47
KNOT	12	24	23	13	15
TENDER AREA	6	13	15	12	9
DISCHARGE/BLEEDING	7	8	16	18	20
NIPPLE CHANGES	3	0	1	3	1
DIMPLING/PUCKERING	2	1	1	1	2
DISCOLORATION	5	3	1	3	4
N =	520	524	406	250	210
MEAN # RESPONSES	1.6	1.7	1.8	1.9	1.9

those not included (p $<$.05 for four Centers). The mean
income category for women included in the followup study
was always higher than those not included (p $<$.05 for two
Centers). The racial distributions were different in each
Center with a higher percentage of Caucasions included
in the followup at four Centers and a higher percentage
of Blacks in one Center (p $<$.05 for five Centers). The
percentage of married women included in the followup study
was four to eleven percent higher than those not included
(p $<$.05 for five Centers). More women in the followup
study were trained at the Center as opposed to offsite
locations (p $<$.05 at three Centers). These differences
indicate some caution is warranted when generalizing results
to the Center population as a whole.

TABLE V

TELEPHONE FOLLOWUP

VISUAL INSPECTION OF BREASTS

(PERCENTAGE OF WOMEN LOOKING AT

BREASTS---MULTIPLE RESPONSES POSSIBLE)

ITEMS LOOKED FOR:	HOSPITAL A	HOSPITAL B	HOSPITAL C	HOSPITAL D	HOSPITAL E
LUMPS*	65	69	72	35	55
BREAST CHANGES	49	33	40	66	55
NIPPLE CHANGES	24	20	23	38	36
DIMPLING/PUCKERING	18	10	8	28	22
DISCHARGE	9	14	19	18	28
RASH SORES	9	13	17	12	8
DEPRESSION/ELEVATION	5	8	2	9	6
ONE BREAST HIGHER	2	4	5	5	4
N =	382	442	358	192	157
MEAN # RESPONSES	1.8	1.7	1.9	2.1	2.1

* NOT COUNTED IN MEAN

The response rate to the telephone followup study was consistently high, ranging from 94% to 98%. The percentage of women included in the followup study, however, varied from Center to Center and ranged from 18% to 45% of total women available. This variation was due to the difference in available women with the older Centers having trained thousands more women than the new Centers.

The followup study was intended to assess BSE behavior one year after Center training, but the logistics were such that the time lapse varied for each woman from 13 to 29 months and for each Center from 13 to 21 months. As has been demonstrated with other health care behaviors/ habits, it is possible that number of months to followup was correlated to reported BSE practice.

TABLE VI

HOSPITALS

THE FIVE HOSPITAL-BASED BET CENTERS WERE LOCATED IN LOS ANGELES
COMMUNITIES THAT REFLECT THE DIVERSITY OF THE ACTION AREA. DUE
TO THE IDIOSYNCRATIC ETHNIC, ECONOMIC, AND SOCIAL COMPOSITIONS
OF THE POPULATIONS, IT IS IMPORTANT TO EXAMINE THE EVALUATION RESULTS
ACCORDING TO THOSE DIVERSE VARIABLES.

● HOSPITAL A: BROTMAN MEDICAL CENTER - 40 MONTHS
  - IN WESTERN PORTION OF ACTION AREA
  - A MEDIUM-SIZED, PRIVATE, COMMUNITY HOSPITAL
    WITH 577 BEDS
  - LOCATED IN A HIGHER SES AREA WITH GROWING POCKETS
    OF LOWER SES MINORITY POPULATIONS

● HOSPITAL B: MARTIN LUTHER KING, JR. GENERAL HOSPITAL - 36 MONTHS
  - IN MIDDLE SOUTHEASTERN PORTION OF ACTION AREA
  - A COUNTY INSTITUTION WITH 394 BEDS
  - LOCATED IN A LOWER TO LOWER MIDDLE SES BLACK AND
    GROWING HISPANIC COMMUNITY

● HOSPITAL C: WHITE MEMORIAL MEDICAL CENTER - 38 MONTHS
  - IN FAR NORTHEASTERN PORTION OF ACTION AREA
  - A SMALL, SEVENTH-DAY ADVENTIST OPERATED INSTITUTION
    WITH 307 BEDS
  - LOCATED IN A LOWER TO MIDDLE LOWER SES HISPANIC
    COMMUNITY

● HOSPITAL D: TORRANCE MEMORIAL MEDICAL CENTER - 21 MONTHS
  - IN SOUTH COASTAL PORTION OF ACTION AREA
  - A BUSY COMMUNITY HOSPITAL WITH 310 BEDS
  - LOCATED IN A MIDDLE TO UPPER SES COMMUNITY

● HOSPITAL E: MEMORIAL HOSPITAL MEDICAL CENTER/LONG BEACH - 19 MONTHS
  _ IN CENTRAL COASTAL PORTION OF ACTION AREA
  - A LARGE COMMUNITY TEACHING HOSPITAL WITH 848 BEDS
  - LOCATED IN AN AREA OF SES CONTRASTS RANGING FROM
    QUITE LOW TO QUITE HIGH

The Los Angeles BET Center experience demonstrated
success with both programmatic outcome and cancer control
process. The documentation of the development and results
of the activities should provide other communities with
guidelines for similar programs (CCC/LA 1982; Wilson, 1981).

The BET Centers have demonstrated that a wide range

of women can be recruited to learn BSE, that many of those women have not practiced BSE previously, and that once learned a large percentage continue to practice for at least one year. The evolution of programmatic procedures, such as staffing patterns, recruitments strategies, and eligibility criteria, resulted in a program that allowed each Center to better serve their local communities. (Lee, 1981). The commitment of hospital administrators and community physicians to the BET Center concept was actualized with the continuation of three Centers past federal funding.

As a community based cancer control program, under the outstanding leadership of Helene Brown, CCC/LA brought together experts from two comprehensive cancer centers (USC and UCLA), the American Cancer Society (five local units), major hospitals and businesses, community medicine and government agencies to develop/implement coordinated and integrated cancer control activities in a large, diverse complex city. The seven year project required ongoing cooperation, creativity and commitment among people and agencies that heretofore had often been competitive and/or had not collaborated. The success of the several CCC/LA activities was primarily due to this cooperative volunteer and staff effort toward achieving the challenging cancer control goals for Los Angeles.

American Cancer Society (1982). "Cancer Facts and Figures." p. 10.
Bailar JC (1976). Mammography: a contrary view. Ann Intern Med 84:77.
Community Cancer Control (1982). "Contractor's Final Report." 3:389.
Eddy DM (1980). "Screening for Cancer: Theory, Analysis, and Design." Englewood Cliffs, NJ: Prentice-Hall Inc.
Gallup Poll (1980). Public attitudes toward cancer and cancer tests. In "CA-A Cancer Journal for Clinicians," American Cancer Society, 3:92.
Haagenson CD (1958). "Carcinoma of the Breast: A Monograph for the Physician." American Cancer Society, p.7.
Hobbs P (1971). Evaluation of a teaching programme of breast self examination. Int J Health Ed 14:564.
Lee CZ (1981). Maybe it will go away: the five most dangerous words in the English language. Family Comm Health 4(3):45.
Leis HP Jr (1967). Differential diagnosis of benign and malignant breast tumors. Geriatrics 22:181.

Shapiro S (1977). Evidence on screening for breast cancer from a randomized trial. Cancer 39:2772.

Shapiro S, Strax P, Venet L, et al (1972). Changes in 5-year breast cancer mortality in a breast cancer screening program. In "7th National Cancer Conference Proceedings," Philadelphia: JB Lippincott Co, p. 663.

Shwartz M (1978). An analysis of the benefits of serial screening for breast cancer based upon a mathematical model of the disease. Cancer 44:1550.

Stillman MJ (1977). Women's health beliefs about breast cancer and breast self-examination. Nurs Res 26:121.

Strax P (1979). Importance of breast self examination (BSE). In Strax P (ed): "Control of Breast Cancer Through Mass Screening," Littleton, Mass: PSG Publishing Co. Inc, p. 153.

Venet L (1979). The clinical examination in mass screening for breast cancer. In Strax P (ed): "Control of Breast Cancer Through Mass Screening," Littleton, Mass: PSG Publishing Co. Inc, p. 157.

Venet L, Strax P, Venet W, et al (1971). Adequacies and inadequacies in breast examinations by physicians in mass screening. Cancer 28:1546.

Wilson R (Ed.) (1981). Family Comm Health, entire edition 4(3):1.

Progress in Cancer Control IV: Research in the Cancer Center, pages 293–303
© 1983 Alan R. Liss, Inc., 150 Fifth Avenue, New York, NY 10011

BREAST SELF-EXAMINATION POST MASTECTOMY:
EMPIRICAL FINDINGS AND THEIR IMPLICATIONS

Prakash L. Grover, Ph.D.
Zili Amsel, Sc.D.
Andrew M. Balshem, B.A.
Barbara Kulpa, M.S.
Paul F. Engstrom, M.D.

The Fox Chase Cancer Center
Philadelphia, Pennsylvania 19111

In the absence of a safe, effective and inexpensive
method for screening for breast cancer, there has been
widespread support for urging women to conduct periodic
breast self-examination for early detection of tumors. In
view of the fact that nearly 80 percent of breast lumps are
detected by women themselves, BSE can be considered
effective only if it helps women identify their tumor at
earlier stage of growth which data show to have a better
relative survival. No specific studies are on record to
provide data on comparative survival of women whose tumors
were detected through BSE versus those whose tumors were
detected accidentally or through other deliberate maneuvers
(e.g. examination by a physician, radiologic examination,
etc.). Several investigators have estimated the benefit
attributable to BSE (Greenwald et al, 1978; Foster et al,
1978; Huguley and Brown, 1981; Feldman et al, 1981) by
examining the stage of disease among patients with breast
cancer, a proportion of whom practiced BSE. They find that
a higher percentage of women who were practicing BSE before
their cancer diagnosis had earlier stages of disease and
had fewer nodes involved. Although the results of these
studies suggest the same conclusion, the estimated magnitude
of effect of BSE on stage of disease at detection varies
substantially. A major problem in comparing the findings
from such studies results from their definition of BSE
practice; while some investigators simply inquire whether
the subjects practiced BSE before their diagnosis,

*Supported by PHS Grant 5-R25-CA23299; and Contract N01-
CN45055.

others define practice in terms of the frequency of their
BSE practice. Furthermore, in most of these studies, the
accuracy with which the subjects practice BSE also remains
an unmeasured variable which could substantially effect
outcomes.

In trying to explain the differences in these studies
in the proportion of women found to practice BSE whose
tumors were identified at earlier stages of disease, Cole
and Austin (1981) conclude that their study samples perhaps
had varying patterns of use of breast cancer detection
services. In particular, they note "among women who use
various other breast cancer detection practices, the incre-
mental effect of BSE is small. However, among women who use
these other services less . . . BSE has a meaningful role to
play." Thus, although the precise quantification of the
effectiveness of BSE has eluded us so far, the recurrent
and relatively consistent results from studies among
different populations in widely varying geographic regions
suggest that BSE plays a role in early detection even if it
is simply a "useful adjuvant to the first line of detection"--
examination by a physician and screening by mammography.

Almost all studies of prevalence, determinants and
effectiveness of BSE have been based on reports from well
women or on the analyses of BSE behavior of cancer patients
prior to their diagnosis. Not much attention has been paid
to the subsequent practice of BSE among women who are
treated for malignancy in one of their breasts, although a
sizeable fraction, 6-15 percent, of these women is expected
to develop cancer in the contralateral breast depending on
their age at diagnosis, histology of the tumor and family
history of cancer (Robbins and Berg, 1964; Hayden, 1975;
Anderson, 1975). Yet we found only two published studies
of the practice of BSE among women who had already received
treatment for cancer in one breast (Hirshfield-Bartek, 1982)
or who were referred to a tertiary cancer care center for
benign or malignant breast disease (Laughter et al, 1982).
Hirshfield-Barteck studied BSE practice of 25 women who had
Stage I or II cancer using the conceptual framework of the
Health Belief Model (HBM). Only personal susceptibility to
cancer was found to have a statistically significant
relationship with frequency of BSE practice. The other
explanatory variables; knowledge about cancer, perceived
benefits from BSE and barriers to its practice were

positively related to BSE practice but not at a statistically
significant level. Laughter et al (1981) studied the BSE
behavior of 142 women referred to the medical and surgical
clinics of M.D. Anderson Hospital and Tumor Institute. Nearly
46 percent of the women who had had a mastectomy (N=76) were
practicing BSE at the time of the study even though nearly
all of them had heard about BSE. No information is available
on their practice of BSE prior to mastectomy.

It may be hypothesized that women who have had breast
cancer would have a high awareness of their personal susceptibility to a bilateral breast cancer, would be aware of its
likely severity and the advantages of early detection. One
would, therefore, expect them to be favorably disposed to
practicing periodic BSE as a means of secondary prevention
of cancer in their remaining breast as well as a recurrence
in the affected side. Data are presented here in examining
this general hypothesis and in considering an explanation of
BSE behavior of a group of women subsequent to their mastectomy.

Materials and Methods

Data for the present paper are part of a larger follow-
up study of women in the Breast Cancer Network registry.
The network constituted the Fox Chase Cancer Center and
eight of its affiliate hospitals in the Delaware Valley
region. The registry includes women who were treated for
a breast cancer at any of the network hospitals during the
years 1975-1978. Of the 1168* female patients treated for
unilateral breast cancer who were sent the questionnaire,
68 percent (or 792)* responded. The disposition of the
remaining sample is as follows:

Refusals	=	171	14.5%
Untraceable	=	84	7.1%
Deceased	=	121	10.3%

---

*12 males with breast cancer have been excluded both from
the target and completed sample figures.

An additional 23 women were found to have undergone a second mastectomy for malignancy in their contralateral breast. Thus, the net sample for analysis consisted of questionnaire responses from 769 women. Data were collected on the socio-demographic characteristics of these women and their pre-and-post mastectomy BSE behavior. Clinical data regarding their tumor and its treatment were obtained from the abstracts of their medical charts.

Findings

Table 1 shows the distribution of the study population on various socio-demographic characteristics. The population is predominantly caucasian, fairly well-educated, and evenly distributed across age groups. Two-thirds of the group were married at the time of the survey and, presumably, living with their spouses.

Table 2 shows the extent of BSE practice among women in the study. Although nearly twice as many women were practicing BSE regularly after mastectomy than before, the proportion of women not practicing BSE post-mastectomy also increased compared to the pre-mastectomy figures. Those who were practicing regularly or not-at-all showed the maximum stability ($\approx 72\%$). Slightly less than a quarter of the non-practicers pre-mastectomy began to practice regularly after mastectomy. But, on the other hand, the fraction which changed from practicing regularly to 'not-at-all' is nearly the same. The major change in the profile of BSE practice is contributed by those who reported practicing BSE irregularly pre-mastectomy; almost as many changed to practicing regularly as those who completely stopped practicing BSE.

Since education and age have often been found to be associated with BSE practice, we looked at the distribution of 'positive' ("not practicing" to "practicing" BSE) and 'negative' changers ("practicing" to "not practicing" BSE) by these two variables. The results are given in Table 3.

It is clear that 'negative' change is inversely related to education and directly to age and 'positive' change is directly related to education and inversely to age. However, it is notable that the degree of change is comparatively larger for age than it is for education.

Table 1

Distribution of Study Subjects by Selected
Socio-demographic Characteristics

	Number	Percent
All subjects	769	100
Race		
Caucasian	721	94
Black	31	4
Other	17	2
Age		
Under 50 years of age	165	22
50-59	211	27
60-69	224	29
70 and older	169	22
Marital Status		
Married	504	66
Widowed	168	22
Separated	19	2
Divorced	22	3
Never Married	56	7
Educational Level		
Less than high school	308	40
High school only	266	35
More than high school	195	25

Table 2

Distribution of Study Subjects by
BSE Practice Pre-and-Post Mastectomy

| | BSE PRACTICE POST-MASTECTOMY | | | |
	Regularly	Irregularly	Never	Total
BSE Practice Pre-Mastectomy				
Regularly	121	8	38	167
Row Percent	*72*	*5*	*23*	
Irregularly	120	28	129	277
Row Percent	*43*	*10*	*47*	
Never	60	22	222	304
Row Percent	*20*	*7*	*73*	
Total	301	58	389	748
	(40%)	*(8%)*	*(52%)*	

Table 3

Percent and Direction of Change in BSE
Practice by Education and by Age

Direction and Percent of Change

	'Negative' Change Y → N	'Positive' Change N → Y
Education	%	%
<High School	22	36
High School	21	46
College	19	48
Age		
<50	13	57
50 - 59	21	49
60 - 69	26	41
>70	23	27

Table 4 shows the association of several explanatory
variables with 'positive' or 'negative' change compared
with 'persistent' non-practice and 'persistent' practice
respectively. While those women who had higher education,
were living with spouse, and who learned BSE through mass
media* were more likely to change from not practicing BSE
pre-mastectomy to practicing BSE post-mastectomy; lower
education, living without spouse and source of BSE training
do not seem to be associated with negative change. Only
age and pathological stage of tumor seem related both to
the 'positive' and 'negative' change in BSE practice.

---

*A relatively high proportion of our sample claimed to
have learned BSE from the mass media than is suggested by
other studies. We suspect that the wide publicity of
mastectomies of Mrs. Betty Ford and Mrs. Happy Rockefeller
as well as the articles carried by so many women's and
home-oriented magazines account for this unusual finding.
However, our data also show that the younger women are
more likely to learn BSE from mass media than the older
women.

TABLE 4
VARIABLES ASSOCIATED WITH CHANGE IN PRE-and-POST MASTECTOMY BSE PRACTICE

Explanatory Variables	Persistent non-practicers vs. Positive Changers (N/N) (N/Y)	Level of Significance	Persistent Practicers vs. Negative Changers (Y/Y) (Y/N)	Level of Significance
Age	Those younger are more likely to change	p < .02	Those older are more likely to change	p < .01
Education	Those with higher education are more likely to change	p < .04	Those with higher education are less likely to change	N.S.
Marital Status	Those with spouse more likely to change	p < .02	Those without spouse are more likely to change	---
Family History	Those with positive history are more likely to change		No significant differences	---
Who Taught BSE	Those who learned BSE from mass media are more likely to change	p < .02	No significant differences	---
Frequency of Prior BSE Practice	- - -		Those practicing irregularly are more likely to switch	p < .02
Reason for Not Practicing BSE Regularly	No significant differences	---	Those saying they: "don't take the time"/ "have physical discomfort"/ "are afraid they will find something," are most likely to change than those who say their doctor examines them.	p < .01
Method of Discovery	Those who discovered their cancer even by casual self-examination are more likely to change	N.S.	No significant differences	---
Pathological Stage of Tumor	Those with early stage Cancers (I,II) are more likely to change	p < .02	Those with stage IV are more likely to change	p < .02

Discussion

Like most other studies of BSE, our study also shows
that BSE practice is positively related to education and
inversely to age; that is true for both pre-and-post
mastectomy periods. However, the observed profile of BSE
practice among the women in our sample is intriguing
considering that detailed guidelines were developed and
distributed among the staff of hospitals in the Network
for early detection, diagnosis and management of breast
cancer as well as for patient education which included BSE
practice post-mastectomy. Two of the areas in which these
guidelines were followed relatively well were patient and
community education. As stated earlier in this paper, it
seems perfectly reasonable to assume that women who have
gone through the experience of developing a breast malignancy
and the procedures for its detection, management and follow-
up would be aware of their susceptibility for recurrence of
cancer in the same breast or developing one in the contralateral breast. They must also have a clear estimate of
its severity as well as the increased probability of survival
if a second malignancy were to be identified at an earlier
stage. Our finding that in spite of these conditions
nearly half the women do not practice BSE suggests that models
of health education such as the Health Belief Model (HBM)
which have had moderate success in explaining health behaviors
such as increasing frequent and accurate BSE in well women
may be inappropriate for women who already have had surgical
removal of a breast. Our data suggest that the overwhelming
focus on beliefs and attitudes should be modified to address
directly a woman's anxiety and fears about her developing a
second breast malignancy and the role she can play in
effecting early diagnosis and increasing her chances of
survival.

Our data also suggest that in an era of rapid information transfer, the public has had rather easy access to
health information from magazines, pamphlets and the
electronic media. For the general public, these sources
of information are inexpensive and presumably credible.
It may be highly beneficial, therefore, to make use of
the mass media more effectively and frequently to educate
and to provide "cues" to women. This can be done recognizing
the important role of physicians and other health personnel
in educating patients and/or reinforcing their practice of
positive health behaviors.

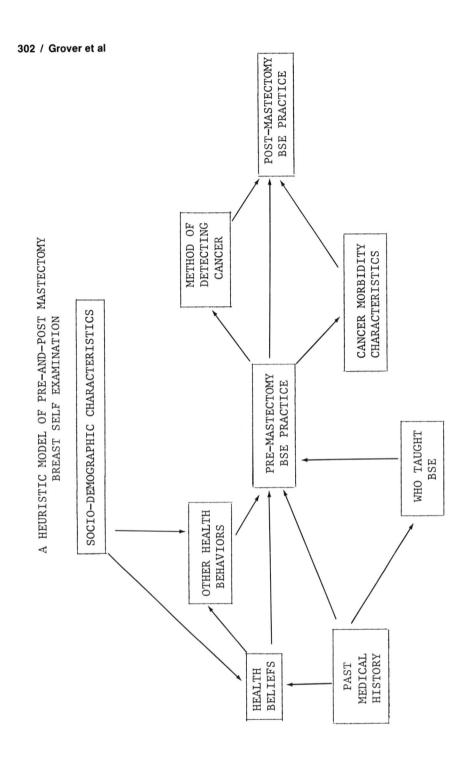

A HEURISTIC MODEL OF PRE-AND-POST MASTECTOMY
BREAST SELF EXAMINATION

Based on findings of our study and our review of literature on BSE, we propose a modified model to explain pre-and-post mastectomy breast self-examination. In this model, health beliefs and practices are conceived to play an important role in explaining breast self-examination practice before the onset of disease and its treatment. Other factors, in addition to BSE pre-mastectomy, particularly those related to the various aspects of the cancer experience, seem to be major determinants of post-mastectomy BSE behavior. Refinement of this model particularly the specification of experiential variables and their psychological and behavioral counterparts could suggest educational strategies to affect instrumental change in women's post-mastectomy BSE behavior.

REFERENCES

Anderson DE (1975). Genetics and breast cancer. In Gallagher HS (ed): Early Breast Cancer: Detection and Treatment. New York, John Wiley & Sons.

Cole PM, Austin H (1981). Breast self-examination: An adjuvant to early cancer detection. American Journal of Public Health, 71(6), pp. 574-576.

Feldman JG, Carter AC, Nicastri AD, Horsat ST (1981). Breast self-examination; relationship to stage of breast cancer at diagnosis. Cancer 47, pp. 2740-2745.

Foster RS Jr, Lang SP, Costanza MC, Worden JK, Haines CR, Yates JW (1978). Breast self-examination practices and breast-cancer stage. The New England Journal of Medicine, 299(6), pp. 265-270.

Greenwald P, Nasca PC, Lawrence CE, Horton J, McGarrah RP, Gabriele T, Carlton K (1978). Estimated effect of breast self-examination and routine physician examination on breast-cancer mortality. The New England Journal of Medicine, 299(6), pp. 271-273.

Hayden CW (1975). The physician, the lump and the mammogram. In Gallagher HS (ed): Early Breast Cancer: Detection and Treatment. New York, John Wiley & Sons.

Hirshfield-Bartek J (1982). Health beliefs and their influence on breast self-examination practices in women with breast cancer. Oncology Nursing Forum, 9(3), pp. 77-81.

Huguley CM, Brown RL (1981). The value of breast self-examination. Cancer 47, pp. 989-995.

Laughter DC, Kean TJ, Drean KD, Esparza D, Hortobagyi G, Judkins A, Levitt DZ, Marcus C and Silberberg Y (1981). The breast self examination practices of high risk women: Implications for patient education. Patient Counseling and Health Education, 3(3), pp. 103-107.

Robbins GF, Berg JW (1964). Bilateral primary breast cancers: A prospective clinicopathological study. Cancer 17, p. 1501.

Progress in Cancer Control IV: Research in the Cancer Center, pages 305–311
© **1983 Alan R. Liss, Inc., 150 Fifth Avenue, New York, NY 10011**

A PRECISE METHOD OF MANUAL BREAST SELF-EXAMINATION

H.S. Pennypacker, Mark Kane Goldstein, Gerald H.
Stein
Center for Ambulatory Studies, University of
Florida. Corporation for Public Medicine, VA
Medical Center, Gainesville, Florida 32602

The seriousness of breast cancer in terms of both morbidity and mortality has been well documented over an extended period. In spite of advances in the treatment of
other forms of cancer, this disorder continues as a major
killer of women and as the leading cause of cancer-related
deaths in women of all ages. The only means presently
available for attenuating the effects of breast cancer lie
in early detection; a number of investigations have consistently shown that the smaller the primary lesion at the time
of detection and treatment, the greater the likelihood of
survival without recurrence and without involvement of the
axillary lymph nodes (Adair, Berg, Joubert, Robbins, 1974;
Fisher, Slack, Bross, 1969; Fisher, Redmond, Fisher, 1980;
Haagensen, 1971; Spratt, Donegan, 1967).

The vast majority of breast cancers are initially discovered by women themselves. Thus, of all the screening
methods available, the one enjoying the most widespread use
is breast self-examination. A number of investigators have
shown retrospectively that regular breast self-examination
is associated with detection of smaller primary lesions
(Feldman, Carter, Nicastri, Hosat, 1981; Foster, Lang, Costanza, Worden, Haines, Tates, 1978; Greenwald, Nasca,
Lawrence, Horton, McGarrah, Gabriele, Carlton, 1978; Huguley,
Brown, 1981; Senie, Rosen, Lesser, Kinne, 1981). Unfortunately, surveys show that only a minority of women practice
breast self-examination (Gallup Organization, 1973) and that
only a tiny fraction of these are proficient when observed
by clinicians (Huguley et al., 1981). For breast self-
examination to realize its potential as an early screen for

cancer on a mass scale, a method must be found to teach the skill so that it is practiced proficiently and frequently by all who learn.

For the past seven years, our group has labored to develop and validate a technology for instructing breast self-examination that meets the criteria set forth above. As a point of departure, we recognized that the skill is essentially one of palpation and that the limits of its proficiency are set by the limits of tactile sensitivity in the human fingertips. Our first task was to determine these limits under laboratory conditions. With the help of our colleagues in Biomaterials Engineering, we perfected a crude silicone model of the female breast that possessed physical load deflection (firmness) characteristics highly similar to human tissue (Madden, Hench, Hall, Pennypacker, Adams, Goldstein, Stein, 1978). We placed tiny ball bearings on a foam pad under this model and asked volunteers to palpate the model and report detections of lump-like objects.

The results of this initial experiment were very encouraging (Adams, Hall, Pennypacker, Goldstein, Hench, Madden, Stein, Catania, 1976). We determined that the size threshold for detection of these simulated lumps through the silicone medium was less than 2 mm; that the threshold decreased slightly with practice, and that once stabilized, was relatively impervious to decay with the passage of time.

In the course of conducting this investigation, we began to learn a few of the details of palpation technique that were involved in accurate detection performance. Our next task was to establish that individuals trained to detect simulated tumors under the silicone models could, using the palpation techniques successful in that task, detect lesions in live breast tissue (Hall, Adams, Stein, Stephenson, Goldstein, Pennypacker, 1980). With the aid of volunteers who had known benign lesions and were willing to serve as stimuli for test purposes, we accomplished this demonstration in the following fashion: Two groups of young women were first asked to palpate individually the breasts of the stimulus women and report any masses detected. One group was then trained using our model and palpation suggestions, the other group passed the time reading. Both groups were again tested using the stimulus women. The group which had received the training nearly doubled their detection rate while the other group showed only a slight, non-significant improvement. Following this, the second group received the training while the first group otherwise occupied themselves. Both groups were again tested with the live women. The group more recently trained demonstrated the same increment in performance as had the originally trained group which, itself, exhibited no decay in proficiency.

These results led to two important conclusions: First, simply practicing palpation (even of breasts with known lesions) is not sufficient to impart substantial skill. Second, the training controlled by the characteristics of the simple silicone model with ball bearings simulating tumors did establish a skill that generalized to the problem of detecting masses in vivo.

The next problem was to refine the training procedure in the laboratory, then evaluate its components against other commonly used methods. A major, though by no means the only, measure of the thoroughness of a breast examination is the amount of surface area palpated. A precise method of this dimension was obtained in the case of searches of the silicone model with the aid of a Periphicon 511 image digitizer mated to an Apple II microcomputer and a video monitor. The camera's field of view was divided into a 32 x 32 matrix of picture elements (pixels). A light emitting diode was taped to the examiner's middle finger. When, in the course of searching the model, the examiner passed the diode into one of the squares in the pixel matrix, that square was lit on the video screen. As a result, the trainer could follow the progress of the examination on line in real time. If the examiner detected a simulated lump in the model, she so indicated by pushing a button which recorded the time and location of the event in the computer file.

Using this apparatus for basic data collection, we compared the before- and after-training performance of five groups which differed according to the type of training they received (Pennypacker, Neelakantan, Bloom, Criswell, Goldstein, Note 1). Group A served as a control and passed the training time reading magazines. Group B received training on their own breast tissue without the aid of silicone models and simulated tumors, Group C read a pamphlet entitled "How to Examine Your Breasts," Group D received training only on the model, and Group E received a combination of the model and real tissue training. After training, all groups were post-tested on the model.

The results consistently showed the superiority of the combination model and real tissue training. A major difference between this method and training with the model alone emerged in the analysis of false positive responding; women trained with only the model gave significantly more false positive responses in testing than did those in whom this tendency was apparently modulated by frequent palpation of their own lump-free tissue. The group trained with only their own tissue as a medium, while not making a large number of false positive responses, were unable to detect the small lump simulations in the test model. This is undoubtedly because the training failed to provide them with a realistic sensation of lumps embedded in simulated tissue. Accordingly, we have come to view this as an absolutely critical component of adequate BSE training; it is not sufficient merely to instruct a woman in the proper technique of palpation, she must also have experience with what her palpations are designed to detect if she is to become proficient and confident of her ability to detect lesions at the earliest possible clinical stage.

In a companion experiment (Neelakantan, Criswell, Pennypacker, Goldstein, Note 2) we compared training provided by the pamphlet with training on the model alone and the combination method in terms of proficiency in performing a breast examination on one's own tissue. Three groups of women were pre-tested on their own tissue, trained according to one of the aforementioned conditions, and them post-tested on the opposite breast. Examination thoroughness was measured with the aid of a grid projected on the woman's torso by an overhead projector. Thus, the area to be examined was platted into numbered 3 cm x 3 cm squares by the projected image and an observer could readily identify by number any square in which palpation occurred. Observers also evaluated each performance with respect to proper use of the flats of the fingers, palpation with small circular motions, application of both light and deep pressure, and the use of a systematic search pattern.

The results of this experiment again showed a clear superiority of the combination model/real tissue training medium in terms of area covered, total number of palpations, and examination duration. Because the woman's own breast was used in pre- and post-testing, no measure of lump detection proficiency could be obtained. Of interest however, was the fact that the pamphlet failed to instruct with respect to either proper palpation topography or application of multiple pressures. In view of these results, it is not surprising that women trained by this popular method fail both to demonstrate clinical proficiency and detect lesions less than 2 or 3 cm in size (Huguley et al., 1981).

In the course of developing this technology for training breast self-examination, we have had occasion to train a total of 428 women as of November 30, 1982. While participating in this training, the women themselves have detected a total of 26 lumps or suspicious masses which have been referred for medical evaluation. Thus, our present hit rate is approximately 6.1%. In a recent screening of 10,418 women, the Breast Cancer Detection Demonstration Project site in Jacksonville, Florida detected with mammography a total of 535 lumps or suspicious masses requiring further evaluation. Their hit rate is approximately 5.3%, not significantly different from ours. This implies that our method of instructing breast self-examination appears as aggressive a screen as mammogrphy while lacking the attendant inconvenience, expense, and risk. It remains for us to develop a technology of mass dissemination if the benefits of our labors are to be translated into reductions in both morbidity and mortality in the population at large.

In the interim, however, we are confident that the majority of women trained by the methods we have developed will, if they practice the skill on at least a monthly basis, enjoy the feeling of relief that comes from assuring themselves that they are free of malignancy. For those few for whom the monthly exam reveals an unexpected change, we offer the consolation that they discovered it at an earlier stage than might have otherwise been the case and all of the prognostic benefits attendant to early detection are theirs to enjoy. Thus, explicit benefit is now available for all women who regularly and proficiently practice breast self-examination.

REFERENCE NOTES

Pennypacker HS, Neelakantan P, Bloom HS, Criswell EL, Goldstein MK (1981) The effects of selected training procedures on acquisition and maintenance of skill in detecting simulated breast cancer. Paper presented at the Seventh Annual Convention of the Association for Behavior Analysis, Milwaukee, Wisconsin, May 29, 1981.

Neelakantan P, Criswell EL, Pennypacker HS, Goldstein MK
(1981) Experimental comparison of breast self-examination training procedures. Paper presented at the
Seventh Annual Convention of the Association for Behavior Analysis, Milwaukee, Wisonsin, May 29, 1981.

REFERENCES

Adair F, Berg J, Joubert L, Robbins G (1974). Long-term
follow-up of breast cancer patients. Cancer 33 1145.
Adams CK, Hall DC, Pennypacker HS, Goldstein MK, Hench LL,
Madden MC, Stein GH, Catania AC (1976) Lump detection
in simulated human breasts. Perception and Psychophysics 20 163.
Feldman JG, Carter AC, Nicastri AD, Hosat MS (1981) Breast
self-examination; relationship to stage of breast cancer at diagnosis. Cancer 47 2740.
Fisher B, Black NH, Bross I (1969) Cancer of the breast –
size of neoplasm and prognosis. Cancer 24 1071.
Fisher E, Redmond C, Fisher B (1980) Pathologic findings
from the national surgical adjuvant breast project
(Protocol No. 4). VI. Discriminants for five-year
treatment failure. Cancer 46 908.
Foster RS, Lang SP, Costanza MC, Worden JK, Haines CR, Tates
JW (1978) Breast self-examination practices and breast
cancer stage. The New England Journal of Medicine 299
265.
Gallup Organization (1973) Women's attitudes toward breast
cancer. New York: Author.
Greenwald P, Nasca PC, Lawrence CE, Horton J, McGarrah RP,
Gabriele T, Carlton L (1978). Estimated effect of
breast self-examination and routine physician examina-
tions on breast-cancer mortality. The New England
Journal of Medicine 299 271.
Haagensen C (1971) "Diseases of the breast" Philadelphia:
W.B. Saunders.
Hall DC, Adams CK, Stein GH, Stephenson HS, Goldstein MK,
Pennypacker HS (1980) Improved detection of human
breast lesions following experimental training. Cancer
46 408.
Huguley CM, Jr, Brown RL (1981) The value of breast self-
examination. Cancer 47 989.
Madden MC, Hench LL, Hall DC, Pennypacker HS, Adams CK,
Goldstein MK, Stein GH (1978) Model breasts for use
in teaching breast self-examination. Journal of Bio-
engineering 2 427-435.

Senie RT, Rosen PP, Lesser ML, Kinne DW (1981)   Breast self-
    examination and medical examination related to breast
    cancer stage.   American Journal of Public Health 71
    583.
Spratt J, Donegan W (1967)   "Cancer of the Breast" Phila-
    delphia: W.B. Saunders

Progress in Cancer Control IV: Research in the Cancer Center, pages 313–322
© 1983 Alan R. Liss, Inc., 150 Fifth Avenue, New York, NY 10011

DETERMINING THE QUALITY OF BREAST SELF-EXAMINATION AND ITS
RELATIONSHIP TO OTHER BSE MEASURES*

Joyce Mamon, Ph.D.[+]
Jane Zapka, Sc.D. [++]

[+]School of Hygiene and Public Health
The Johns Hopkins University
Baltimore, Maryland 21205

[++]Division of Public Health
University of Massachusetts
Amherst, Massachusetts 01003

BACKGROUND

Female breast cancer is a major health concern. It remains the most common type (27%) of cancer among women. In
1981, about 110,000 new cases were diagnosed and an estimated 37,000 deaths were recorded from this condition.[1]
The age-adjusted breast cancer death rate (1978) was 23.1
per 100,000 population or almost to 20% of the death rate
for all cancers combined.[2]

Since there is no known method of primary prevention
for breast cancer, secondary prevention remains the most
significant approach to reducing mortality from breast cancer. There is considerable evidence that prognosis can be
improved if a malignancy is detected in the early stages
of disease.[3-4]

Breast self-examination (BSE) has been widely promoted
as a method for early breast cancer detection; the National
Cancer Institute (NCI) and American Cancer Society (ACS)
have consistently recommended that women of all ages perform monthly BSE in addition to other periodic clinical

*Supported in part by the National Cancer Institute, Contract
N01-CN-95439.

screening methods.[5-7] However, the efficacy of breast self-examination (BSE) as a screening method for early detection of breast cancer, is a controversial issue. Part of this controversy relates to the types of measures used to examine the impact of BSE. Studies to date have primarily focused on BSE frequency/regularity. Recently attention has begun to focus on quality of BSE performance. It is being examined in order to determine whether it is a more sensitive and appropriate measure of BSE performance than frequency and regularity. Information on quality of BSE performance and its relationship to BSE frequency and regularity and other breast self-examination measures will provide a basis for determining what components of BSE performance are necessary to evaluate in order to adequately test the efficacy of BSE in early breast cancer detection.

Those studies which have examined quality of BSE performance[8-18] have varied in the number and type of criteria used to evaluate quality of breast self-examination. General agreement on content validity appears necessary. Additionally, some studies have attempted to measure quality of performance using a written instrument or interview. The assumptions examined in this study ware that the relationships of self-reporting to actual performance must be thoroughly investigated. Also the interrelationships of quality to other BSE measures need examination. Otherwise, it is inappropriate to evaluate quality of BSE using data collection methods that do not include some direct observation of BSE technique.

METHODS

The data were collected during a 3-year BSE demonstration evaluation program at a large mid-atlantic cost public university. There were two major phases to the data collection: baseline surveys and evaluation surveys. A total of 600 female students participated in a baseline community telephone interview prior to the demonstration program[19], 1682 women participared in the subsequent evaluation, one thousand women were exposed to the educational program (experimental), 682 were not exposed (comparisons). During the educational program, students were encouraged to talk to their mothers about BSE. As part of the project evaluation, 100 mothers were interviewed by telephone prior to the intervention (baseline survey) and 199 mothers were

interviewed by telephone 6 months after the educational
program.

   A subsample of the students in the evaluation (N=91)
participated in a validation substudy at posttest.[20] This
substudy examined the amount of congruence between written
reporting of quality of BSE performance and demonstration
of performance (clothed) in front of a trained observer.
The criteria used for scoring BSE performance were based on
American Cancer Society and National Cancer Institute recommendations regarding steps a woman should do while performing BSE. Nineteen (19) items were used in the measurement
of BSE quality. These are shown in Figure 1. For both the
self-reporting and demonstration of BSE quality, each of
these steps was scored as being done (1) or not (0); the
possible range was 0-19. All items were equally weighted.

Figure 1

Nineteen Steps Used in Measurement of BSE Quality

Lying Down Position

1) place hand behind head
2) place prop under shoulder
3) use opposite hand
4) press with finger pads
5) check for abnormalities
6) check armpit area
7) squeeze nipple for discharge
8) cover entire breast area
   using either circular
   motion or ladder method

Upright Position

1) use opposite hand
2) press with finger pads
3) check for abnormalities
4) check armpit area
5) squeeze nipple for
   discharge;
6) cover entire breast area
   using either circular
   motion or the ladder
   method;
7) raise arm above head

Mirror Position

1) place arms at side
2) raise arms over head;
3) press palms of hands on hips or in
   in front of chest
4) check visually for abnormalities

Results of the validation substudy indicated that of the nineteen steps included in the BSE quality measure only 5 items had high levels of sensitivity and specificity between written reporting of BSE performance and demonstration. These five items are mentioning of 3 positions (lying down, upright and mirror), squeezing the nipple and covering the armpit area.[20] The congruence levels between the written survey and the actual demonstration for these items were 96%, 81%, 82%, 72%. 72% respectively. These items were then used in the development of a five-item quality index score.

No statistical difference in the nineteen item index score were found between the student baseline population (via telephone) and the comparison groups who participated in the validation substudy (via written survey and demonstration). Therefore, telephone reporting was considered a comparable method to written reporting. This paper examines the relationship of telephone self-report of BSE quality with other BSE behaviors reported in the literature. Also factors of age, race, and socioeconomic status have been reported as related to breast cancer and preventive behaviors. These factors need to be investigated with respect to measurement of BSE quality.

The relationship pf BSE quality to other BSE behaviors include: frequency/regularity of performance, amount of time spent performing BSE and number of BSE positions performed. In this study, frequency of BSE performance is defined by four categories: (1) never performed BSE, (2) have performed BSE but not currently not within the past six months), (3) perform BSE currently but not regularly (within the past six months but less often than monthly) and (4) perform BSE currently and regularly (monthly or more often within the past six months). An estimate of the amount of time spent performing BSE was obtained by asking each respondent to estimate the number of minutes it takes her to examine her breasts. It has been estimated that if conducted adequately, BSE should take at least five minutes.[21] The reported time estimate was then categorized into (1) less than five minutes or (2) five minutes or more. Number of positions ranges from 1 to 3 for those who have ever performed BSE, that is, the lying down, upright and in front of mirror positions.

RESULTS

Examination of a students persons scores on the two quality measures is provided in Table 1. For the nineteen item quality score, the average score for college women is less than one-fifth of a perfect score. In contrast, using the validated five-item quality score that has been determined to reflect more accurately demonstration, the average score in self-report is 1.6; which is about one-third of the perfect score of five. Both scores reflect that at baseline, students have considerable deficiencies in terms of quality of performance. However, the level of deficiency is overestimated using the nineteen step quality score. Examination of an older population, in this case mother's of student subjects, exhibited a similar pattern.

Table 1 also provides data of these two quality measures by the major factors which have been found to be related to breast cancer and prevention behaviors. For categories within race, no significant differences were found with either measure for students or their mothers. Significant differences in the 5 item index score, albeit at a lower level, were found for students' age and income. For mothers' age, the 5 item score detected a higher level of significance, with older mothers (50-64 years) reporting lower quality. For mothers', only the use of the 19 item score resulted in significant differences for income levels.

The second aspect examined in this paper is the strength of association or lack of it, between quality of BSE practices and other BSE measures more frequently used to examine BSE performance. Tables 2 and 3 present the interrelationships of these measures for the students and mothers surveyed at baseline. An ordinal measure of association, Tau_c, is reported. Examination of the associations between the 29 item index and the 5 item validated measure shows it is only moderate in size. This supports the argument that the use of nonvalidated measures may lead to spurious conclusions. This is substantiated further by the differences in the size of the association between the two quality indices and the other BSE measures. This is particularly true for the older population (i.e. mothers).

Table 1: Comparison of BSE Quality Scores based Upon 19 Recommended Steps versus 5 Item Validated Score

	N	19-Step Quality of BSE Measure			5-Step Quality of BSE Measure		
		$\overline{X}$	s.e.	Sig.	$\overline{X}$	s.e.	Sig.
Students	430	3.7	.04	NA[+]	1.6	.12	NA
Race:							
White	362	3.7	.12		1.6	.04	
Black/Other	66	3.9	.33	NS	1.6	.16	NS
Age:							
17-34	390	3.6	.12		1.6	.04	
35-49	35	5.3	.56	.001	2.1	.20	.01
Income:							
< $10,000	28	4.2	.48		1.9	.18	
$10,000-14,999	17	3.2	.37	.01[*]	1.4	.16	.05[*]
$15,000-24,999	88	3.6	.25		1.6	.09	
$\geq$ $25,000	232	3.8	.17		1.6	.06	
Mothers	73	4.4	.28	NA[+]	2.0	.11	NA
Race:							
White	41	4.4	.36		2.0	.15	
Black/Other	32	4.4	.44	NS	2.0	.17	NS
Age:							
35-49	43	4.8	.36		2.2	.14	
50-64	30	3.8	.41	.10	1.7	.16	.02
Income:							
< $10,000	3[++]						
$10,000-14,999	7	6.0	.88	.10[*]	2.6	.43	
$15,000-24,999	13	4.5	.63		2.3	.21	
$\geq$ $25,000	35	4.3	.38		2.0	.15	NS

[+]Not Applicable
[++]Cell size too small for statistical analysts
[*]Designates group which differs significantly from women in $\geq$ $25,000 group.

Table 2.   Associations of BSE Performance Measures:
Students' Baseline Telephone Survey (N)

	Y_1	Y_2	Y_3	Y_4	Y_5
Frequency/Regularity of BSE (Y_1)	1.00				
Number of BSE Positions Performed (Y_2)	.06 (408)	1.00			
Time Spent Performing BSE (Y_3)	− .05 (425)	.11* (409)	1.00		
19 Step Quality of BSE Performance Measure (Y_4)	.09 (408)	.55* (431)	.11 (409)	1.00	
Validated Quality of Performance Index (5 Steps) (Y_5)	.08 (408)	.65* (431)	.08 (409)	.53* (431)	1.00

Table 3.   Associations of BSE Performance Measures:
Mothers' Baseline Telephone Survey (N)

	Y_1	Y_2	Y_3	Y_4	Y_5
Frequency/Regularity of BSE (Y_1)	1.00				
Number of BSE Positions Performed (Y_2)	− .05 (76)	1.00			
Time Spent Performing BSE (Y_3)	.35* (72)	.08 (76)	1.00		
19 Step Quality of BSE Performance Measure (Y_4)	.15 (76)	.53* (79)	.34* (76)	1.00	
Validated Quality of Performance Index (5 Steps) (Y_5)	− .01 (76)	.70* (79)	.15 (76)	.66* (79)	1.00

* Significance $\leq$.01

As is also evidenced in these tables, the validated quality index measure does not have a strong association to frequency/regularity of BSE performance or to amount of time spent performing BSE. Number of BSE positions is the only other BSE measure that has a moderately large association to the five-step validated quality score. The size of this association was expected to be large, given that the quality measure is composed of the three positions as well as two other items. The associations in Table 3 are for the older age population, the mothers. The sizes of the associations are different for quality as it relates to the other BSE measures but they follow the same order of magnitudeaas the correlations of the students; with quality having the strongest association with number of positions and the smallest association with regularity of performance.

DISCUSSION

The data presented provide support for the importance of examining quality of BSE performance and ensuring that:

1)   the criteria used for determing quality are clearly identified; and

2)   that if the measure does not include direct observation it is critical to be able to assess how the reporting method reflects reality (i.e. actual demonstration).

In this paper, the analysis of a quality measure began with the ideal components identified by ACS and NCI. Some components were not highly congruent with behavior; many items were reported incorrectly (false negatives as well as false positives) on the self-report of BSE quality. The results of the level of quality performance varied significantly, thus indicating that when using an indirect measure of BSE, its concurrent validity with demonstration must be determined.

This study does not address the issue of which criteria should be used as the ultimate criterion standard for BSE quality. Without a prospective study that examines components of quality and its impact on lump detection, it is impossible to arrive at a definitive answer regarding which criteria need to be included in a BSE quality score.

Since no definitive quality measure can be delineated at the present time, it is even more imperative that studies systematically report what criteria are used to measure BSE quality.

Findings on the relationships of quality of BSE to other BSE measures also indicate that quality is a distinct dimension of BSE behavior. This paper contends that it is the most critical dimension to eventually determine the effectiveness of BSE educational efforts and ultimately the efficacy.

ACKNOWLEDGEMENTS

The authors would like to acknowledge programming assistance from Kathryn C. Docie.

REFERENCES

American Cancer Society (1981). Cancer facts and figures. New York: American Cancer Society, Inc., p. 11.

National Center for Health Statistics (1982). Vital Statistics of the United States, 1978, Vol II, Part B. DHHS Publ. No. (PHS) 82-1102. Public Health Service, Washington, U.S. Government Printing Office, 1982.

Shapiro S (1977). Evidence on screening for breast cancer from a randomized trial. Cancer 39:2772.

Greenwald P, Nasca PC, Lawrence CE, Horton J, McGarrah, RP, Gabriele T, Carlton K (1978). Estimate effect of breast self-examination and routine physicians' examination on breast cancer mortality. N Eng J Med 299:271.

Department of Health and Human Services (1981). Recommendations of the National Cancer Institute and the American Cancer Society on screening for breast cancer of asymptomatic women (memorandum). National Institutes of Health, Public Health Service.

National Cancer Institute (1981). Breast Exams, What you should know? (NIH Pub. No. 82-1000), Bethesda.

American Cancer Society (1980). Cancer facts and figures, New York: American Cancer Society, Inc., p. 15.

Crosson K, et al (1978). Health education research in preventive oncology: A study of factors influencing the practice of breast self-examination. The Fox Chase Cancer Center, Grant N01-CN-45055, NCI, DHEW.

Lynch I, et al (1978). Mobile cancer screening: Epidemiologic and cancer control model. In Prevention and detection of cancer, Newbergs H (ed) Part II, Vol. I.

Grady KE, Kegeles SS, Lund AK (1980). Experimental studies to increase BSE-preliminary findings. In Progress in clinical and biological research. Volume 83, C. Mettlin, GP Murphy (eds). Issues in cancer screening and communications. New York: Alan R. Liss, Inc.

National Cancer Institute (1980). National survey on breast cancer: A measure of progress in public understanding. NIH Pub. No. 81-2306. Public Health Service, Washington, Government Printing Office.

Trotta P (1980). Breast self-examination: Factors influencing compliance. Oncology Nurse Forum 7:13.

Huguley CM, Brown RL (1982). The value of breast self-examination. Cancer 47:989.

Laughter D, et al (1981). The breast self-examination practices of high risk women: implications for patient education. Pat Coun Health Ed, p. 103.

Adams CK, et al (1976). Lump detection in simulated human breasts. Precept Psychophysics 29:163.

Hall DC, Goldstein MK, Stein GH (1977). Progress in manual breast examination. Cancer 49:364.

Hall DC et al (1980). Improved detection of human breast lesions following experimental training. Cancer 46:408.

Howe HL (1980). Proficiency in performing breast self-examination. Pat Coun Health Ed 4:1521.

Zapka J, Mamon J (1982). Integration of theory practitioner standards, literature findings and baseline data: A case study in planning breast self examination education. Health Educ Quarterly (Winter).

Mamon J, Zapka J (Forthcoming). Determining validity of measuring the quality of breast self-examination: Comparisons of written questionnaire with demonstration.

Lieberman,S (1977). Study of the Effectiveness of alternate breast cancer education programs. Lieberman Research, Inc., New York.

Progress in Cancer Control IV: Research in the Cancer Center, pages 323–329
© **1983 Alan R. Liss, Inc., 150 Fifth Avenue, New York, NY 10011**

THE RELATIONSHIP BETWEEN BREAST SELF-EXAMINATION FREQUENCY,
TECHNIQUE, AND BREAST LUMP DETECTION

Annlouise Assaf, M.S., K. Michael Cummings, Ph.D.
Debra Walsh, M.A.

Roswell Park Memorial Institute
Buffalo, New York 14263

The importance of early diagnosis of breast cancer has
been emphasized in the literature in recent years. Breast
self-examination (BSE) has been widely advocated as a useful early detection tool. However, the effectiveness of
breast self-examination as a screening method for breast
cancer has been the cause of much controversy. Several
retrospective studies have indicated that frequent performance of breast self-examination is associated with more
favorable clinical and pathological stages of breast cancer
(Feldman et al. 1981; Foster et al. 1978; Greenwald et al.
1978; Mahoney et al. 1979). Other retrospective studies,
however, have failed to find this association (Senie et al.
1981; Smith et al. 1980). One reason for the discrepancy in
these studies may be that the woman's ability to properly
perform BSE has not been assessed.

A recent study by Howe examined the association between
BSE frequency, BSE technique and lump detection. She found
that technique was a better indicator of a woman's ability
to detect lumps in a simulated breast model than was frequency of BSE practice (Howe 1980). Moreover, Howe found
that many women who report practicing BSE do not do the
procedure correctly. The present study re-examines the
questions of BSE frequency and technique as they relate to
a woman's ability to detect lumps in silicone breast models.
This study also evaluates the effectiveness of different
methods of training women to properly perform BSE.

The study was conducted in Buffalo, New York at the
Roswell Park Memorial Institute Prevention Detection Clinic.

The study population consisted of three hundred and eighty-eight women between the ages of 18 and 70 who were seen in the Clinic for a routine cancer screening examination. The mean age of the participants was 51 years. Subjects were predominantly white, married, middle class women. Eighty percent had at least a high school education.

The study utilized a post-test only control group design to evaluate the effects of the three different approaches for training women to perform BSE. These teaching approaches were: (1) presenting women with a pamphlet detailing the proper technique for BSE; (2) having women view a 6½ minute video presentation on BSE technique and presenting them with a pamphlet detailing proper BSE technique; and (3) having women practice BSE on a breast model with simulated breast lumps under the supervision of a nurse-teacher until they had mastered the technique and presenting them with a pamphlet detailing proper BSE technique. Each woman was seen for a follow-up interview three months after her initial visit and training session. It was during this interview that BSE frequency, BSE technique, and lump detection were measured.

BSE frequency was defined as the number of times per month that the woman reported practicing breast self-examination in the three months following her initial clinic visit and BSE training session. This measure was categorized into four groups: (1) never; (2) less than once a month; (3) once a month; and (4) more than once a month. Each woman was asked to demonstrate her BSE technique by palpating two silicone breast models. These models were modified to each contain two simulated breast lumps ranging in size from 0.5cm to 4.0cm. Lump detection accuracy was measured as the total number of lumps found by the woman during these two exams. BSE technique was determined by having the interviewer observe and record the steps used by each woman as she examined the two silicone breast models. These steps included: (1) feeling all parts of the breast; (2) pressing down firmly and deeply; (3) using an acceptable pattern of palpation; (4) using the pads of the fingers during palpation; (5) squeezing the nipple area; and (6) beginning the examination at the top of the breast (12 o'clock). The total number of steps performed correctly during the two exams was calculated to form a measure of BSE technique. The possible range of scores on this measure was from zero to twelve. For purposes of these analyses, our measure of BSE technique was divided into four categories: (1) no steps done dorrectly; (2) one to four steps done correctly; (3) five to eight steps done correctly; and (4) nine to twelve steps done correctly.

Since the BSE training interventions which were tested in this study may confound the associations between BSE frequency, technique, and lump detection, analyses were done separately on each experimental group. These analyses showed that associations between BSE frequency, technique, and lump detection did not vary significantly among the different BSE training groups. Therefore, the results presented in this paper are for the combined groups.

Table 1

BSE FREQUENCY BY LUMP DETECTION

| BSE practice last three months | Total Number of Lumps Correctly Detected | | | | |
	None	One	Two	Three	Four
Never (n=62)	19%	26%	18%	24%	13%
< Once a month (n=112)	13	28	15	21	23
Once a month (n=94)	3	20	22	29	26
> Once a month (n=117)	11	26	15	27	21

As shown in Table 1, reported frequency of BSE practice is not associated with the number of lumps correctly detected in the silicone breast models. Only one quarter of the women who reported practicing BSE once a month were able to detect all four breast lumps. Forty-five percent of these regular BSE practicers were only able to find two lumps or less. Women who reported practicing BSE more than once a month had even lower lump detection accuracy than those practicing only once a month.

Table 2

BSE TECHNIQUE BY LUMP DETECTION

Number of BSE steps done correctly	Total Number of Lumps Correctly Detected				
	None	One	Two	Three	Four
None (n=79)	28%	49%	15%	8%	0%
One to Four (n=129)	10	30	24	27	9
Five to Eight (n=143)	6	13	13	31	37
Nine to Twelve (n=35)	0	3	17	29	51

Table 2 shows that the number of lumps a woman is able to detect in a silicone breast model is positively related to the number of BSE components she performs correctly. More than half of the women who performed the greatest number of correct steps in their exam (i.e. had the best BSE technique) found all four lumps. More than a quarter of the women who did not do any of the correct steps were not able to find any lumps.

Table 3 shows that reported frequency of BSE practice is not strongly associated with the number of BSE steps a woman performs correctly. While those who report not practicing BSE were least likely to perform the technique properly, there is little difference in the number of BSE steps performed between those women who report practicing BSE less than once a month and those who report practicing BSE once a month or more.

If BSE is to become an effective early detection tool for breast cancer, it appears that women need to be trained how to do the procedure correctly. Our results indicate that frequent examination will not compensate for improper technique.

Table 3

BSE FREQUENCY BY BSE TECHNIQUE

| BSE practice last three months | Number of BSE Steps Done Correctly | | | |
	None	One to Four	Five to Eight	Nine to Twelve
Never (n=63)	33%	38%	27%	2%
< Once a month (n=113)	20	29	42	9
Once a month (n=94)	16	25	44	15
> Once a month (n=117)	19	41	32	8

A second part of our study examined different methods of training women to perform BSE. Table 4 indicates that the women who received individual training and practice on the silicone breast models performed a significantly higher number of correct steps in their exams three months after their training than did the women who received their training via a pamphlet or a video presentation. Table 5 shows that the same relationship exists between method of BSE training and number of breast lumps correctly detected.

In summary, we have found that many women who report practicing BSE regularly do not do the technique properly. Secondly, the technique used in breast self examination appears to be a better indicator of ability to detect lumps in a breast model than is frequency of BSE practice. Finally, it appears that BSE technique is affected by the type of training a woman receives. Since BSE proficiency is influenced by the method of training a woman receives, it is imperative to continue working on the development of an effective method of BSE training. The findings from the present study seem to indicate that training methods which rely on passive or vicarious learning are not effective in teaching women how to do BSE properly. The opportunity for practice and positive reinforcement seems to be important to the BSE learning process.

Table 4

BSE TECHNIQUE BY BSE TRAINING METHOD

Number of BSE Steps Done Correctly

BSE Training Method	None	One to Four	Five to Eight	Nine to Twelve
Pamphlet Only (n=142)	38%	37%	23%	2%
Video and Pamphlet (n=123)	15	42	38	5
Nurse Training and Pamphlet (n=121)	6	20	53	21

Table 5

LUMP DETECTION BY BSE TRAINING METHOD

Total Number of Lumps Correctly Detected

BSE Training Method	None	One	Two	Three	Four
Pamphlet Only (n=142)	15%	35%	15%	25%	10%
Video and Pamphlet (n=123)	14	32	20	17	17
Nurse training and pamphlet (n=121)	3	7	17	33	40

Mean Number of Lumps Correctly Detected: Pamphlet = 1.79
Video = 1.92
Nurse = 2.89

Feldman JG, Carter AC, Nicastri AD, Hosat ST (1981). Breast self-examination, relationship to stage of breast cancer at diagnosis. Cancer 47:2740.

Foster RS, Lang S, Castanza M, et al. (1978). Breast self-examination practice and breast cancer stage. N Engl J Med 299:265.

Greenwald P, Nasca P, Lawrence C, et al. (1978). Estimated effect of breast self-examination and routine physicians examinations on breast cancer mortality. N Engl J Med 299:271.

Howe HL (1980). Proficiency in performing breast self-examination. Patient Counseling and Health Education 4th Quarter:151.

Mahoney LJ, Bird BL, Cooke GM (1979). Annual clinical examination: The best available screening test for breast cancer. N Engl J Med 301:315.

Senie RT, Rosen PP, Lesser ML, Kinne DW (1981). Breast self-examination and medical examination related to breast cancer stage. Am J Public Hlth 71:583.

Smith EM, Francis AM, Polissar L (1980). The effect of breast self-exam and physician examinations on extent of disease at diagnosis. Prev Med 9:409.

Progress in Cancer Control IV: Research in the Cancer Center, pages 331–339
© **1983 Alan R. Liss, Inc., 150 Fifth Avenue, New York, NY 10011**

VALIDATION OF BREAST SELF-EXAMINATION PRACTICE RELATED TO
FREQUENCY AND COMPETENCY OF BSE

David D. Celentano, Sc.D.

School of Hygiene and Public Health
The Johns Hopkins University
Baltimore, MD   21205

INTRODUCTION

Mortality from breast cancer among women in the United
States has remained fairly constant and high over the last
four decades and remains a cause of great concern (Petrakis
et al. 1982). While a large proportion of available cancer
control resources have been directed at pretreatment evaluation, treatment, and rehabilitation of women with breast
cancer, early detection has also received attention, particularly through promotional campaigns directed at both
providers and consumers to adopt certain preventive health
behaviors. One of the more widespread secondary prevention
measures which has received considerable support from those
in cancer control and in the medical community at large has
been breast self-examination (BSE). The BSE procedure has
been widely recommended for most women (Eddy 1980), and it
is hoped that proper BSE conducted at regular intervals
will lead to earlier detection of breast abnormalities, and,
hopefully, to reduced mortality. Despite the widespread
acceptance of BSE as a useful cancer control measure, there
is no concensus in the current literature on the relationship of BSE to the detection of breast abnormalities, to
stage at diagnosis, or to patient survivorship.

THE EVIDENCE FROM THE LITERATURE

The relatively large and growing literature on BSE
shows that there are a number of reports that women who have
breast cancer commonly detect abnormalities themselves.

Other reports show that physicians are more effective at detecting breast abnormalities and tumors. Greenwald et al. (1978) reported that breast cancer patients who performed BSE were more likely to detect their tumors while performing BSE rather than by accidental discovery or during a routine physical examination. Huguley and Brown (1981) reported that women who did monthly BSE were more likely to detect tumors themselves during routine breast checks than by accident as compared to women who did not report conducting BSE. Smith et al. (1980) also found similar findings, although one cannot determine whether patients in this study discovered their tumors purposively through BSE or accidentally. On the less optimistic side, Mahoney et al. (1979) followed a cohort of women for six years to ascertain the sensitivity and utility of a number of cancer screening measures, of which BSE was one technique included. The women were all taught BSE and judged competent (although no criteria of competency were given). During the study interval 128 new lesions were detected, although approximately two-thirds were discovered only during routine physical examination, with the remainder being found during BSE (23%) or accidentally (11%).

With respect to the relationship between BSE and stage of disease at diagnosis, the evidence is mixed. Three groups of investigators (Foster et al. 1978; Greenwald et al. 1978; Huguley and Brown 1981) found smaller tumors, on average, to be associated with doing BSE or with more frequent performance. Smith et al. (1980) and Senie et al. (1981), however, failed to show similar relationships. Cole and Austin (1981) suggest that BSE can best be useful when no other detection practices are used. While this conclusion warrants study (none of these reports have data directly addressing the issue), another factor which might account for the lack of consistency in findings is that the determination and measurement of the BSE practice itself varies considerably in the various investigations. In some of the reports BSE practice as a dichotomous outcome is considered, while others report on the frequency of BSE, the regularity of BSE or the monthly timing of the behavior. Of potentially greater interest is a remaining question: Are the women who report performing BSE conducting the procedure in the recommended way? While women may report doing BSE, what they are actually doing may bear little resemblance to the concensus recommendations on correct procedure. Only one of the five studies cited ascertained the validity of the

BSE technique, although no methodology was given. The study presented here is focused at determining the extent to which women are competent in performing BSE using a methodology based on self-reported behavior. This measure was related to a number of criterion variables related to BSE to give a validation of the behavior.

METHODS

A telephone survey of one sector of Baltimore, Maryland was conducted in 1981 to ascertain the prevalence and correlates of behavioral risk factors in the population as well as to assess the current preventive health behaviors and participation in cancer control programs. Geographically, this area lies in northeast Baltimore and has a population of 75,000 persons, is two-fifths black, and contains a mixed socioeconomic population, ranging from a large poverty community to an affluent fringe suburb. To obtain a sample of households, a sampling frame was constructed using a current 'reverse' telephone directory, and a systematic sample of telephone-serviced households was drawn for study. A sample of 308 women, representing a response rate of 85% of eligible households, was obtained, and interviews lasting approximately 25 minutes were conducted by trained female interviewers who were quite experienced in conducting cancer control interviews (Celentano et al. 1982).

During the course of the interview, data on sociodemographic factors, health care utilization patterns, knowledge and attitudes towards cancer screening, and a number of questions on BSE were included. The specific questions on BSE included: (1) current BSE practice; (2) how and from whom they learned BSE (and whether they were asked to demonstrate their competency to their teacher); (3) their perceived confidence in performing BSE; and (4) a description of exactly how and in what position(s) they actually perform the technique. It is this indicator which was used to ascertain BSE competency.

The measure of BSE competency described here is an adaptation of the NCI measure of BSE behavior used in the 1979 national survey of women (Zdep et al. 1981) which incorporated ACS recommendations on the correct technique for performing BSE. The NCI "thoroughness score" (Table 1) was the basic indicator of competency used, consisting of the simple sum of six steps. However, these scores incorporate both position and technique, often blurring the distinction between the specific procedures relevant for the different positions. The measure used here (Table 2) is a score which is based upon 4-6 steps for each of three positions: (1) lying down; (2) standing up (often "in the shower"); and (3) the "mirror" position. The reliability of the measure reached acceptable limits, having internal consistency reliability of approximately 0.70.

TABLE 1

NCI "THOROUGHNESS SCORE"

1. Circular Motion; feel around; examine nipples
2. Lying down; lying on pillow
3. Upright; in shower
4. Arm over head; behind head
5. Under arms
6. Looking

TABLE 2

"COMPETENCY SCORES"

Lying Down:
1. Hand behind head; prop
2. Opposite hand
3. Fingers flat-finger tips
4. Small circular motions; outward-inward; around
5. Check nipple - discharge
6. Armpit area, underarm

Upright:
1. Two-three fingers; flat
2. Opposite hand; arm up
3. Circular motion; outward-inward; all around
4. Breast changes, soreness
5. Armpit area, underarm
6. Check nipple

Mirror:
1. Arms at sides
2. Raise arms overhead
3. Look - nipple abnormality, dimpling, discoloration
4. Press palms on hips, fex chest muscles

Sophistication:
1. Fingers flat
2. Armpit, underarm mentioned
3. Nipple changes, discharge

RESULTS

86% of the women reported that they had performed BSE at some point, and approximately 76% (or 235 women) reported that they had done BSE at least one time during the preceding twelve months. It is this sample that serves as the group for examining the relation between self-reported BSE behavior, frequency of BSE, and related factors.

The distributions across the BSE position scores and the overall summed competency measure showed little overt awareness of the correct methods of performing BSE in this sample (Table 3) The average competency score was only 4.2 out of a possible range of 19 points. Nearly 20% of the women who reported performing BSE could name only one step, and nearly one-half (43%) could name fewer than four steps. Indeed, only a handful of women (6%) could name eight or more of the proper BSE steps. Thus, the knowledge of the BSE procedure is quite low in this sample as measured by self-reports.

TABLE 3
BSE COMPETENCY SCORES

Position	Mean Score	S.D.	Range
Lying Down	1.93	1.54	0-6
Standing Up	0.85	1.33	0-6
Mirror	0.14	0.58	0-4
Sophistication	1.24	0.62	0-3
Competency	4.16	2.29	0-19

BSE competency scores were correlated with a number of factors considered to be important to BSE ability (Table 4). Women who performed BSE at the recommended frequency (i.e., monthly) had significantly higher competency scores than women who performed BSE less frequently. Further, women who report that they were taught BSE by a health professional (e.g., by a physician - most commonly - or a nurse) were significantly higher on the BSE measures than those who were not personally taught how to perform BSE. This latter group most commonly report having read about BSE in a women's magazine or having seen a film. Of the women who reported having been taught BSE (approximately one-half of the sample) there were no differences in competency whether or not they had been asked to demonstrate their proficiency to the instructor. When the amount of time usually taken to perform BSE was analyzed, no differences in BSE scores could be detected, thereby putting into question some of the findings reported earlier. If women are (or can be) motivated to perform BSE but they do not spend sufficient time doing the procedure, they are not very likely to detect any abnormalities that may exist nor notice any of the more subtle changes that occur over time. Finally, perceived confidence in their ability to do BSE was associated with higher competency scores as well as to more frequent BSE.

TABLE 4

PREDICTORS OF BSE COMPETENCY AND FREQUENCY[a]

CHARACTERISTIC	(N)	$\overline{X}$ COMPETENCY	t	$\overline{X}$ FREQUENCY	t
Taught BSE:					
Yes	(148)	4.50		1.49	
No	(87)	3.59	3.01**	1.62	2.00*
BSE Confidence					
Some, Very	(175)	4.46		1.48	
Little, None	(60)	3.28	3.53**	1.70	2.99**
BSE Frequency					
Monthly	(109)	4.59			
Semi-Monthly	(126)	3.79	2.69**	--	--

[a] Frequency coded 1=monthly, 2=less frequently than monthly
* $p < .05$ ** $p < .01$

Overall, neither age or race was associated with BSE competency, although when competency was dichotomized at the median (a score of 4 on the overall measure), women with higher scores were significantly younger than women who had lower scores (46 and 54 years, respectively). No socioeconomic differentials could be detected, whether measured by annual income, educational attainment or occupational prestige. Multiple regression analyses were conducted with both BSE Competency and BSE frequency as dependent variables. For BSE Competency, only having been taught BSE by a health professional and perceived confidence in the

BSE technique were significant predictors (R^2=0.09, p <.01). For BSE frequency, only perceived confidence and race (being white) were significant variables (R^2=0.10, p <.01). In neither analysis were utilization factors, knowledge and attitudes about preventive care or cancer, knowledge of the cancer symptoms and signs, perceived susceptibility to cancer, or socioeconomic status factors of importance.

CONCLUSIONS

On the basis of these data there is some evidence that a valid methodology for ascertaining BSE competency has been developed. Certainly, there are some indications of construct validity, although some of the hypothesized relations failed to attain significance. The lack of correlation of BSE competency or frequency to the amount of time spent in performing the BSE technique is particularly critical from a health education perspective. Of greatest importance is the documentation that while a large number of women may report performing BSE, few are actually aware of and can describe the proper method for performing BSE. Indeed, there is evidence that this is not an artifact of the methodology itself, for verbal ability was not found to be a variable related to BSE competency (given education and occupational prestige as proxy measures of verbal ability).

The findings of this study offer evidence that some of the contradictory findings relating BSE practice to both tumor detection and to stage of disease at diagnosis may be due to unreliable and invalid measurement of the key independent variable -- BSE itself. Given the great care that is often the hallmark of good clinical epidemiological studies in selecting cases and standardizing treatment and follow-up, so too must the ascertainment of BSE as a factor related to breast cancer. The same attention to determining BSE should be given as that of symptoms and history.

The implications for health education are self-evident. As with most complex behaviors, it is essential to determine the extent of knowledge rather than merely determining the presence or absence of a self-report. Given the problems of acquiescence associated with ascertaining preventive health practices, greater vigilance needs to be paid to eliciting behavior related to BSE.

REFERENCES

Celentano DD, Shapiro S, Weisman C (1982). Cancer preventive screening behavior among elderly women. Prev Med 11: 454.

Cole P, Austin H (1981). Breast self-examination: an adjuvant to early cancer detection. Am J Publ Health 71:572.

Eddy D (1980). Guidelines for the cancer-related checkup; recommendations and rationale. Cancer J Clin 30:194.

Foster RS, Lang SP, Costanza MC, Worden JK, Haines CR, Yates JW (1978). Breast self-examination and breast cancer stage. N Engl J Med 299:265.

Greenwald P, Nasca PC, Lawrence CE, Horton J, McGarrah RP, Gabriele T, Carlton K (1978). Estimated effect of breast self-examination and routine physician examinations on breast-cancer mortality. N Engl J Med 299:271.

Huguley CM, Brown RL (1981). The value of breast self-examination. Cancer 47:989.

Mahoney LJ, Bird BL, Cooke GM (1979). The best available screening test for breast cancer. N Eng J Med 301:315.

Petrakis NL, Ernster VL, King M-C (1982). Breast. In Shottenfeld D, Fraumeni JF (eds): "Cancer Epidemiology and Prevention," Philadelphi: W.B.Saunders, p 855.

Senie RT, Rosen PP, Lesser ML, Kinne DW (1981). Breast self-examination and medical examination related to breast cancer stage. Am J Publ Health 71:583.

Smith EM, Francis AM, Polissar L.(1980). The effect of breast self-exam practices and physician examinations on extent of disease at diagnosis. Prev Med 9:409.

Zdep SM, Kilkenny MJ, Jaworski CM, Spiller GG, Stryker JG, Willey AL, Keeney DA (1981). "Breast Cancer: A Measure of Prdgress in Public Understanding," NIH Publication No. 81-2291. Bethesda: National Cancer Institute.

ACKNOWLEDGEMENTS

I wish to thank Drs. Carol Weisman, Margaret Dear, Joyce Mamon and Deborah Holtzman for their suggestions, Professor Sam Shapiro for his guidance and ideas, and Dr. T.P. Waalkes of the Johns Hopkins Oncology Center for his support. This work was supported in part by Grant CA20322 from the National Cancer Institute.

Progress in Cancer Control IV: Research in the Cancer Center, pages 341–350
© 1983 Alan R. Liss, Inc., 150 Fifth Avenue, New York, NY 10011

MULTISITE CANCER SCREENING OF WOMEN IN A RURAL POPULATION

Ned D. Rodes, M.D., Charles W. Blackwell, M.D.,
Dinah K. Pearson, B.A.
Cancer Research Center
P.O. Box 1268
Columbia, Missouri 65205

The Cancer Research Center, Columbia, Missouri, was selected, in 1974, as the site for one of 27 Breast Cancer Detection Demonstration Projects (BCDDP) in the United States. Several features made the Cancer Research Center project unique, but the longterm, sustained participation of the women and the high level of cooperation by Missouri physicians are two outstanding features.

Consequently, the Cancer Research Center expanded the program in 1979, naming it the Women's Cancer Control Program (WCCP). This new program offers screening for cancers of the breast, colorectum, and uterine-cervix, as well as for hypertension. Since the Cancer Research Center has retained its BCDDP core staff for the WCCP, the cumulative experience and resulting expertise lend credibility, reliability, and consistency to the total effort, especially to breast cancer screening, which the Cancer Research Center has pursued continuously since 1974.

THE BREAST CANCER DETECTION DEMONSTRATION PROJECT

The experience of the 27 national Breast Cancer Detection Demonstration Projects has established the value of the combination of physical examination and mammography in the detection of curable cancers (Beahrs, Shapiro, Smart, McDivitt 1979; Gohagan, Rodes, Ballinger, Blackwell, Butcher, Darby, Pearson, Spitznagel, Wallack 1982; Pearson, Blackwell, Sullivan, Rodes 1980). One hundred thirty-six

(136) cancers were detected by the Cancer Research Center's BCDDP in 10,000 participants during five years of screening. Mammography was the sole mode of detection in 56% of the cases, 30% were found by mammography and physical examination, 14% by palpation alone.

The Cancer Research Center has followed 152 cases of breast cancer among the BCDDP participants for at least five years; some have been observed for nine years. The 152 cases include 136 detected by the BCDDP and 16 not found by screening. Only 15 of the women have died: 12 of advanced breast cancer, three of other causes. The 12 either had clinical symptoms when screened or were among the 16 whose cancers were not detected in the BCDDP.

The expected annual incidence of breast cancer in the United States is .7/1000. At the Cancer Research Center, the prevalence rate was 6/1000 and the annual incidence rate ranged from 2/1000 to 3/1000. The large yield of breast cancers is probably due to several factors: 1) the volunteer, self-selected, high-risk group of women; 2) improved mammographic technique; 3) lead time and length of bias inherent in screening (Smart, Beahrs 1979).

THE WOMEN'S CANCER CONTROL PROGRAM

One objective of the BCDDP was to provide basis for continued screening. Therefore, the Cancer Research Center initiated the Women's Cancer Control Program to screen for the three most prevalent cancers. Breast, colorectal, and uterine-cervix cancers comprise 56% of all cancers in women in the United States.

To be eligible to participate in the WCCP, women must be at least 35 years-of-age and asymptomatic at the time of their initial visit. During fiscal years 1980-82, 6,735 women were screened at least one time and the total number of annual visits through June, 1982, reached 14,664. The WCCP staff examines more than 30 women per day, five days a week. Participants come from 112 of Missouri's 115 counties.

Each woman is offered the opportunity to participate in all screening tests annually: breast, palpation

and mammography; colon, Hemoccult II; uterine-cervix, Pap
smear; and blood pressure. However, she may decline any of
the examinations and is not obligated to return for annual
visits.

At the time of the initial visit, each woman provides
the name of her private physician. If any of the test
results are abnormal, the private physician and the participant are notified. Although the WCCP staff is always
available for consultation, the woman and her physician
handle all arrangements for diagnostic tests and treatment. The WCCP staff follows each case to determine what
action has been taken. The medical staff determines the
appropriate time for the next WCCP appointment.

Because of the lag-time involved in receiving
pathology reports and other followup information, only the
first three years of the program are discussed.

Colorectal Cancer Screening

The prognosis for individuals with colorectal cancer
is related directly to the stage of the disease at the time
of diagnosis. Patients with Duke's Stage A, confined to
the mucosa, have a five-year survival rate of almost 90%.
Only 27% of the patients with metastasis to the regional
lymph nodes live five years (Hardcastle, Balfour, Amar
1980). The survival rate is somewhat better for patients
with cancers of the colon than for those with rectal
cancers (Winawer, Sherlock, Miller 1979).

Almost all cancers of the colon and rectum bleed
intermittently. Screening for colorectal cancers is
possible, therefore, by using the simple, inexpensive
guaiac-impregnated slides (Hemoccult). This test is
effective and renders the fewest "false positives" when
women who are screened follow a simple meat-free,
high-fiber diet for 48 hours and then collect samples from
three consecutive bowel movements (Fazio 1979). The false
negative rate is reduced when these specimens are examined
promptly after collection. Ideally, the specimens should
be examined on the day of the final collection, but never
more than four days after the collection of the third
specimen.

The WCCP offers the Hemoccult II test as part of each participant's annual visit. With her appointment letter, each woman receives a Hemoccult II kit and detailed instructions regarding diet and collection of specimens. The participant is encouraged to start the diet five days prior to her scheduled appointment so that the final specimen collection will occur on the day of the appointment. Ninety-five percent of the participants complete the procedure, finding it aesthetically satisfactory. Although not all women have three bowel movements during the three-day period, more than 99% of the slides are prepared properly.

During the 14,664 annual visits, almost 14,000 sets of Hemoccult II slides were submitted for evaluation. Test results from slides prepared by 454 women were interpreted as positive; that is, at least a trace of blood was present on one or more of the slides. Most women submit six slides, two slides from each of three consecutive bowel movements.

Whenever a Hemoccult II test result indicates blood, the medical staff notifies the participant and her private physician, recommending colonoscopy and barium enema for further workup. These recommendations are based on a randomized, controlled study of occult blood in stool specimens that is being conducted on 48,000 asymptomatic people between the ages of 50 and 80 years (Nivatvongs, Gilbertsen, Goldberg, Williams 1982).

The WCCP follows each participant who needs a colonic workup to learn which, if any, diagnostic procedures are performed. Table 1 presents the diagnostic procedures and Table 2 identifies the diagnosis. Many WCCP participants are not given thorough followup tests. Without doubt, some early colon cancers and neoplastic polyps are undiagnosed.

Studies show that when asymptomatic individuals over the age of 40 years are screened, approximately 1% will have positive test results. When these people are subjected to thorough colonic workups, approximately 10% are found to have cancer. An additional 30%-40% have neoplastic polyps (Vanneman 1980).

TABLE 1

Diagnostic Procedures Performed on 454 Women Whose
Hemoccult Test Results Were Positive

No Workup		183
Participant did not contact physician	10	
Participant refused workup	8	
Physician decided workup unnecessary	28	
Hemoccult II test repeated - negative	121	
Hemoccult II test repeated - positive	16	
Diagnostic Workup Performed		261
At least colonoscopy and barium enema	59	
At least colonoscopy	18	
At least barium enema and procto- sigmoidoscopy	68	
At least barium enema	68	
At least proctosigmoidoscopy	32	
At least upper gastrointestinal test	3	
Other diagnostic studies	13	
Incomplete Followup Information		10

TABLE 2

Diagnosis For 261 Women Who Had Colonic Workup

Malignant	10
Benign polyps	26
Diverticulosis	41
Hemorrhoids	26
Other benign conditions	42
No definitive diagnosis	116

Screening for Breast Cancer

Breast cancer screening is the primary focus of the
WCCP. The physical inspection and palpation of the breasts
includes having the participant place her hands on her hips
while seated. The nurse asks her to press her hands down
firmly, flex her chest muscles, then to elevate her arms
over her head. The examiner visually inspects the breasts

for symmetry of shape, size, and contour, checking the
nipples and skin surface.

Next, the woman is placed in a supine position. Her
arm is placed above her head on the side to be examined.
The nurse firmly palpates the breast tissue in a clockwise
motion with her fingers flat, using her four fingertips on
both hands. The palpation begins at the outermost portion
of the breast at the 12 o'clock positon and progresses in
continuous circles toward and including the nipple.
Finally, the nipple is gently milked to check for
discharge. If a discharge is found, a Pap smear is obtained. The axillary and supraclavicular regions are
examined for evidence of bulging, edema, discoloration, or
retraction. As the nurse examines the participant, she
explains her findings while teaching the woman how to
examine her breasts. If a mass or thickening is present,
the nurse carefully measures it and records its texture,
mobility, and shape. Finally, she diagrams the area.

The mammogram has been the major factor in earlier
detection of breast disease during the past two decades.
Evidence from the Breast Cancer Detection Demonstration
Projects shows that good quality mammography is the most
important modality for detecting clinically occult breast
cancers (Beahrs, Shapiro, Smart, McDivitt 1979). Not only
is mammography capable of detecting preclinical lesions, it
is also beneficial in the differential diagnosis of
clinically evident or questionable breast abnormalities.

Either technique of mammography (film or Xerox)
produces high quality diagnostic images. The Cancer
Research Center uses the Xerox process exclusively because
the radiologist prefers its speed, ease of interpretation,
and reliability.

At the Cancer Research Center two views are routine:
the recumbent mediolateral and the cephalocaudad.
Occasionally, additional views may be necessary.

Through June, 1982, the WCCP had made 250 specific
recommendations for breast biopsies. Pathology reports
have been received on 80% of the cases. There were six
aspirations, 132 benign diseases, and 53 breast cancers.
Almost 30% of the biopsies performed revealed cancer. The

prevalence and incidence rates of breast cancers are
indicated in Tables 3 and 4.

TABLE 3

Prevalence of Breast Cancer in 2988 New Participants

21 Breast Cancers (Prevalence)
    Family history - 6 women
    Diagnosis - 15 infiltrating, 6 intraductal
    Nodes - 15, no cancer; 2 women with 1 cancerous
        node, 3 with 3, 1 with 9
    Lesion Size - 1 lesion $\leq$ 1cm, 5 were 1-2cm,
        4 were 2-3cm, 2 were 3cm,
        9, not indicated
    Detection modality - 20 mammography,
        14 physical examination
    Surgery - 15 modified radical mastectomies,
        3 simple mastectomies, 2 radical
        mastectomies, 1 excisional biopsy

TABLE 4

Incidence of Breast Cancers in 3747 Previously Screened
Participants

32 Breast Cancers (Incidence)
    Family history - 6
    Diagnosis - 29 infiltrating, 3 intraductal
    Nodes - 21, no cancer; 4 women with 1 cancerous
        node, 2 with 2, 2 with 3, 1 with 4,
        1 with 5, 1 with 8
    Lesion size - 7 lesions $\leq$ 1cm, 11 were 1-2cm,
        5 were 2-3cm, 1 was 5cm,
        8, not indicated
    Detection modality - 31 mammography,
        24 physical examination
    Surgery - 21 modified radical mastectomies,
        7 radical mastectomies, 3 simple
        mastectomies, 1 excisional biopsy

Although it is neither a detection modality nor part
of routine screening, the WCCP has performed diagnostic
ultrasound on all women with palpable or mammographic

breast masses since April, 1981. While ultrasound is not
always beneficial, it is useful in many cases to distin-
guish cystic from solid lesions.

Screening for Cancers of the Uterine-Cervix

Eighty percent of the annual screening visits in the
WCCP include cervical Pap smears. Of almost 12,000 Pap
smears done by June 30, 1982, 20 were interpreted as
Classes III through V.

Of the 15 Class III Pap smears, five later had follow-
up smears interpreted as Class I. One woman had a cervical
mass excised and diagnosed as an endocervical polyp
containing Nabothian cysts, with chronic endocervicitis.
Five women had cervical biopsies interpreted as benign.
Cytology reports indicated one case of Nabothian cysts; two
of cervicitis; one of focal mild dysplasia, which was
treated with cryosurgery; and one of moderate dysplasia.
Four women had cancer. Three had carcinoma in situ; one
had a Grade III adenocarcinoma. She had radiation therapy
and surgery. One of the four had a vaginal hysterectomy;
the other three had abdominal hysterectomies with bilateral
salpingo-oophorectomies. None had a family history of
uterine cancer. Two of the four, ages 40 and 56, had had a
normal Pap smear within one year prior to the Class III
smear. One woman, age 58, had had a Class III smear six
months prior to her WCCP visit. The fourth woman was 65
years-of-age and had never had children. The Pap smear in
the WCCP was her first.

Both women who had Class IV Pap smears underwent D&C
with directed biopsies of the cervix and endometrium.
Neither had cancer.

All three women with Class V Pap smears had hysterectomies with bilateral salpingo-oophorectomies. One woman's
disease was benign, the other two were carcinoma in situ.
These two women were 48 and 53 years-of-age. One had had a
Pap smear the previous year. The other had not had a Pap
smear for three years prior to her initial WCCP visit. One
had no family history of uterine cancer, but the other
had two sisters who had had cancer of the cervix.

FUTURE PLANS

Missouri physicians have been supportive of the WCCP and the participants have been enthusiastic. New participants enroll in the WCCP almost every day and the vast majority return for annual appointments. The WCCP has had no difficulty in attracting an adequate screening population and, thus far, has required little promotion.

Although the State of Missouri has provided the largest portion of funding, the Cancer Research Center intends to make the program more self-supporting. Participants are being asked to contribute a larger portion of the screening costs. However, women who cannot make a contribution still go through the project. At present, efforts are being made to provide screening for empolyee groups. The WCCP has a contract to examine women with symptomatic breast diseases for the state cancer center. Third parties are billed for diagnostic procedures done on women who are referred to the WCCP by their private physicians. The WCCP also receives contributions from philanthropic organizations, such as the Missouri Order of the Eastern Star.

The early cancer detection programs at the Cancer Research Center have 1) verified that a large number of curable cancers can be detected in asymptomatic women and 2) served as demonstration projects to educate practicing physicians about costs and applicability of clinical methods for early cancer detection.

Beahrs OH, Shapiro S, Smart C, McDivitt RW (1979). Summary report of the working group to review the National Cancer Institute-American Cancer Society Breast Cancer Detection Demonstration Projects. J Nat Cancer Inst 62:647.
Fazio VW (1979). Early diagnosis of anorectal and colon carcinoma. Hosp Med, vol 15, Jan.
Gohagan JK, Rodes ND, Ballinger WF, Blackwell CW, Butcher HR, Darby WP, Pearson DK, Spitznagel EL, Wallack MK (1982). "Early Detection of Breast Cancer: Risk, Detection Protocols, and Therapeutic Implications." New York: Praeger Press.

Hardcastle JD, Balfour TW, Amar SS (1980). Screening for symptomless colorectal cancer by testing for occult blood in general practice. Lancet 1:791.
Nivatvongs S, Gilbertsen VA, Goldberg SM, Williams SE (1982). Distribution of large bowel cancers detected by occult blood test in asymptomatic patients. Dis Colon Rectum 25:420.
Pearson DK, Blackwell CW, Sullivan WK, Rodes ND (1980). Breast cancer screening: a six-year experience. Mo Med 77:713.
Smart CR, Beahrs OH (1979). Breast cancer screening results as viewed by the clinician. Cancer 43:851.
Vanneman WM Jr (1980). Toward the control of colon cancer. Geriatrics 35:51.
Winawer SJ, Sherlock P, Miller DG (1979). Current diagnosis of large bowel cancer. Cont Ed 13:56.

This investigation supported in part by grant no. RR-05824 from the National Cancer Institute, National Institutes of Health, DHHS, and by the Missouri Order of the Eastern Star.

Progress in Cancer Control IV: Research in the Cancer Center, pages 351–360
© **1983 Alan R. Liss, Inc., 150 Fifth Avenue, New York, NY 10011**

RISK FACTORS AND PHYSICIAN DELAY IN THE DIAGNOSIS OF
BREAST CANCER

Mary Lou Finley, Ph.C.
Anita Francis, Ph.D.
Social Epidemiology Program
Fred Hutchinson Cancer Research Center
Seattle, Washington 98104

The early detection, diagnosis, and treatment of breast
cancer has been a focus of cancer control efforts for several decades. As a part of that effort, research attention
has been focussed on screening programs, breast self examination, and patient delay in seeking medical care. (Shapiro et al. 1972, Reeder et al. 1980, Antonovsky, Hartman
1974). These are important concerns. However, physician
delay, i.e., delay during the diagnostic process, has
received relatively little attention.

Previous studies have identified the problem of physician delay and reported the frequency of its occurrence;
delays exceeding one month were found in 8% to 30% of breast
cancer cases (Leach, Robbins 1947; Dennis et al. 1975; Finley, Francis 1982). However, few studies have identified
factors which contribute to delay. Some patient and illness
characteristics have been examined; delay was found to be
somewhat longer in patients whose symptoms did not include a
lump (MacArthur, Smith 1981; Paganini-Hill, Ross 1981), and
race was found to be related to delay, with black patients
more likely to experience delay (Dennis et al. 1975). These
studies, however, provide only a beginning for the examination of this question.

We would suggest that the relationship between risk
factors and delay is a promising area for research. No
previous studies have focussed on this question, though
Dennis et al. (1975) did examine the relationship of
patient's age to physician delay; no association was found.

If physicians utilize risk factors to identify potential cases during the diagnostic process, we would expect
that the physician's index of suspicion would be higher for
patients with one or more risk factors, and that these patients would be diagnosed more promptly. Concomitantly, patients who were not considered at high risk of the disease
would be more likely to experience delays in diagnosis, as
the physician would be less suspicious of the presence of
cancer in these individuals. However, if risk factors are
not associated with delay, this would suggest a lack of attention to these factors by diagnosing physicians, and
would indicate that more attention to risk factors could be
an important means for decreasing delay in diagnosis.

This argument rests on the assumption that physician
delay is largely the result of physician decision-making
during the diagnostic process, rather than patient noncompliance or problems in scheduling. There has been little
previous research on this question. However, an earlier report from this project found that most delay during the
diagnostic interval is due to diagnostic problems, with patient noncompliance and scheduling accounting for delay in
only a small proportion of cases (Finley and Francis, 1982).

In this study, then, we will examine the association
between risk factors and delay in diagnosis, in an effort
to determine if these warning signals are being utilized by
physicians. Risk factors selected for inclusion were those
which are well-established in the epidemiological literature,
and which we could reasonably expect primary care physicians
to utilize in their practice (Leis 1977; Vorherr 1980;
American Cancer Society 1981). Risk factors examined include age, previous breast cancer in the opposite breast,
family history of breast cancer, age at birth of first
child, nulliparity, age at menarche and age at menopause.

METHODS

The data for this study were collected as part of a
larger research project on patterns of care for breast cancer patients. Participants for the study were identified
through a population-based cancer registry for an urban
county in the western U.S. Those meeting the following
criteria were eligible to participate: newly diagnosed pri-

mary breast cancers; diagnosis microscopically confirmed; diagnosed between January, 1977 and October, 1978; age 30-79; county residents; diagnosed or treated in a hospital located in the county; female.

454 patients were interviewed out of an eligible population of 887. Twenty-three percent of the eligible patients were excluded because they were not identified by the tumor registry until after the completion of the study. The registry's procedure for identifying cases was undergoing change at the time of the study and information was not obtained from some hospitals until quite late. Other patients were not included due to physician refusals (16%), patient refusals (8%), and inablilty to locate the patient, including patients who were deceased, had moved, etc. (3%).

Participants in the study were compared with those in the total eligible population. Study participants were significantly less likely to have an advanced stage of disease at diagnosis; this could be expected, however, as patients with advanced disease are more likely to be too ill for an interview. There were no significant differences on other disease variables (such as tumor size, number of positive lymph nodes, and extension of tumor) or on the demographic variables (age, race, marital status).

Patients were interviewed two to four months following surgery or other treatment, and asked an extensive list of questions concerning detection, medical care, and risk factors. Medical records data collected by the tumor registry were consulted for problemmatic cases.

The length of the diagnostic interval, i.e., the number of days from first contact with a physician to date of biopsy, was calculated for each patient. Physician delay was defined as occurring in cases in which the diagnostic interval exceeded thirty days.

Chi square tests were used to examine the relationships between dependent and independent variables.

RESULTS

Age

The incidence of breast cancer is substantially higher in older women. For example, the incidence rate rises from 57 cases per 100,000 for women aged 35-39 to 282 cases per 100,000 for women aged 65-69 (Young et al., n.d.). Thus we would expect that physicians would be more likely to suspect cancer when breast symptoms are present in an older woman. This expectation is strengthened by the fact that benign breast disease and cyclic breast symptoms — the main conditions which can be confounded with breast cancer — are more commonly found in premenopausal women (Leis, 1977).

As expected, we found that age was negatively related to delay in diagnosis, with older women less likely to experience delay (p=.004). These results are displayed in Table 1.

Table 1: Age of Patient and Physician Delay

Age of patient	TOTAL No. of cases (n=454)	PHYSICIAN DELAY No. of cases (n=135)	Percent
30-39 years	33	14	42%
40-49 years	72	29	40%
50-59 years	143	47	33%
60-69 years	128	33	26%
70-79 years	78	12	15%

$$X^2_4 = 15.69 \ (p=.004)$$

Other Risk Factors

Each of the other six risk factors was then examined separately to determine if it was associated with delay in diagnosis. The results are presented in Table 2.

Only one factor, family history of breast cancer, was significantly associated with delay in diagnosis, and this association was not in the predicted direction. Patients with a family history of breast cancer were more likely to experience delay in diagnosis. This finding will be discussed in more detail below.

Table 2:   Risk Factors and Physician Delay

		% of cases with Physician Delay	Significance
Previous breast cancer			
No	(n=434)	30%	n.s.
Yes	(n= 19)	26%	
Family history of breast cancer			
No	(n=279)	28%	p=.03
Yes	(n= 71)	42%	
Nulliparity			
No	(n=351)	28%	n.s.
Yes	(n= 90)	37%	
Age at first parity 30 or more*			
No	(n=298)	30%	n.s.
Yes	(n= 60)	18%	
Age at menarche 10 or less			
No	(n=428)	30%	n.s.
Yes	(n= 19)	42%	
Age at menopause 55 or more**			
NO	(n=292)	27%	n.s.
Yes	(n= 40)	20%	

*Excludes nulliparous women
**Excludes women who have not reached menopause

We found that age was significantly associated with three risk factors, with older women more likely to have the risk factors (previous breast cancer in the opposite breast, age at first parity, and, by definition, age at menopause). These associations raised a question about the meaning of the finding that age and delay are negatively associated: is this an actual relationship, or is it an artifact of the difference in frequency of other risk factors for differing age groups? To examine this question, relationships for each age group were examined separately. Age groups were defined as patients under 50 years of age and 50 years of age and older. When age was controlled for in this manner the relationships between the other risk factors and delay were unchanged, with the exception of the family history variable.

When age was controlled for on the family history variable, we found that the relationship was significant only for the under 50 age group (X^2=4.58, p=.03) although there was still a trend in the same direction for women over 50 years of age (X^2=1.57, p=.21).

Risk Factor Index

Risk factors can be viewed as potential signals to the physician. The presence of at least one risk factor should serve as a warning, and one would expect that as the number of risk factors increases, delay in diagnosis would be even more likely to decrease. In order to examine this possibility, we created a Risk Factor Index calculated by counting the number of risk factors reported by each patient. Age was excluded from the index.

No association was found between the Risk Factor Index and physician delay. The results of this analysis are displayed in Table 3. Only one case had three risk factors; it was excluded from the table.

When age was controlled for, the results were unchanged; delay was not related to the Risk Factor Index for any of the age groups. Age was controlled for by two methods: first, by dichotomizing into under 50 years and 50 years and over, and secondly, by using ten year age intervals.

Table 3: Risk Factor Index and Physician Delay

Number of Risk Factors	TOTAL No. of cases (n=454)	PHYSICIAN DELAY No. of cases (n=135)	Percent
0	212	60	28%
1	186	55	29%
2	55	20	36%

Family History of Breast Cancer

Because of the unexpected finding that patients with a family history of breast cancer were significantly more likely to experience delay in diagnosis, additional analysis

was performed to examine the relationship in more detail.
Though our previous findings indicated that most physician
delay is due to diagnostic problems, it seemed possible that
this might be an exceptional group. Perhaps patients with
family members who have had breast cancer are more fearful
and tend to not comply with physician instructions for return appointments, thus prolonging the diagnostic interval
themselves.

In order to explore this question, we examined the components of the diagnostic interval for this subset of patients. The days in the diagnostic interval had been coded
into three categories, defined as follows:
a) Diagnostic problems: days following an appointment
at which the physician ahd instructed the patient to "watch
and wait" or had dismissed the case.
b) Patient noncompliance: days due to the patient not
returning for an appointment when instructed to do so.
c) Scheduling: days due to waiting for an appointment.

An examination of the components of the delay interval
for these cases revealed a pattern similar to that for all
delay cases. These findings are displayed in Table 4.
Diagnostic problems were most important; patient noncompliance (see items b,d, and f) exceeded 30 days in only one
case.

Table 4: Delay Components: Factors Contributing 30 Days
or More to the Diagnostic Interval
(Delay Cases with Family History of Breast Cancer)

	No. of cases	Percent
a. Diagnostic problems	20	67%
b. Patient noncompliance	0	0%
c. Scheduling	3	10%
d. Diagnostic problems + patient noncompliance	1	3%
e. Diagnostic problems + scheduling	5	17%
f. Patient noncompliance + scheduling	0	0%
g. Combination of 3 components	1	3%
	n=30	100%

NOTE: Categories (d) - (f) include two components which each
contributed 30 days or more to the diagnostic interval.

DISCUSSION

In summary, this study found that age had a strong negative association with physician delay, with older women
less likely to experience delay, as expected. Other risk
factors were not found to be associated with delay in diagnosis, either when considered separately or when combined
into a Risk Factor Index, with the exception of family history of breast cancer, which was not related in the predicted direction. These findings were unchanged when age
was controlled for, indicating that the lack of association
between risk factors and delay exists for all age groups
and is not an artifact of the tendency for older women to
have more risk factors. The family risk factor variable remained significant only for the under 50 age group.

The findings on the relationship between age and delay
are not consistent with those previously reported by Dennis
et al. (1975); they reported no association. Differences in
the results of these two studies may be due to differences
in the two samples. Dennis et al. used a hospital-based sample of breast cancer patients treated with radical mastectomy in New York. Because the sample is hospital-based, its
results may be less generalizable. The New York study does
not indicate whether the population of patients treated with
radical mastectomy is representative of the total hospital
population of breast cancer patients or represents a particular subgroup which might have had an unusual diagnostic
experience.

Confidence in our results regarding the lack of association between other risk factors and delay is strengthened
by the finding that there is no association either when the
risk factors are considered separately, or when they are
combined into a Risk Factor Index. Particularly striking
is the finding that delay is just as likely for older women
with more than one risk factor. This suggests quite strongly that risk factors other than age are not taken into
account during the diagnostic process. Confidence in these
findings is further strengthened by utilizing in the analysis only those risk factors which we could reasonably expect
primary care physicians to use in diagnosis.

It is difficult to explain the finding that younger
patients with a family history of breast cancer are signif-

icantly more likely to experience delay in diagnosis, particularly when the delay is largely the result of physician
decisions. It is unlikely that physicians would knowingly
slow the diagnostic process for these patients. A finding
of no association would be more plausible; that would suggest that many physicians simply do not take information
about family history into account in making diagnostic decisions. As we cannot suggest a mechanism for this association, we would suggest that the finding could represent a
chance occurrence. Further investigation is needed before
this finding can be considered conclusive.

Implications for Further Research and Cancer Control

This study suggests that further attention to risk factors during the diagnostic process could play a role in decreasing delay. However, it should be noted that only 54%
of the breast cancer patients in this study had one of the
six risk factors in the Risk Factor Index. More attention
to these risk factors during diagnosis could minimize delay
for some women with breast cancer but not for all. Further
research examining a wide range of explanatory variables is
needed in order to improve understanding of additional factors affecting delay in diagnosis.

The research design for this study did not allow us to
pinpoint the specific nature of the problem in diagnosis.
That is, does this lack of association between most risk
factors and delay occur because physicians are unaware of
breast cancer risk factors, do not collect risk factor information from their patients, or do not utilize risk factor information in making their decisions about when to refer patients to biopsy? Or, is this finding due to patients'
supplying inaccurate information on risk factors to their
physicians? Research based on information from physicians
about the diagnostic process will be necessary in order to
answer these questions.

Though further research is needed to confirm and ampli-
fy the findings of this study, this avenue of investigation
has clear implications for cancer control. Minimizing delay in diagnosis is one aspect of achieving early treatment
for breast cancer. This study suggests that giving greater
consideration to risk factors during diagnosis would be one
method for reducing delay for breast cancer patients. Fur-

ther research on other factors associated with delays in
diagnosis could suggest other approaches for decreasing delay. Cancer control research efforts can perform a valuable
service by conducting further research on delay in diagnosis
and then developing education programs for physicians based
on the findings.

REFERENCES

American Cancer Society (1981). "Cancer Facts and Figrues,"
    New York: American Cancer Society.
Antonovsky A, Hartman H (1974). Delay in the detection of
    cancer: review of the literature. Hlth Ed Monographs 2
    (2):98.
Dennis CR, Gardner B, Lim B (1975).   Analysis of survival
    and recurrence vs. patient and doctor delay in treatment
    of breast cancer. Cancer 35:714.
Finley ML, Francis AM (1982). Patterns of diagnostic delay
    in breast cancer patients. Presentation for the 13th
    International Cancer Congress, UICC, Seattle, Washington.
Leach JE, Robbins GF (1947). Delay in the diagnosis of
    cancer. JAMA 135:5.
Leis HP (1977). The diagnosis of breast cancer. CA - a
    Cancer J for Clinicians 27:209.
MacArthur C, Smith A (1981). Delay in breast cancer and
    the nature of presenting symptoms. Lancet 1:601.
Paganini-Hill A, Ross RK (1981). Breast lumps and consul-
    tation delays. Lancet 1:995.
Reeder S, Berkanovic E, Marcus A (1980). Breast cancer de-
    tection behavior among urban women. Pub Hlth Reports
    95:276.
Shapiro S, Strax P, Venet L (1978). Periodic breast cancer
    screening in reducing mortality from breast cancer.
    JAMA 215:1777.
Vorherr H (1980). "Breast Cancer: Epidemiology, Endocrin-
    ology, Biochemistry and Pathobiology." Baltimore-Munich:
    Urban and Schwartzenberg.
Young JL, Percy CL, Ardyce JA, Berg JW, Cusano MM, Gloeckler
    LA, Horm JW, Lourie WI, Pollack ES, Shambaugh EM (n.d.).
    "Cancer Incidence and Mortality in the United States,
    1973-77." National Cancer Institute Monograph #57.

    Supported in part by PHS Grant #2-R18-CA16404, award-
ed by the National Cancer Institute, DHHS.

Progress in Cancer Control IV: Research in the Cancer Center, pages 361-368
© **1983 Alan R. Liss, Inc., 150 Fifth Avenue, New York, NY 10011**

FAMILY PHYSICIANS' BELIEFS ABOUT CANCER SCREENING TESTS

K. Michael Cummings, Ph.D., M.P.H.
Curtis Mettlin, Ph.D.
Roswell Park Memorial Institute
Louis Lazar, M.D.
Millard Fillmore Hospital
Kenneth B. Frisof, M.D.
Wayne State University

Results of several clinical and epidemiological studies provide evidence demonstrating the efficacy of many tests used for the early detection of cancer (American Cancer Society 1980). Despite the availability of effective screening tests, the American Cancer Society estimates that one-third of the 430,000 people who died of cancer in 1982, might have been saved by earlier diagnosis and prompt treatment (American Cancer Society 1981). Thus, it appears that mortality from cancer might be substantially reduced simply by applying available technology to detect cancer in an early stage of disease to a larger segment of the population.

Researchers have found that regular contact with a health care provider is the most consistent predictor of whether a person has been screened for cancer (Celentano 1982; Warnecke, Graham 1976; Warnecke 1980). However, even among persons who regularly visit physicians, many do not receive specific cancer screening tests (Warnecke 1980).

Little is known about the opinions and uses of cancer screening tests by practicing physicians. Herein, we present data from a survey of family physicians in New York State which assessed opinions about various cancer screening tests and recommendations for using each test in asymptomatic patients of different ages. Information was obtained on six cancer screening tests: Pap test; physical breast examination; mammography; digital rectal examination; stool guaiac slide test; and proctosigmoidoscopy. Family physicians were

selected for study because they are in an opportune position
to provide information and services to affect early cancer
detection by virtue of their frequent contact with a large
segment of the adult population (Rosser 1978; Schuman 1979;
Williams 1982). Findings from this study may be useful in
identifying areas in which educational programs are needed
to better inform primary care physicians about the rationale
and proper uses of different cancer screening tests.

Materials and Methods

The study population consisted of 509 board certified
family physicians randomly selected from a list of 1,212
physicians from New York State included in the 1981 Directory
of Board Certified Family Physicians. Data were collected
using a mailed questionnaire.

In January 1982, questionnaires were sent to physicians
in the sample along with a cover letter explaining the aims
of the study and a prepaid return envelope. Nonrespondents
were sent another questionnaire and a letter urging their
participation in the survey four weeks and ten weeks following
the initial mailing. Of the 509 physicians in the sample,
57 were dropped because the mailing address used was incorrect,
or because the questionnaire was returned in the mail with no
forwarding address. Of the 542 remaining physicians, 270
completed and returned questionnaires yielding a response
rate of 60 percent.

Eighty-eight percent of physicians who responded to the
survey were male. The age range of respondents was from 28
to 76 years with an average age of 48 years. Fifty-five
percent had a private solo practice, 23 percent were members
of a private group practice, 13 percent worked either full or
part-time in a hospital, five percent were members of a
prepaid group practice, and four percent worked in another
setting such as a public health clinic or nursing home. The
median number of patients seen by each physician in an
average week was 100, with about two percent of patients
being treated and/or followed for cancer.

Questionnaire

Half of the physicians in the sample were sent a
questionnaire which included a section asking them about
their recommendations for how frequently an asymptomatic

woman should have a Pap test, breast physical examination, and mammogram. The other half of the sample received a similar questionnaire which included a section asking them about their recommendations for how frequently an asymptomatic person should have a digital rectal examination, stool guaiac slide test, and proctosigmoidoscopy. Recommendations for screening were obtained for persons in each of three age groups: 20 to 40 years of age; 41 to 50 years of age; and over 50 years of age. Physicians who indicated that they would not recommend a screening test were asked to give their reasons for not recommending the test.

All physicians were asked to indicate for five cancer sites, how much of a difference in length of survival they think it makes if the cancer is detected early. In addition, all respondents were asked to rate the effectiveness of six screening tests in detecting early stage cancer.

Results

Recommended Screening Frequency

Nearly all physicians who responded to our survey recommended the Pap test for women over the age of 20, with the majority recommending an annual Pap test. Sixty-six percent of physicians recommended that women under age 40 have a yearly Pap test. For women 41 to 50 years of age, 77 percent recommended an annual Pap test, with an additional 14 percent recommending the test every two years. For women over age 50, 61 percent recommended an annual Pap test, 18 percent recommend the test every two years, 16 percent recommended the test every three years, and five percent recommended the test every three to five years.

All of the physicians who responded to our survey recommended that women over age 20 have a physical breast examination, with the majority recommending a yearly breast exam. Eighty-five percent of physicians recommended that women under age 40 have a yearly physical breast exam. For women over age 40, 96 percent of physicians recommended a yearly physical breast examination.

Table 1 shows the responses for the recommended frequency of having a mammogram for asymptomatic women of different ages. Although the recommended frequency for mammography increased with the patients' age, a substantial

number of physicians did not recommend a mammogram for
patients of any age. Concerns about the safety and
reliability of the procedure, the low probability of detecting
breast cancer through screening, and cost were the most
common reasons given for not recommending mammography.

Table 1

Recommended Frequency of Having a Mammography for Women
of Different Ages

Recommended Frequency of Having a Mammogram	Age Groups		
	20-40 years (n=132)	41-50 years (n=136)	Over 50 years (n=137)
Once every 6 months	-	-	-
Once every year	-	3%	8%
Once every 2 years	4%	10%	14%
Once every 3 years	2%	12%	14%
Once every 3 to 5 years	5%	15%	14%
Once for baseline	4%	7%	5%
When indicated	18%	18%	16%
Not recommended	67%	35%	29%

The recommended frequency for having a digital rectal
examination increased with the person's age. Only 13 percent
of physicians recommended a yearly digital rectal exam for
persons under age 40. Twenty-two percent of physicians did
not recommend a digital rectal exam for persons under age
40. The main reason given for not recommending a rectal
exam for persons under age 40 was the low probability of
detecting cancer in this age group. For persons 41 to 50
years of age, 65 percent of physicians recommended a yearly
digital rectal exam, with an additional 25 percent recommending the exam every two years. For persons over age 50,
nearly all physicians (97 percent) recommended a yearly digital
rectal exam.

The recommended frequency for having a test for stool occult blood also increased with the person's age. Fifteen percent of physicians recommended that persons under age 40 have a stool guaiac slide test; 30 percent did not recommend the test for persons under age 40. The main reason given for not recommending the test in persons under age 40 was the low probability of detecting cancer in this age group. For persons 41 to 50 years of age, 66 percent of physicians recommended having a stool guaiac slide test once a year. For persons over age 50, nearly all physicians (95 percent) recommended having a stool guaiac slide test done annually.

The recommended frequency of having proctosigmoidoscopy also increased with the persons age. Fifty-five percent of physicians did not recommend proctosigmoidoscopy for persons under age 40, and 17 percent reported that they would use the examination only when indicated by symptoms of disease. For persons 41 to 50 years of age, 67 percent of physicians recommended proctosigmoidoscopy, but only 11 percent suggested that the exam be done on a yearly basis. For persons over age 50, 31 percent of physicians recommended that their patients receive a proctosigmoidoscopic exam annually, with an additional 45 percent recommending the exam at least once every three to five years. For persons under age 40, the most frequently mentioned reason for not recommending proctosigmoidoscopy was the low probability of detecting cancer in this age group. For persons over age 40, concern about the cost of the exam was the most frequently cited reason for not recommending the procedure.

Opinions About the Effectiveness of Cancer Screening Tests

Table 2 shows the responses regarding physicians' beliefs about the benefits of early cancer detection for five cancer sites. With the exception of prostate cancer, the majority of physicians indicated that early cancer detection makes a great deal of difference in patient prognosis.

Table 2

Physicians' Beliefs About the Benefits of Early Cancer Detection
for Five Cancer Sites

Cancer Site	A Great Deal of Difference	Some Difference	Little or No Difference
Cervical (n=269)	90%	9%	1%
Breast (n=268)	71%	28%	1%
Colon (n=269)	75%	23%	2%
Rectum (n=269)	75%	23%	2%
Prostate (n=268)	43%	46%	11%

Note: Number of respondents indicated in parentheses

Table 3

Physicians' Beliefs About the Effectiveness of Various
Screening Tests in Detecting Early Stage Cancer

Screening Test	Very Effective	Fairly Effective	Somewhat Effective	Not Very Effective
Pap test for the detection of cervical cancer (n=267)	61%	34%	4%	1%
Physical breast examination for the detection of breast cancer (n=266)	20%	62%	17%	1%
Mammography for the detection of breast cancer (n=265)	34%	54%	9%	3%
Digital rectal examination for the detection of colorectal cancer (n=267)	12%	50%	31%	7%
Digital rectal examination for the detection of prostate cancer (n=265)	17%	48%	30%	5%
Stool guaiac slide test for the detection of colorectal cancer (n=267)	21%	59%	17%	3%
Proctosigmoidoscopy for the detection of colorectal cancer (n=267)	37%	47%	15%	1%

Note: Number of respondents indicated in parentheses

Physicians' opinions about the effectiveness of various screening tests in detecting early stage cancer are shown in table 3. Only the Pap test was rated as "very effective" by a majority of physicians. Mammography was rated as slightly more effective in detecting early stage breast cancer than physical breast examination. Among the screening tests for colorectal cancer, proctosigmoidoscopy was rated as most effective followed by the stool guaiac slide test and digital rectal examination.

Discussion

Inclusion of cancer specific tests as part of a periodic medical examination is one way to ensure that a large segment of the population is regularly screened for cancer. Since primary care physicians do the majority of periodic medical exams that are done in doctor's offices today, they are in a good position to affect early cancer detection. However, little is known about the opinions and uses of cancer screening tests by practicing physicians.

The findings from this study are encouraging in that they show that most family physicians believe that early cancer detection can favorably influence patient prognosis. Moreover, of the six cancer screening tests asked about in our survey, the majority of physicians rated each as either "very" or "fairly" effective in detecting cancer in an early stage of disease. Consistent with these beliefs, most of the physicians responding to our survey recommended that their asymptomatic patients routinely receive these cancer screening tests, with the frequency of screening usually increasing with the persons age. With the exception of mammography, most of the physicians surveyed either exceeded or were in agreement with the guidelines for cancer screening frequency in asymptomatic persons recently published by the American Cancer Society (American Cancer Society 1980).

Perhaps the most striking results from this study were our findings regarding physicians' opinions and recommended uses of mammography. Despite the fact that most physicians (88 percent) rated mammography as either "very" or "fairly" effective in detecting early stage breast cancer, few recommended routine screening with mammography in asymptomatic women. Even in women over age 50, 45 percent did not recommend mammography or recommended using mammography only when the patient is suspected of having breast disease. Only eight percent of physicians recommended that women over the age of 50 have a mammogram every year.

It appears that the reluctance of some physicians to recommend mammography in screening asymptomatic women is due to a lack of awareness of improvements in mammographic technology enabling reduction of radiation dose and increased accuracy in detection of breast cancer. This finding suggests a need to better educate primary care physicians about the use of mammography in screening asymptomatic women for breast cancer, especially with regards to its safety and reliability. In addition, physicians may need to be better informed about factors which influence the quality of mammographic examination such as the type of equipment used and the expertise of the radiologist responsible for interpreting the results of the examination.

References

American Cancer Society (1980). Guidelines for the cancer-related check-up: recommendations and rationale. Ca-A Journal for Clinicians 30:194.

American Cancer Society (1981). "Cancer Facts and Figures, 1982." New York: American Cancer Society, p 3.

Celentano DD, Shapiro S, Weisman CS (1982). Cancer preventive screening behavior among elderly women. Prev Med, 11:454.

Rosser WW (1978). Screening in family medicine: the current situation. J Fam Pract, 6:503.

Schuman SH (1979). Prevention: the vital and unique role of the family physician. J Fam Pract, 9:97.

Warnecke RB, Graham S (1976). Characteristics of blacks obtaining Papanicolaou smears. Cancer, 37:2015.

Warnecke RB (1980). Intervention in black populations. In: Mettlin C, Murphy GP (eds): "Cancer Among Black Populations," New York: Alan R. Liss, Inc., p 167.

Williams P (1982). How primary care physicians can improve cancer survival: early diagnosis, prevention. The Clinical Cancer Letter, 5:2.

III. TREATMENT, REHABILITATION, AND DATA MANAGEMENT

Progress in Cancer Control IV: Research in the Cancer Center, pages 371-378
© 1983 Alan R. Liss, Inc., 150 Fifth Avenue, New York, NY 10011

CRITERIA SETTING AND ADHERENCE TO CRITERIA FOR MANAGING CERVICAL, BREAST AND ENDOMETRIAL CANCER AMONG COMMUNITY PHYSICIANS

Wesley C. Fowler, Jr., M.D.

Department of Obstetrics-Gynecology and the Cancer Research Center, University of North Carolina Chapel Hill, North Carolina, 27514

Anne C. Freeman, M.S.P.H.

The Cancer Research Center University of North Carolina Chapel Hill, North Carolina, 27514

Barbara S. Hulka, M.D.

Department of Epidemiology and the Cancer Research Center, University of North Carolina Chapel Hill, North Carolina, 27514

Arnold D. Kaluzny, Ph.D.

Dept of Health Policy and Administration and the Cancer Research Center University of North Carolina Chapel Hill, North Carolina, 27514

Shirley P. O'Keefe, M.S.P.H.

The Cancer Research Center University of North Carolina Chapel Hill, North Carolina, 27514

Michael J. Symons, Ph.D.

Dept of Biostatistics and Cancer Research Ctr University of North Carolina Chapel Hill, North Carolina, 27514

In April, 1980, faculty at the University of North Carolina at Chapel Hill, working with physicians in five North Carolina communities, began a cancer control demonstration project, funded by the National Cancer Institute. The purpose of the project is to study patterns of care in breast, cervical and endometrial cancer in different types of practice settings in an effort to improve current cancer treatment. Cancer is the second leading cause of death in North Carolina with a crude death rate in 1980 of 165.1 per 100,000 population (North Carolina Department of Human Resources, 1980). The American Cancer Society (1981) estimated 19,000 new cases of cancer in North Carolina in 1981. Of these, breast cancer represents the second highest number of new cases and the third highest number of deaths, while uterine and cervical cancer, excluding carcinoma in situ, accounted for 1,900 new cases and 275 deaths. From 1979 to 1980, the death rate from cervical cancer in North Carolina rose 29.2 percent and for black women rose 84 percent, in contrast to a decline in previous years (North Carolina Department of Human Resources, 1980).

The basic assumptions of the project are that (a) a cancer knowledge transfer problem exists, and that (b) addressing the problem could improve the treatment provided to cancer patients. Existing models of technology transfer (Zaltman, 1973; Rogers, 1971; Havelock, 1969) suggest that acceptance of new knowledge occurs when individuals see a difference between their current practice and the accepted norm. When such evidence is presented to them, they are stimulated to change their behavior. This project combines basic research in the patterns of care provided by physicians, evaluation of resulting data, and presentation of that data to physicians in an effort to encourage acceptance of current cancer treatment.

Five areas in the state, part of the North Carolina Area Health Education Centers Program, were chosen to be three study sites and two comparison sites. The study sites were (1) a University-affiliated hospital, (2) an urban hospital, and (3) a combination of rural hospitals in eastern North Carolina. The comparison sites were two large community hospitals.

Briefly stated, the study required the establishment

of diagnosis and treatment plan criteria for breast, cervical and endometrial cancer by each study area. This was followed by a review of medical records of participating physicians for the period January 1, 1977 through December, 1980. Physicians in each area were then provided with a description of their patient management profile compared to the criteria developed for their area. Information was given only to the individual physician with no identification of patients or other physicians. A meeting was held in each study site to review the group results and answer questions. Physicians located in comparison sites participated in the chart review but were not provided with a description of their patient management profile. This phase of the study is now complete.

After twelve months, records of new patients seen since the previous data collection will be reviewed in all sites. Analysis will be done to see whether in the study sites physicians' treatment patterns changed based on the information they were given in the feedback.

Community participation has been a critical element in this project. Prior to the grant application, faculty at the University met with key physicians in the communities to discuss their interest in the project. These physicians then reviewed the grant application and presented the project to other members of the medical staff in their communities for approval. A letter of intent to participate in the project accompanied the grant application. A practicing physician in each site agreed to direct the work performed in his area. He developed a steering committee to establish the criteria for his area and chaired the discussions. University faculty and staff attended these meetings, but it was made clear from the outset, that the community physicians would decide on the criteria for their area and that practice patterns of individual physicians would be compared to criteria for that area and not to a set of criteria imposed from outside.

CRITERIA SETTING PROCESS

The steering committees began their criteria setting task with a sample set of criteria compiled from already existing criteria such as the American College of Radiology's Patterns of Care and the Grand Rapids' Cancer Control Program Criteria for Patient Management. A draft criteria list was then prepared for each disease by the committee in each of the three study areas.

These draft criteria were distributed to all practicing physicians in the area who care for patients with these types of cancer. Each was asked to comment on the criteria and their relevancy to his/her practice. Broad participation in the criteria setting process was considered vital to the ultimate success of the project and every effort was made to elicit responses from physicians. The final response rate for those physicians receiving feedback varied from 30% for the gynecological cancer criteria in hospital #2 to 100% for the breast cancer criteria in hospital #3 and for the gynecological criteria in hospital #1.

All comments from physicians were then compiled and reviewed by each steering committee. After a usually lively debate, final versions of the criteria were established for each area. These final lists were arranged into five categories of criteria: history, physical examination, diagnosis, pretreatment evaluation, and treatment plan.

DATA COLLECTION

The criteria lists formed the basis for an abstract form which was developed and pretested. All records of women diagnosed as having breast, endometrial or cervical cancer from January 1, 1977 through December, 1980 in four of the five area hospitals were reviewed. In situ cancer, cases women who were pregnant at the time of diagnosis, and women who had received treatment at another hospital were excluded from the study. The fifth hospital has a large number of patients and a small number of physicians so each physician's patient load was randomly sampled. The review resulted in 1378 abstracts being completed: 768 breast, 287 cervical and 323 endometrial.

The data collected included basic demographic and diagnostic information, data needed to assign a portion of the patient's care to a physician, evaluation of criteria performance, and detailed information on history, physical examination, diagnostic method, test results, stage of disease, and treatment plan. The major problems encountered in the data collection were difficulties in identifying cases in one hospital and unanticipated answers to several data items. The later problem meant the addition of codes and the recoding of "other" category answers.

FEEDBACK

Physicians at the study site hospitals were provided with a description of their own individual patient management profile compared to the criteria for their area and compared to the group performance of the physicians in their area. This feedback to physicians was designed in three steps to have the largest possible impact on modification of behavior.

The first part of the feedback was a color bar graph for each cancer type showing the physician's performance on groups of criteria compared to that of all the physicians in the same area. Two weeks later, each physician received a detailed report showing performance on specific criteria compared to the group's performance.

Shortly thereafter, a seminar was held at which the group results were presented and their relation to patient care was discussed. Participation in the seminars varied from 13.2% to 45.7% of the physicians who received feedback. Since some physicians received data on only one patient and rarely see such patients, this percentage of participation is not surprising.

RESULTS

Comparisons of the criteria setting process across the three study areas show a slight difference on the number of criteria chosen. The biggest differences for cervical cancer are between hospital #3 and the other two hospitals, especially in the pretreatment evaluation and history categories.

TABLE 1.
NUMBER OF CRITERIA ACROSS HOSPITALS

	Hospitals		
	1	2	3
History	13	13	8
Physical Examination	10	11	8
Diagnosis	5	5	5
Pretreatment Evaluation	16	18	9
Treatment Plan	3	2	2
TOTAL	32	36	20

Some specific differences in the criteria were as follows: for cervical cancer one hospital required a drawing of the lesion while others did not, in another example only one hospital required a follow up schedule to be recorded in the chart. For breast cancer one hospital did not require information on family history of breast cancer or age or race of patient, one hospital made a drawing of the lesion optional while the others required it, only one hospital required CEA levels or consideration of breast reconstruction.

Adherence to the criteria varied considerably for some criteria across hospitals and very little for other criteria. Some examples of the types of variation are in Table 2.

In retrospect it is clear that some of the adherence problems resulted from overly strict criteria, e.g., requiring supraclavicular, cervical and axillary nodal status to be recorded for breast cancer. Another problem that is inherent in this type of medical records review is that procedures are done or questions asked without the results or answers being recorded in the chart. Some history and physical examination data were taken in the physician's office and never transferred to the hospital chart. Another difficulty was incomplete descriptions of procedures. For instance, the criteria for endometrial cancer required a "TAH BS&O with pelvic and periaortic node evaluation (by palpation or, preferably, by biopsy) and cytologic washings" for the treatment plan for several stages of disease. Often the procedure was called only a "TAH BS&O" and no further information could be retrieved from the operative note or pathology report even though the surgeon may have done it all.

TABLE 2
ADHERENCE TO CRITERIA

	HOSPITALS					
	1		2		3	
Criteria	Total # of pts	Percent Adherence	Total # of pts	Percent Adherence	Total # of pts	Percent Adherence
Breast cancer						
lesion size	146	88	211	77	51	73
estrogen receptors	117	61	213	16	53	23
bone scan	140	77	88	80	43	35
Reach to Recovery visit	89	83	189	33	47	2
Cervical cancer						
Pap smear history	99	32	72	26	48	10
results of latest previous Pap smear	99	56	72	27	48	25
Endometrial cancer						
hormone use history	96	63	76	36	64	6
uterine sounding	96	95	76	63	64	77

Despite these methodological problems we did find substantive differences in the adherence to the criteria in the different practice settings. Keeping in mind the potential problems with medical records, it appears from this study that there is a need to transfer new, accepted technologies to practicing physicians.

The project is now in an early analysis phase, waiting for the twelve months' time to elapse before the second data collection effort. The results of that record review will indicate whether or not the feedback method used had an impact on physician practices and, ultimately, on patient care.

REFERENCES

North Carolina Department of Human Resources (1980). "Leading Causes of Mortality, North Carolina Vital Statistics 1980, Vol. 2." Raleigh:Division of Health Services, Public Health Statistics Branch.

American Cancer Society (1981). "1981 Cancer Facts and Figures." New York:American Cancer Society.

Zaltman G, Duncan R, Holbek J (1973). "Innovation and Organizations." New York:Wiley-Interscience.

Rogers E, Shoemaker F (1971). "Communication of Innovation: A Cross Cultural Approach." New York: The Free Press.

Havelock R G (1969). "Planning for Innovation through Dissemination and Utilization of Knowledge." Ann Arbor:University of Michigan.

Progress in Cancer Control IV: Research in the Cancer Center, pages 379–390
© 1983 Alan R. Liss, Inc., 150 Fifth Avenue, New York, NY 10011

COMPLIANCE WITH CHEMOTHERAPY: THEORETICAL BASIS AND
INTERVENTION DESIGN

Jean L. Richardson, Dr.P.H., C. Anderson Johnson, Ph.D.,
Judith Selser, R.N., Leonard A. Evans, Ph.D., Connie
Kishbaugh, R.N., B.S., Alexandra M. Levine, M.D.,
Div. of Hematology, Dept. of Medicine, Los Angeles
County-USC Medical Center and Comprehensive Cancer
Center and Health Behavior Research Institute,
University of Southern California, Los Angeles, CA

Advances in cancer treatment are measured by the comparative effectiveness of research protocols in obtaining
tumor response. Yet the assessment of treatment effect is
usually made with no attention to the influence of treatment
compliance. Although great care may be taken to design the
protocol, measure physiological effects, randomize subjects,
and conduct national collaborative trials, any given finding
may be in question simply because the level of compliance
with treatment has not been measured. In other words, whenever home medications are prescribed, we, as health professionals, do not know the effect of the given treatment
because we do not know how much of the medication was
actually taken. Furthermore, clinicians who are interested
in patient care must understand how compliance can be improved
so that a given patient may gain the full benefit of treatment
(Levy, 1982). Research on patient non-compliance should
address 1) the consequences of non-compliance, 2) the extent
of non-compliance, 3) the factors associated with non-compliance, and 4) the management of non-compliance (Stone,
1979). These issues will herein be discussed as they relate
to a study of compliance with chemotherapy in patients with
hematologic malignancies, which is currently being conducted
at the University of Southern California.

THE CONSEQUENCES OF NON-COMPLIANCE

Compliance in patients with hematologic malignancies is
especially important because, in many instances, these cancers are curable, or controllable for long periods of time
with appropriate treatment and management. Compliance with

This investigation was supported by PHS Grant No. CA31151
Awarded by the National Cancer Institute DHHS.

medical instructions may mean the difference between long-term
survival or death from disease. For example, with a protocol
such as MOPP for Hodgkins Disease, the treatment response has
been reported to be an 80% complete response rate and 50% cure
rate in Stage IV disease (DeVita, 1970). However with MOPP,
the Nitrogen Mustard (M) and Oncovin (O) are parenterally administered by a health professional, while the Prednisone (P) and
Procarbazine (P) are self-administered. The reported treatment
response may well be based on high protocol adherrence for MO
but low adherrence for PP. The potential treatment response
may thus be substantially higher if, in fact, all patients com-
plied with treatment. This concern for the actual dose response
has also been indicated by Bonadonna and Valgussa (1981) in a
study of dose response in the adjuvant treatment of breast cancer with CMF (cyclophosphamide, methotrexate, and fluorouracil).
In particular, they cited the repeated observation of non-compliance by elderly women receiving oral cyclophosphamide as a
problem in assessing the actual effectiveness of the variations
in CMF dosing.

For many cancer drugs therapeutically effective blood
dosage levels may be high while the half-life is short, requiring frequent and regular administration to sustain therapeutic levels. Discontinuation of allopurinol for example,
results in a drop from steady state to undetectable plasma
levels in less than two days (Kramer and Feldman, 1979). Under-
medication may render treatment potentially ineffective whereas
overmedication may be dangerous due to the toxicity of certain
medications.

THE EXTENT OF NON-COMPLIANCE

Although the issue of compliance has received considerable
attention in the management of other chronic diseases, it has
been largely ignored in the case of cancer research. Only one
study has been published which indicates that among children wit
acute leukemia or lymphoma, 33% were non-compliant and among
adolescents a surprisingly high number, 59%, were non-compliant
with orally, self-administered prednisone. Such a high rate of
non-compliance may contribute considerably to the wide variance
in the response of children with the same disease and on the
same therapy.

It may be reasonable to expect the rate of compliance
among cancer patients to approximate the rate of compliance
reported from studies of other diseases. Non-compliance

rates of 30 to 80% have been found across a wide range of treatments, diseases, and individual characteristics (Haynes, 1979a; Marston, 1970). Estimates differ depending on what is measured (compliance with long term versus short term treatment regimens), who is measured (children, adolescents, young adults, the elderly), and the degree of rigor with which compliance is defined (total defaulting, partial defaulting or scheduling efforts). In a recent extensive review by Sackett and Snow (1979) "rates of compliance with different long-term medication regimens for different illnesses in different settings tend to converge to approximately 50%."

FACTORS ASSOCIATED WITH NON-COMPLIANCE

Unfortunately there is no clear way to determine at the outset of treatment, which patients are more likely to be compliant and which patients are not. Studies have shown that physicians are unable to judge which of their patients are adherring to self medication regimens (Kasl, 1975) and tend to overestimate the level of compliance (Charney, 1972). In general, age, sex, educational level, socio-economic status, religion, race, marital status, and other demographic variables have been poor or inconsistent predictors of compliance (Becker, 1975; Haynes, 1979b). Similarly illness and treatment variables have been shown to be poor predictors of compliance with treatment. Duration of disease, length of hospital stay, severity of disease, and extent of disability, have not been shown to predict compliance with treatment. As Becker (1975) maintains, any patient is a potential non-complier. Only the complexity of treatment regimens has been demonstrated to consistently result in lower levels of compliance. This is a particularly important finding for compliance with chemotherapy since these treatment regimens can be very complex, lengthy, do not guarantee positive results, and may actually cause severe side effects.

Although the relationship between side effects and non-compliance, seems intuitively obvious, it has not yet been convincingly established. Controlled studies have found no difference in the frequency of side effects for compliers and non-compliers and when patients were asked about their reasons for non-compliance, side effects are infrequently mentioned (Haynes, 1979b). Yet this bears further investigation with cancer patients because the profound side effects with chemotherapy may well have a considerable effect compared with less obvious and less probable side effects

associated with other drugs. Nausea and vomiting may preclude normal activities for one or two days each week, loss
of hair may interfere with social interaction, and bone
marrow suppression may result in infections or bleeding that
can be potentially life-threatening.

Traditionally, non-compliance has been seen as a failure
on the part of the patient. Physicians report that they
respond to the patient's non-compliance with tactics that
usually include further explanations, admonitions, authoria-
trian tactics, fear appeals, threats, increased interaction
to encourage compliance, and finally withdrawal (Davis, 1966;
Hayes Bautista, 1976).

There are many problems with these approaches to improving
compliance. First, interventions are typically based on a
belief that non-compliance is due to lack of confidence by
the patient that the treatment is effective. Second, the
intervention is usually provided after the undesirable behavior has already been learned. To be effective, the
intervention must overcome what may already be a learned
habit of non-compliance.

Raising fear levels among cancer patients as a means
of stimulating compliance may be especially open to question.
The word "cancer" in itself evokes fears of death, pain,
disability, and other negative consequences. To further
increase fear levels by indicating the certainty of those
outcomes if compliance is not obtained may serve to immo-
bilize the patient's ability to comply with the regimen
(Janis, 1967). Research by Leventhal (1971) and Rogers
(1975) indicates that fear may reduce compliance unless the
patient has specific strategies which they are confident
they can perform correctly and which they believe are effective to counter the fear producing event. Although some
studies have shown that admonitions may improve compliance
(Schmidt, 1977; Svarstad, 1976) the preponderance of information indicates that scolding patients decreases compliance.
The effects of scare tactics are shortlived and the arousal
of fear can evoke behavior that is opposite of the behavior
desired (Gillum and Barsky, 1974). When fear inducing information must be given to patients, steps should be taken
to offset the adverse consequences of fear by teaching skills
useful for successful compliance and instilling perceptions
of self confidence (Bandura, 1982).

THE MANAGEMENT OF NON-COMPLIANCE

In the compliance study at USC, educational, behavioral, and psychosocial interventions are being tested for their effect on compliance with chemotherapy among patients with hematologic malignancies. These will be referred to as the Education Program, the Shaping Program, and the Home Structuring Program. From previous reports, we have reason to believe that each of these interventions will improve patient compliance to some degree.

All patients assigned in random blocks to experimental interventions receive the individualized instructional program. In addition they receive either the shaping procedure in the hospital, the social/environmental supports enhancing procedure at home, or both. Randomly assigned blocks of patients who receive no compliance enhancement interventions provide the experimental control group.

Education Program

Although at first consideration, it would appear that high levels of knowledge about a disease and its therapy would result in higher levels of patient compliance with that therapy, the literature is, at best, equivocal. In his comprehensive review of the compliance literature, Haynes (1979) concludes that there is no relationship between knowledge and compliance. At the very least, understanding the prescribed regimen, including when and how much medications to take, is probably a necessary if not sufficient condition for compliance.

Providing information about ways to cope with situations emotionally and behaviorally has been shown to have beneficial effects for persons in dealing with stressful surgical procedures such as cardiac catheter insertion (Kendall, 1979), and post-surgical recovery (Langer, 1975). Egbert (1964) found that patients who were given brief presurgical messages about sensory information (pain they would feel) and behavioral coping (relaxation, proper turning in bed) had lower levels of post surgical narcotic use. Other studies have shown that sensory information may be more beneficial in reducing discomfort during endoscopy than procedural information (Johnson, Morrissey and Leventhal, 1973).

The education program consists of an interactive slide/

tape teaching session conducted by project nurses designed to inform the patient about his disease, its treatment and the patient's responsibilities in treatment. After each of these three areas is discussed, the nurse engages the patient in a structured exchange in which the patient reveals his level of understanding about the disease and treatment. The patient is also encouraged to ask additional questions.

In keeping with good educational principles (Green, 1979), the material is presented in an easily understood manner, with explanations phrased at about the fourth grade level (i.e., think of your bone marrow as a factory that produces blood cells). All information is repeated (first by slide/tape, then in the nurse patient interaction, and finally with a supplementary pamphlet). Specific suggestions are made (drink four extra glasses of water, juice or other liquid per day).

In our educational program six types of information are provided. These include:

Factual information: facts and prognosis ("Leukemia is a cancer of a type of white blood cell").

Procedural information: specific events that will happen ("Your doctor will take a sample of your blood").

Sensory information: forewarning about sensations that might occur ("If your stomach cells are affected by chemotherapy, you may develop nausea and vomiting.").

Behavioral instructions: actions the patients should take as part of self management ("Take all of your medicine regularly and on schedule in the morning.").

Motivational aids: suggestions to increase the salience of the behavior to be performed ("You are the most important person in your own health care").

Emotional coping: guides to mechanisms of coping ("We know you may be feeling a little afraid or sad now. This is normal for someone in your situation, but it may help to talk to us about your feelings.").

Shaping Program

Ultimately hospitalized patients must actually assume responsibility for self-medication away from the hospital. Yet the entire time that patients are hospitalized they are prevented from taking responsibility for self-medication. Pills are usually passively administered without discussion, or any decision on their part. Yet immediately upon discharge, the patient is expected to self medicate correctly. If the medication schedule is complex, occurs more than once a day, or must be maintained for an extended period of time, the patient will probably fail.

Shaping is a procedure in which a complex behavior is broken down into successive steps. Each step is then taught and reinforced and the individual is moved closer to the desired final behavior. The patient self-medication shaping program is a specific strategy designed to increase appropriate medication use at home. Patients participating in this program are required to have direct involvement in their medication, treatment, and education while in the hospital. In a test of an in-hospital self-medication program for hypertension patients the level of compliance (0-2 day deviation in medication control) obtained was 30% in the control group and 71% in the experimental group (Johnson and Beardsley, 1978).

Patients gradually assume responsibility for administering their own medications by progressing through three levels; Level I, patients select medications and nurses select the administration times; Level II, patients select medications and request medications on schedule with close nurse supervision; and in Level III, patients have their medication at their bedside and essentially administer their drugs in the same manner as they would at home. At all three levels nurses monitor patient medication administration, encourage correct use and correct inappropriate use. Thus patients become active participants in the program and are able to practice taking medications before being discharged.

Practice, together with systematic reinforcement by nurses, provides not only the skills for compliance, but also establishes confidence that one is capable of performing the tasks in question. Practice increases self-efficacy and intentions to perform the behavior in question.

Home Structuring

The purpose of the home visit is to increase levels of social and environmental supports for complying with treatment regimens. Structuring the home environment is tailored to the patient's needs and resources.

Project nurses arrange to visit the patient at home one week after discharge. A discharge poster, provided to each patient during the home visit, indicates side effects and appropriate responses, self-medication schedules, appointment reminders, and criteria for self referral for medical care. Prior to the visit, patients are asked to identify a person with whom they interact frequently, who has been supportive of them in the past, and who is someone that they believe they can look to for help in the future. Patients are encouraged to invite that person to meet with them and the project nurse on the day of the home visit.

There is a significant number of studies indicating a positive correlation between social support and health (e.g. Berkman and Syme, 1979), or the loss of social support and illness (Parkes, 1969). Studies have indicated that social support may play a role in "buffering" stress (Turner, 1981; Gore, 1978). A correlation between social support and recovery from myocardial infraction has been tested and found to increase home-medication compliance (Caplan, 1976). Similarly social support from the spouse has been shown to improve the long term results of a weight loss program (Brownell, Heckeman, Westlake, et al., 1977). Support from professionals has also been shown to improve the post-surgical recovery of mastectomy patients (Bloom, 1978).

The design of interventions to improve social support is difficult because the mechanism for the influence of social support on adaptation to illness is unclear. The construct has only recently been separated into dimensions that may provide meaningful approaches for measurement and intervention design. For example, Bloom (1982) specifies five dimensions: maintenance of social identity, emotional support, material aid and services, information, and social affiliation.

In this study we have defined certain problems in the home that can hinder compliance and that can be addressed using behavioral and cognitive strategies that involve both the patient and a support person. In particular, the strategies involve cueing, contracting, problem solving and maintaining pleasant activities.

Cueing: The patient and support person decide together which everyday occurrences or habits could be linked to pill taking (such as brushing teeth, morning coffee, etc.). In effect the desired behavior is linked to an already learned behavior to increase the probability of occurrence.

Contracting: The patient and support person decide upon and describe in writing a role for the support person in symptom recognition and response.

Problem solving: The patient and support person identify and develop a solution to a barrier to compliance (such as lack of transportation for clinic visits). In addition, they devise solutions for four hypothetical vignettes involving symptom recognition and mood disturbances.

Maintaining pleasant activities: Patients are encouraged to participate in pleasant activities in order to keep a positive mental attitude. Patients are assisted by the nurse and support person in conducting an inventory of activities they find enjoyable and assessing whether they can continue the activity, alter it in ways that are manageable, or substitute a similar activity (Lewinsohn, Munoz, Youngren, and Zeiss, 1978).

SUMMARY

An experimental chemotherapy compliance enhancement program has been developed based on theory and findings from social psychology and learning theory. The essential ingredients are individualized instruction, behavior shaping and enhancement of social and environmental supports. The differential effects of these interventions upon compliance, as measured both by patient self-reports and by objective pharmacokinetic assays, are being tested.

Bandura A (1982). Self-efficacy mechanism in human agency. Amer Psych 37:122.
Becker MH, Maiman LA (1975). Sociobehavioral determinants of compliance with health and medical care recommendations. Med Care 13:10.
Berkman L, Syme SL (1979). Social networks, host resistance, and mortality: A nine year follow-up study of Alameda County residents. Am J Epid 109:186.

Bloom JR (1982). Social support systems and cancer: A con-
  ceptual view. In Cohen J, Cullen JW, Martin LR (eds):
  "Psychosocial Aspects of Cancer." New York: Raven Press.
Bloom JR, Ross RD, Burnell GM (1978). Effect of social
  support on patient adjustment following breast surgery.
  Patient Counsel Health Educ 1:50.
Bonadonna G, Valaquessa P (1981). Dose-response effect of
  adjuvant chemotherapy in breast cancer. N Engl J Med 43:169.
Brownell KD, Heckerman CL, Westlake RJ, Hayes SC, Monti R
  (1977). Couples training and spouse cooperativeness with
  behavioral treatment of obesity. Presented at the eleventh
  annual convention of the association for the Advancement of
  behavioral therapy, Atlanta.
Caplan RD, Robinson E, French JR, Caldwell JR, Shinn M (1976).
  Adhering to Medical Regimens: Pilot Experiments in Patient
  Education and Social Support Report, Institute for Social
  Research Ann Arbor, Michigan
Clarney E (1972). Patient-doctor communication: Implications
  for the clinician. Ped Clin N Amer 19:263.
Croog S, Levine S, Lurie Z (1968). The heart patient and the
  recovery process: A review of the directions of research
  on social and psychological factors. Soc Sci Med 2:111.
Davis MS (1966). Variations in patients' compliance with
  doctor's orders: Analysis of congruence between survey
  responses and results of empirical investigations.
  J Med Educ 41:1037.
Devita VT, Serpick AA, Carbone PP (1970). Combination chemo-
  therapy in the treatment of advanced hodgkins disease.
  Ann Int Med 73:881.
Dunbar JM, Marshall GD, Hovell MF (1979). Behavioral strate-
  gies for improving compliance. In Haynes RB, Taylor DW,
  Sackett DL (eds): "Compliance in Health Care," Baltimore:
  The Johns Hopkins University Press, p 174.
Egbert LD, Battiti GW, Welch CE, Bartlett MK (1964). Reduc-
  tion of post-operation pain by encouragement and instruc-
  tion of patients. N Engl J Med 270:825.
Gillum RF, Barsky AJ (1974). Diagnosis and management of
  patient non-compliance. JAMA 228:1563.
Gordis L (1979). Conceptual and methodological problems in
  measuring patient compliance. In Hayes RB, Taylor DW,
  Sackett DL (eds): "Compliance in Health Care," Baltimore:
  The Johns Hopkins University Press p 23.
Gore S (1978). The effect of social support in moderating
  the health consequences of unemployment. J Health Soc
  Beh 19:157.
Green LW (1979). Educational strategies to improve compliance

with therapeutic and preventive regimens: The recent evidence. In Haynes RB, Taylor DW, Sackett DL (eds): "Compliance in Health Care," Baltimore: The Johns Hopkins University Press p 157.

Haynes BR, Taylor DW, Sackett DL (1979a). "Compliance in Health Care," Baltimore: Johns Hopkins University Press.

Hayes-Bautista DE (1976). Modifying the treatment: Patient compliance, patient control and medical care. Soc Sci and Med 10:233.

Haynes RB (1979b). Determinants of compliance: The disease and the mechanics of treatment. In Haynes RB, Taylor DW, Sackett DL (eds): "Compliance in Health Care," Baltimore: The Johns Hopkins University Press p 49.

Janis IL (1967). Effects of fear arousal on attitude: Recent developments in theory and research. In Berkowitz L (ed): Adv in Exptl Soc Psych Vol 3. New York: Academic Press.

Johnson CA and Beardsley RS (1978). Life style as a mediator of post-discharge adherence to a hypertension treatment regimen following an in-hospital behavioral modification program. Prev Med 7:95.

Johnson JE, Morrisey JF, Leventhal H (1973). Psychological preparation for an endoscopic examination. Gastrointestinal Endoscopy 19:180.

Kasl SV (1975). Issues in patient adherence to health care regimens. J of Human Stress 1:5.

Kendall PC, Williams L, Pechacek TF, Graham L, Shisskak C, Herzoff N (1979). Cognitive-behavioral and patient education interventions in cardiac catheterization procedures: The Palo Alto medical psychology project. J Consult Clin Psych 47:49.

Kramer WG, Feldman S (1977). Apparent metabolism of allopurinol by blood: A preliminary report. Res Comm Chem Path Pharmacol 19:781.

Langer E (1975). Reduction of psychological stress in surgical patients. J Exptl Psych II 155.

Lewinsohn PM, Munoz RF, Youngren MA, Zeiss AM (1978). "Control Your Depression," Englewood Cliffs, New Jersey: Prentice Hall, Inc.

Leventhal H (1971). Findings and theory in the study of fear communications. In Berkowitz L (ed): Adv in Exptl Soc Psych Vol 5 New York: Academic Press.

Levy SM (1982). Biobehavioral interventions in behavioral medicine: An overview. Cancer 50:1936.

Marston MV (1970). Compliance with medical regimens: a review of the literature. Nurs Res 19:313.

Parkes CM, Benjamin B, Fitzgerald BG (1969). Broken heart:

a statistical study of increased mortality among widowers. Br Med J 4:740.

Rogers RW (1975). A protection motivation theory of fear appeals and attitude change. J of Psych 91:93.

Sackett DL, Snow JC (1979). The magnitude of compliance and non-compliance. In Haynes RB, Taylor DW, Sackett DL (eds): "Compliance in Health Care," Baltimore: The Johns Hopkins University Press, p 11.

Schmidt DD (1977) Patient compliance: The effect of the doctor as a therapeutic agent. J of Fam Practice 4:853.

Smith SD, Rosen D, Trueworthy RC, Lowman JT (1979). A reliable method for evaluating drug compliance in children with cancer. Cancer 43:169.

Stone GC (1979). Patient compliance and the role of the expert. J of Soc Issues 35:34.

Svarstad B (1976). Physician-patient communication and patient conformity with medical advice. In Mechanic D (ed): "The Growth of Bureaucratic Medicine." New York: John Wiley and Sons, Inc.

Turner RJ (1981). Social support as a contingency in psychological well-being. J Health Soc Beh 22:357.

Progress in Cancer Control IV: Research in the Cancer Center, pages 391–400
© **1983 Alan R. Liss, Inc., 150 Fifth Avenue, New York, NY 10011**

IMPORTANT GAPS IN PATIENTS' KNOWLEDGE PRIOR TO CHEMOTHERAPY*

Wendy L. Jones, Ph.D., Barbara Rimer, Dr.P.H.,
Paul F. Engstrom, M.D., Michael Levy, M.D., Ph.D.,
Anthony Paul, M.D., Robert Catalano, Pharm.D.,
Ruth Peter, R.N.
The Fox Chase Cancer Center
Philadelphia, PA 19111

INTRODUCTION

The overall goal of the informed consent process is to give patients sufficient information about medical recommendations that they may make informed choices. The informed consent process is of particular importance in the case of cancer patients because many of the treatments recommended to them are unfamiliar and some are experimental. Based on the most recent Federal regulations, an informed decision is one made by a patient who understands the nature of the proposed treatment, its risks and benefits, the possible alternatives to the proposed treatment and the right to withdraw from treatment (Federal Register 1981). These regulations reflect the patients' right to information and their responsibility to use this information in the decision-making process. Underlying these regulations are both ethical and practical issues. For a variety of reasons, it is important that patients be able to identify the drugs they are taking, the side effects of these drugs and the appropriate methods of managing side effects which may occur.

There have been few studies of informed consent practices and even fewer studies that investigate consent with regard to the cancer patient. Some recent research (Gray et al. 1978; Grunder 1980; Morrow 1978) indicates that consent forms are written at such a high level as to preclude

*Supported by grants from the American Cancer Society
(IN-140) and National Institutes of Health (CA23321).

their understanding by most lay readers. Morrow (1978) concluded that the forms from five national clinical trials
were only slightly less difficult to read than the New
England Journal of Medicine.

Studies by Dodd and Mood (1979) showed important areas
of cancer patient misunderstanding about the names of their
drugs, risks and side-effects. An information visit by a
nurse following the consent interview significantly improved
the patients' recall of this information. Morrow (1978)
found that recall of consent information by cancer patients
could be significantly improved by allowing patients to
retain the form overnight before signing.

Cassileth (1980) found significant misinformation about
treatment in a sample of cancer patients. For example, one
day after signing consent forms, only 60% of the patients
could correctly answer questions about the nature and
purposes of treatment. Epstein and Lasagna (1969) concluded
that patient understanding was inversely related to the
length of the consent form, and a study at the University
of Washington (Schultz 1975) found that only 52% of patients
were judged to be adequately informed.

Increasingly, issues related to informed consent have
been discussed in the medical and lay press. Nevertheless,
there has been little investigation either of what actually
occurs in the process of informed consent or with what other
outcomes, such as satisfaction and compliance, consent is
associated. Although many studies document patients' lack
of knowledge after signing consent forms, it is not possible
to identify the cause(s) of their insufficient knowledge.
Perhaps physicians did not discuss required information
(Meisel and Roth 1980); perhaps, patients did not read or
understand the forms which they signed; or perhaps, patients
did not hear or understand verbal communications.

This led Meisel and Roth (1981) to conclude that,

"there is a strong need for clinical studies which
examine the relationship not merely between disclosure and decisions, or understanding and
decision but the complex relationship between what
patients are told, what they understand, if and
how they use it in making a decision, and whether
they consent to treatment."

Recognizing the need for further research in the area
of informed consent, researchers at the Fox Chase Cancer
Center are investigating the extent and causes of patients'
insufficient knowledge about cancer treatments. Preliminary
results from this investigation are reported here. The
major study aims are (1) to test a method of recording the
process of informing patients about chemotherapy and
(2) to investigate patients' understanding of the information
which they were provided by professionals.

CONCEPTUAL FRAMEWORK

The design for this study was devised from the conceptual framework of patient decision-making, shown in
Figure 1. This conceptualization is based on a modified
version of the health belief model (Rosenstock 1974),
Green's PRECEDE model (1980), complementary behavioral
theory (Fishbein and Ajzen 1975, 1980) and research findings
(Haynes 1979; Jones 1981). Predisposing, modifying and
enabling factors are seen to affect the patients' decision-
making process. Another factor influencing this process is
the patients' emotional state. This factor is bracketed in
our conceptualization because emotional distress is known
to be common among cancer patients and because there are no
well-accepted measures of this distress. In this study, the
patients' emotional state is included only insofar as it is
behaviorally displayed during consultations with professionals
or study interviews (and may influence decision-making).
The outcome of the patients' decision-making process is
measured by their intent to comply with recommended treatment, satisfaction with the information process and
commencement of recommended treatment.

METHODS

Data for the preliminary analyses reported here were
gathered from an inception cohort of 95 patients with lung
and colo-rectal cancers who were advised to undergo chemotherapy during a six-month period in 1982. Selected socio-
demographic characteristics of the sample are shown in
Table 1. The majority of respondents were age 60 or over,
male, and had completed between 9 and 12 years of education;
most of these respondents were accompanied by a friend or
relative during the observed consultation. All eligible

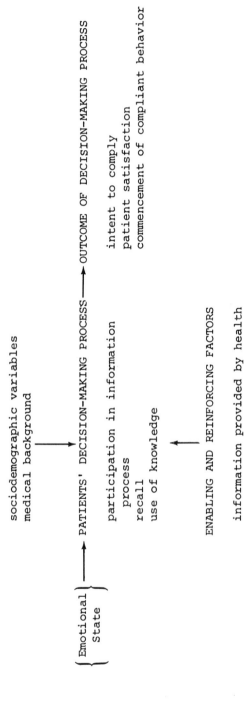

Figure 1. Conceptual Framework of the Patients' Decision-Making Process

Table 1

Selected Sociodemographic Characteristics of the Sample

Characteristic	Percent of Sample (n=95)
Age:	
Under 60	40
60 and over	59
Missing data	1
Sex:	
Female	41
Male	59
Education:	
No high school (< 9 years)	12
Some high school (9-12 years)	58
More than high school (> 12 years)	27
Missing data	3
Others present during consultation:	
Friend(s) and/or relative(s) accompanied patient	64
No one accompanied patient	36

patients were informed about the study and were asked to participate. In accordance with the decision of the Institutional Review Board, oral consent was obtained and patients were free to withdraw from participation or to refuse to answer any of the study questions. No patient refused to participate.

Data were gathered through observation of the consultations between patients and professionals and in subsequent interviews with the patients. When the attending physician was ready to recommend chemotherapy to a patient, one of the researchers (W. J. or B. R.) was notified. The researcher observed the consultation and interviewed the patient. Both the observation record and interview questions related to the DHHS guidelines (Federal Register 1981) for information to be communicated during the consent process, for example, description of purpose, risks, benefits and alternatives.

Simple enumerative analyses were carried out on these study data. These were descriptive analyses and preliminary investigations of associations between variables, using standard BMDP programs. These investigations included two-way cross tabulations of respondents' sociodemographic characteristics and the observation/interview data. A *chi*-square test of significance was used to test the null hypothesis of no relationship between variables. The tentative null hypothesis was rejected and an association between variables accepted when the probability of achieving the calculated *chi*-square statistic by chance was .05 or less.

These methods have been used to generate two types of findings. First, there are descriptive data which document the process of informing patients about recommended chemotherapy and the extent of patients' misunderstanding about the regimens recommended to them. Of more importance, since we have documented what patients actually were told, we have been able to investigate the kinds of information patients remembered, the kinds they forgot, and misunderstood. Primarily, the significance of this study derives from the combination of observation and interview data, which allows an examination of previously unanswered questions about the consent process.

RESULTS

The results of our preliminary analyses are summarized in Table 2. Our research indicates that most patients consenting to chemotherapy do not know important facts regarding their regimens. The observation records preclude blaming the patients' lack of knowledge on the possibility that the information was not presented. In each case, the observer at these consultations documented that these issues were discussed. In fact, the professionals observed in the study did an admirable job of transmitting complex information.

As shown in Table 2, at the time of consent most patients in the sample do not know the names of their drugs. This is an important deficiency, because patients may need to communicate this information to an emergency room physician or an out-of-town doctor. Given the polypharmacy which is characteristic of most older people (Pfeiffer 1980), these patients, especially, should be able to identify medications to prevent drug interaction problems. The fact that 36% of patients do not know their chemotherapy schedules could create compliance problems for patients who must take pills at home or come to the clinic for scheduled treatments. One of the most serious problems stems from the inability of patients to identify the major side effects of chemotherapy. This may be especially relevant for patients living alone who must be able to recognize symptoms as side effects which should be reported to physicians and/or cared for at home. Frequently, patients have trouble remembering the conditions under which physicians or nurses should be notified about side effects. Additionally, a large majority (73%) cannot remember what they are expected to do to prevent or control side effects. This is a problem since nearly all cancer treatments have some adverse side effects (Chabner 1981).

Preliminary analyses reveal a significant relationship between male gender and not knowing how to prevent side effects ($x^2 = 4.1$, p = .04). There is a significant relationship between having read the consent form and knowing drug names ($x^2 = 6.75$, p = .03), and a suggestive relationship between careful reading of the consent form and knowing the correct schedule ($x^2 = 5.4$, p = .06).

Table 2

Preliminary Results from the Informed Consent Study
at the Fox Chase Cancer Center

Observation or Interview Topic	Percent of Sample (n=95)
Names of drugs:	
knows drug names	24
does not know drug names	76
Chemotherapy schedule:	
knows correct schedule	64
does not know schedule	36
Side effects:	
knows major side effects	12
does not know all major side effects	88
Management methods:	
knows at least one recommended management method	27
does not know any recommended management method	73
Reading of consent form (patient's self-report):	
read very carefully	30
scanned	33
did not read	37
Understanding of consent form (patient's self-report):	
understood very well	60
understood somewhat	35
did not understand	5

DISCUSSION

The preliminary study findings suggest that patients either misunderstand or fail to remember important facts or instructions about chemotherapy regimens to which they have agreed. Since their lack of knowledge cannot be explained by professionals' failure to inform patients, those who seek to improve patients' knowledge must develop better education strategies and materials to supplement the standard process of informing patients about recommended chemotherapies. If the goals of the informed consent process are to be achieved, professionals must do more than comply with the legal requirements for disclosure of information. These study findings highlight the challenge and the difficulty of providing patients with new, technical and often frightening information in a form which is understandable and useful for patients' decision-making and for their compliance with treatment regimens.

REFERENCES

Alfidi R (1973). Informed consent and special procedures. Clev Clin Q 40:21.
Cassileth BR, Zupkis RV, Sutton-Smith K, March V (1980). Informed consent - Why are its goals imperfectly realized? N Engl J Med 302:896.
Chabner BA, Myers CE (1982). Clinical pharmacology of cancer chemotherapy. In DeVita VT, Helman S, Rosenberg SA (eds): "Cancer: Principles and Practice of Oncology." Philadelphia: J. B. Lippincott, p 158.
Dodd M, Mood D (1981). Chemotherapy: helping patients to know the drugs they are receiving and their possible side effects. Cancer Nurs 4:311.
Epstein L, Lasagna L (1969). Obtaining informed consent. Arch Intern Med 123:682.
Federal Register (1981). 46:8366.
Fishbein M, Ajzen I (1975). "Beliefs, Attitudes, Intentions and Behaviors," Reading, MA: Addison-Wesley.
Fishbein M, Ajzen I (1980). "Understanding Attitudes and Predicting Behavior," Englewood Cliffs, NJ: Prentice Hall.
Gray B, Cooke R, Tannenbaum A (1978). Research involving human subjects. Science 201:1094.
Green LW, Kreuter MW, Deeds SG, Partridge KB. "Health Education Planning," Palo Alto, CA: Mayfield.

Grunder TM (1980). On the readability of surgical consent forms. N Engl J Med 302:900.

Haynes RH (1979). Determinants of compliance: the disease and the mechanism of treatment. In Haynes RB (ed): "Compliance in Health Care," Baltimore: Johns Hopkins University.

Jones WL (1981). "Report of the Patient and Family Needs Assessment," Philadelphia: Fox Chase Cancer Center (unpublished report).

Meisel A, Roth L (1982). What we do and do not know about informed consent. JAMA 246:2473.

Morrow G, Gootnik J, Schmale A (1978). A simple technique for increasing cancer patients' knowledge of informed consent to chemotherapy. Cancer 42:793.

Pfeiffer E (1980). Pharmacology of aging. In Lesnoff-Caravaglia G (ed): "Health Care of the Elderly: Strategies for Prevention and Intervention," New York: Human Sciences.

Rosenstock I (1974). The health belief model and preventive behavior. Health Ed Mono 2:354.

Schultz A, Pardee GP, Ensinck JW (1975). Are research subjects informed? West J Med 123:76.

Progress in Cancer Control IV: Research in the Cancer Center, pages 401–410
© **1983 Alan R. Liss, Inc., 150 Fifth Avenue, New York, NY 10011**

RECENT PROGRESS AND RESULTS OF MODERN RADIATION THERAPY IN
MEDULLOBLASTOMA

H. W. Chin, M.D.,Ph.D. and Y. Maruyama, M.D.

Department of Radiation Medicine
University of Kentucky
Lexington, Kentucky 40536

Considerable progress was achieved in the management
of medulloblastoma during the past 10 years. This was associated with improved techniques of diagnosis and treatment
for this tumor. Until the era of megavoltage radiotherapy,
the prognosis of this disease was extremely poor and there
were few cures. In addition to the accurate radiographic
localization of tumor and improved neurosurgical techniques,
the use of optimum radiation therapy becomes of major importance in the control of the tumor. Today a majority of medulloblastomas are potentially curable by radiotherapy although for the advanced cases, even optimum radiotherapy may
not significantly alter the natural history of the disease.
With the application of modern radiotherapy using megavoltage machines, 5-year cure rate in medulloblastoma cases can
be around 70 percent (Berry 1981; Chin 1981; Bongartz 1979;
Hirsch 1979; Hope-Stone 1970; Pichler 1981). For the early
stages of medulloblastoma, roughly 90 percent 5-year cures
could be expected if accurately staged and adequately treated. In spite of those exciting achievements, the outlook is
confusing to the family doctor or general practitioner since
textbooks are still outdated and survival is variably quoted
from series to series.

In 1925 Bailey and Cushing identified medulloblastoma
as a disease entity and differentiated it from other gliomas
or sarcomas of the posterior fossa. Medulloblastomas are
rapidly growing cellular tumors that occur most often in the
middle cerebellum. In Bailey and Cushing's series (1925),
the estimated average length of evolution of medulloblastoma
cases was about twelve months from onset of the disease.

After operation, only six to nine months lapsed before recurrence. Since surgery alone was not enough to control medulloblastoma, Cushing and Bailey used roentgen rays to attempt to improve clinical results. Based on their experience, Bailey et al (1928) stated "Roentgen ray therapy was able to retard the growth of medulloblastoma for a considerable period" as early as 1928. The addition of roentgen therapy to surgery resulted in considerable improvement in survival. The average survival time increased to thirty-four months compared to six months with surgery alone. Because roentgen ray therapy at that time was in its infancy, it was still not possible to destroy the tumor completely or cure the patients.

Until the 1960's the radiotherapy techniques were still in the developmental stage. With the introduction of Cobalt-60 and megavoltage energies in the 1960's the outcome began to change favorably. Five year survival rates as high as 75% have been quoted in 1970's (Hope-Stone 1970). In contrast to the growing evidence for curability, some believed that survival rates of approximately 40% at five years and 30% at 10 years probably represented the best that could be achieved (Bloom 1977). This is perhaps because survival data were often drawn from patients who were treated with variable radiation doses. In addition, the evolution of modern techniques of optimum radiotherapy had not been appreciated by many radiation centers and suboptimal radiotherapies were still in use in many medical centers.

MODERN RADIATION THERAPY AND INFLUENCE OF OPTIMUM
RADIOTHERAPY ON SURVIVAL IN MEDULLOBLASTOMA

Since Bailey's experience with roentgen therapy in early 1920's medulloblastoma has been proven to be the most radiosensitive of all intracranial tumors. The tumor is generally not amenable to complete surgical resection and radiotherapy for medulloblastoma remains cornerstone of treatment in the cure of the disease. Until the advent of megavoltage energies for radiation therapy the treatment results were poor and it was widely believed that medulloblastoma was a hopeless disease. While radiation therapy in the past was inadequate and accomplished little beyond temporary arrest of tumor progression, modern megavoltage radiation is now able to overcome the physical limitation of radiation dose distribution in poorly penetrating kilovoltage X-rays. The evolution from the kilovoltage to the megavoltage radiotherapy eliminated a dose-limiting factors, i.e., skin tolerance, and larger irradiation doses could be safely delivered to tumors without adverse effects to the surrounding normal tissues. The number of long-term disease free survivors began to increase, and in late 1970's favorable reports of greater than 70% five-year survival rates appeared (Berry 1981; Chin 1982; Bongartz 1979; Hirsch 1979; Cumberlin 1979; Pichler 1981; Tokars 1979).

Table 1. Comparison of past and present survival results

```
*  Average survivals from onset
        1930 (Cushing)     : 8-9 months
        1928 (Bailey et al): 12 months (surgery alone)
                            34 months (with postop radiation)
*  3-year survival rates
        1949 (Lampe et al) : 28 percent
        1953 (Paterson et al): 54 percent
            (Richmond)     : 50 percent
*  5-year survival rates (Kilovoltage)
        1958 (Paterson)    : 41 percent
        1966 (Bouchard)    : 27 percent
        1969 (Bloom   )    : 32 percent
*  5-year survival rates (Megavoltage)
        1970 (Hope-Stone)  : 75 percent
        1979 (Hirsch et al): 72 percent
        1981 (Chin,Maruyama):78 percent
        1981 (Pichler et al):74 percent
        1981 (Berry et al) : 74 percent
        1982 (Duffner et al):74 percent
```

These historical trends and changes in survival are shown in Table 1. It shows progressive changes and improvement in survival of patients with medulloblastoma from the time when the initial Roentgen X-ray was used by Bailey and Cushing (1928) to the era of orthovoltage irradiation (Lampe 1949), and to the era of megavoltage radiation therapy.

The first reports on the importance and dose-dependence of tumor control began recently. Two years ago, the authors (Chin & Maruyama 1981) reported our experience at the University of Kentucky, that showed significantly improved survivals at five years when an adequate and optimum dose of radiotherapy was applied after surgical resection. Compared to the low dose radiotherapy group, our report revealed that approximately 80% five-year survival was possible if high tumor dose was given to the primary tumor site in the posterior fossa. A great number of reported series in the literature were reviewed and supported similar findings of improved survival with high dose irradiation (Berry 1981; Bongartz

1979; Chin 1981; Cumberlin 1979; Duffner 1982; Hirsch 1979;
Hope-Stone 1970; Pichler 1981). In addition we found that
there was a relationship between radiation tumor dose and
survival rate (Chin & Maruyama 1982). Comparative data (Fig.
1) collected from recent literature supported our view of a
radiation dose dependent tumor control relationship in medulloblastoma (Cumberlin 1979; McFarland 1969; Smith 1973).

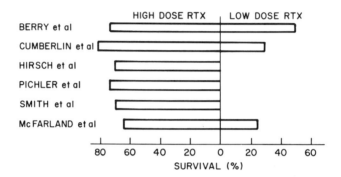

Fig. 1. Comparison of five-year survival results according
to high vs. low dose radiotherapy shows definite and remarkable improvement in survival with high dose megavoltage
radiation therapy.

The treatment results in relation to radiotherapeutic
techniques are shown in Fig. 1. Five-year survival in patients with medulloblastoma has improved from less than 50% for
low-dose radiotherapy to around 70% with high-dose megavoltage irradiation. It should be noted that all stages of disease are included in each of these series, and they represent differing proportions of various stages. Depending on
the proportion of early or advanced stages, there were difference in survival rates from series to series. Modern high
dose radiotherapy yielded roughly 70% five-year survivals.

From the preliminary analysis of our data at the University of Kentucky we observed significant differences in
survival of patients treated with doses more or less than
5000 rad of tumor dose to the posterior fossa. In Figure 2,
further detailed analysis of our experience assesses whether
any group of patients treated by high dose radiotherapy shows
a significantly better survival. The treatment data of

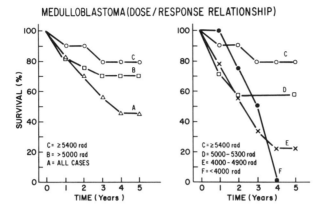

Fig. 2. Analysis of survival of patients with medulloblastoma
of all stages, treated at University of Kentucky Medical
Center; subdivided according to radiation tumor dose. (A) High
dose radiation groups (left), (B)Four different radiation dose
groups (right).

different radiotherapeutic groups were pooled to construct
survival curves using Cutler's life table method. These show
a progressive improvement in survival results with increment
of total tumor dose. In Fig. 2 (A) various survival outcomes
are shown according to radiation tumor doses used in the treatment of the patients with medulloblastoma. Curve A included
all 30 patients who received widely varied tumor doses ranging
from 3700 rad to 6000 rad. The 5-year survival rate was 45%
comparable to figures reported in the past. Curve B represented the patients who received high dose radiotherapy of at
least 5000 rad of tumor dose to the posterior fossa with dose
ranging between 5000 rad to 6000 rad. Five-year survival rate
increased to 70% when tumor dose of 5000 rad to 6000 rad was
used. Curve C consisted of the patients who received a tumor
dose of 5400 rad and more. With the higher tumor dose, five-
year survival rate was further increased to 79%. In Fig. 2
(B) the patients were subdivided into four radiation groups;
Group C received more than 5400 rad to the posterior fossa;
Group D between 5000-5300 rad; Group E between 4000 and 4900
rad; and Group F less than 4000 rad. There show a close
correlation between radiation tumor dose and survival outcome.
Improvement in survival was seen in the high dose radiotherapy

groups treated with more than 5000 rad. Further increment in survival was obtained with the best results at a radiation dose of at least 5400 rad to the posterior fossa. In contrast to the highest tumor dose group (Curve C), the moderate tumor dose group (5000-5300 rad) had only a 60% 5-year survival rate. Low dose radiotherapy was not effective in the treatment of medulloblastoma. Less than 4000 rad was totally ineffective and there were no 5-year survivor. From these survival curves, it appears that optimum radiotherapy should potentially be able to cure the disease in a majority of cases. Inadequate radiotherapy has been unable to alter the natural course of medulloblastoma as presented in Fig. 2 (Curves E and F). A literature review revealed comparable survival results to ours which attests that modern optimum radiotherapy has become the primary modality for cure of medulloblastoma (Berry 1981; Van Eys 1981; Tokars 1979; Smith 1973; Hirsch 1979; Bongartz 1979).

Of a number of factors influencing the prognosis of medulloblastoma, the most important factor is the stage of the disease at presentation. There were two presentations of medulloblastoma that behaved distinctly in the natural history of disease, and also in the response to the radio-

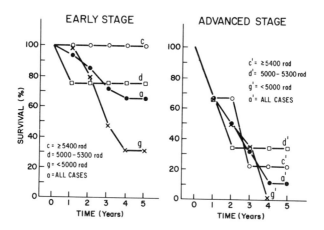

Fig. 3. Analysis of survival of patients with medulloblastoma according to clinical stage and radiation dose at the University of Kentucky Medical Center; (A) early stage groups (left), and (B) advanced stage groups (right).

therapy (Chin & Maruyama 1982). Since the majority of
patients who had clinical evidence of irreversible hydrocephalus did not survive more than four years, the presence
of clinical hydrocephalus requiring shunting has been classified as a more advanced stage of disease. As shown in Fig.
3 (A) early stage medulloblastomas responded favorably to
radiotherapy, and if adequate radiotherapy was given almost
100% 5-year survivals were possible (Curve c). In sharp
contrast, the curves for advanced medulloblastoma cases in
Fig. 3 (B) showed significantly poorer survivals even with
high-dose optimum radiotherapy. The authors observed no
significant difference in survival of patients in these
advanced groups whether treated with high or low dose radiotherapy. The curves (Fig. 3, B) fell steeply regardless of
the radiation dose. The results of radiotherapy in advanced
stages were disappointing and there were few patients surviving at five years.

The treatment results in childhood medulloblastomas
with those of the whole group are shown in Fig. 4. Fig. 4
(A) and (B) show very similar survival curves. We did not
observe a remarkable difference in survivals between childhood and all age groups. More important may be an advanced
or early stage for the tumor.

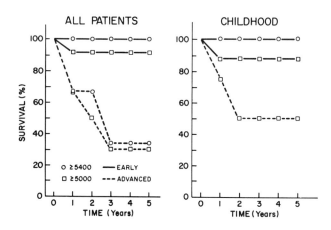

Fig. 4. Comparison of survival results from two age groups;
all ages (A) and childhood (B), for patients with medulloblastoma treated with high-dose radiotherapy, at University
of Kentucky Medical Center.

From our studies, we believe that the view that all brain tumors are fatal diseases is an erroneous one. Our results show that medulloblastomas are highly radioresponsive and potentially curable disease if adequate and proper postoperative radiotherapy is used. Adequate staging studies are important as favorable results are seen in their early stage, whereas poor results are seen with advanced stages.

Conclusions: The Curability of Medulloblastoma and Future Prospects

It is evident that modern megavoltage radiotherapy has substantially increased survival of patients with medulloblastoma. The survival rates have been consistently high since the adaption of optimum irradiation technique. Many patients treated in their early childhood have survived into their teens or young adult stage with no subsequent symptoms or signs of tumor. Hynes (1955) stated "when remission of signs and symptoms persists for ten or more years, without the need of continued treatment, it is proper to describe such remission as apparent cure". In our series, all patients who have survived more than five or ten years have had no evidence of residual or recurrent disease. Although further and careful observations will be needed for at least ten years or longer, the analyses of the survival curves have provided unambiguous indication that optimum radiation therapy does indeed not only significantly prolong survival of the patients with medulloblastoma but at the same time would be able to cure the disease in substantial proportion of early stage cases. For advanced cases, however, it seems unlikely that substantial survival improvement can be achieved from optimum radiotherapy. Thus, future research for advanced medulloblastomas should be directed to a search for new approaches to examine the efficacy of a variety of new treatment modalities. Another focus in future studies should be a development of practical staging system which is very important in formulating therapeutic approaches as well as in predicting the prognosis. Finally, in dealing with this relatively uncommon tumor, large medical centers of excellence in neuro-oncology care can produce better outcomes compared to those where such interest is lacking.

Bailey P, Cushing H (1925). Medulloblastoma cerebelli: a common type of midcerebellar glioma of childhood. Acta Neurol Psychiat 14:192.

Bailey P, Sosman MC, van Dessel A (1928). Roentgen therapy of gliomas of the brain. Am J Roentgenol 19:203.

Berry MP, Jenkin RDT, Keen CW, Nair BD, Simpson WJ (1981). Radiation treatment for medulloblastoma: a 21-year review. J Neurosurg 55:43.

Bloom HJG, Wallace ENK, Henk JM (1969). The treatment and prognosis of medulloblastoma in children. Am J Roentgenol 105:43.

Bloom JHG (1977). Medulloblastoma: prognosis and prospects. Int J Rad Oncol Biol Phys 2:1031.

Bongartz EB, Bamberg M, Nau HE, Schmitt G, Bayindir C (1979). Optimum therapy in medulloblastoma. Acta Neurochirurg 50:117.

Bouchard J (1966). "Radiation Therapy of Tumors and Diseases of the Nervous System." Philadelphia: Lea and Febiger, p 111.

Chin HW, Maruyama Y (1981). Results of radiation treatment of cerebellar medulloblastoma. Int J Rad Oncol Biol Phys 7:737.

Chin HW, Maruyama Y (1982). Prognostic factors in medulloblastoma. Am J Clin Oncol 5:359.

Chin HW, Maruyama Y (1983). Early response and long term results in the radiotherapy of childhood medulloblastoma. J Neuro-Oncol (in press).

Cumberlin R, Luk KH, Wara WM, Sheline GE, Wilson CB (1979). Medulloblastoma treatment results and effect on normal tissues. Cancer 43:1014.

Cushing H (1930). Experiences with the cerebellar medulloblastomas: a critical review. Acta Pathol Microbiol 7:1.

Duffner PK, Cohen ME, Flannery JT (1982). Referral patterns of childhood brain tumors in the state of Connecticut. Cancer 50:1636.

Hirsch JF, Renier D, Czernichow P, Benveniste L, Pierre-Kahn A (1979). Medulloblastoma in childhood: survival and functional results. Acta Neurochirurg 48:1.

Hope-Stone HF (1970). Results of treatment of medulloblastomas. J Neurosurg 32:83.

Hynes, JF (1955). Radiocurability of malignant lymphoma. Acta Unio Internat Coutra Canerum 11:514.

Jenkin RDT (1969). Medulloblastoma in childhood: radiation therapy. Canad Med Assoc J 100:51.

Lampe I, MacIntyre RS (1949). Medulloblastoma of the cerebellum. Arch Neurol Psychiat 62:322.

McFarland DR, Horowitz H, Saenger EL, Bahr GK (1969). Medulloblastoma-a review of prognosis and survival. Brit J Radiol 42:198.

Mealey J, Hall PV (1977). Medulloblastoma in children: survival and treatment. J Neurosurg 46:56.

Paterson E, Farr RF: Cerebellar medulloblastoma: treatment by irradiation of the whole central nervous system. Acta Radiol 39:323.

Paterson R (1963). "The Treatment of Malignant Disease by Radiotherapy." 2nd Ed London: Edward Arnold Ltd, p 451.

Pichler E, Kogelnik HD, Reinartz G, Karcher KH, Zaunbauer F, Jurgenssen OA, Koos W, Kundi M (1981). Ergebnisse der therapie des medulloblastoms in den letzten 15 jahren. Strahlentherapie 157:508.

Richmond JJ (1953). Radiotherapy of intracranial tumors in children. J Fac Radiol 4:180.

Smith RA, Lampe I, Kahn EA (1961). The prognosis of medulloblastoma in children. J Neurosurg 18:91.

Smith CE, Long DM, Jones TK, Levitt SH (1973). Medulloblastoma: an analysis of time-dose relationships and recurrence patterns. Cancer 32:722.

Tokars RP, Sutton HG, Griem MI (1979). Cerebellar medulloblastoma: results of a new method of radiation treatment. Cancer 43:129.

Van Eys J, Chen T, Moore T, Chek W, Sexauer C, Starling K (1981). Adjuvant chemotherapy for medulloblastoma and ependymoma using IV vincristine, intrathecal methotrexate and intrathecal hydrocortisone: a Southwest Oncology Group Study. Cancer Treat Rep 65:681.

Progress in Cancer Control IV: Research in the Cancer Center, pages 411–415
© **1983 Alan R. Liss, Inc., 150 Fifth Avenue, New York, NY 10011**

EVALUATION OF A COORDINATED COMMUNITY APPROACH TO HOSPICE
SERVICES: AN ABSTRACT

M. E. Grobe, D. M. Ilstrup, D. L. Ahmann, J. C.
Miller, M. Gillard, H. Haycock, D. Jacobsen
Mayo Comprehensive Cancer Center

Mayo Clinic, Rochester, MN 55905

BACKGROUND

Since the Hospice concept was first introduced to North
America in the 1970s, both the concept and the conviction
that certain hospice models are intrinsically beneficial have
been widely accepted.

In 1979 prior to changing our service to terminally ill
cancer patients and their family members, we believed it was
necessary to examine our practice and our community in order
to answer some basic questions. First, did patients and their
families perceive a lack of or need for a coordinated, family-
centered approach to services? Then, if there was a need for
a change, were the prescribed hospice models of care appropriate and transferable to a largely rural, three-county area in
Southeastern Minnesota?

To answer these questions, we conducted a two-pronged
assessment: 1) an examination of the needs of our local advanced cancer patients and their families, and 2) a survey of
existing human services available to these patients and their
families (Grobe 1982).

The 1979 needs assessment involved structured interviews
of 30 adult advanced cancer patients who were no longer recipients of specific anti-cancer therapy and 28 affected family
members of deceased cancer patients. Twenty-nine affected
family members of deceased cancer patients identified by
death certificates and chosen by random selection also participated.

Data from this descriptive study has been reported in various journals and scientific forums (Grobe 1982, Grobe 1980, Grobe 1981). Our programmed interventions based on the 1979 study results included the appointment of a coordinator to assess the specific service needs of our local cancer patients in any phase or stage of disease and assist these adult patients and their family members by primarily providing information about and facilitating assistance from various community resources. This assistance is provided in an anticipatory rather than crisis-oriented manner in order to enable the patient to remain home as long as possible, if he so desires.

Another outcome of the 1979 study was the development and distribution of a glossary of supportive services, for one of the major problems discovered in the studies was that neither patients nor health care providers were aware of the range of existing supportive services in the community. A further responsibility of the Patient Care Coordinator has been to sensitize the array of medical specialists and allied health professionals to the needs of our local cancer patients and their family members, and to educate the public and professionals in the area about resources available to help cancer patients.

STUDY DESIGN/SUBJECTS

To evaluate the effectiveness of these program interventions, the original needs assessment descriptive study was replicated, in part. In 1982, 76 affected family members of deceased cancer patients were interviewed using the same structured format of the 1979 study. Participant selection, however, was stratified so that patients who were enrolled in the Hospice Program were proportionately represented. Of the 76 participants in 1982, 30 had been on the Program, that is the family had been direct recipients of the Patient Care Coordinator's services, and 46 had not participated in the Program, but may have benefited indirectly from the professional education and glossary distribution throughout the community. The same procedures used in 1979 for death certificate review and random selection were applied within each strata.

Proportionately the samples were similar with respect to the sex and age of patients, location of patient's residence, and location of patient's death. Proportionately, the 1982 sample reflected more lung cancer patients, more married patients, more patients with college educations and fewer patients with extremely low incomes. The educational characteristics of family member respondents were proportionately quite similar in both samples. In the 1982 sample, more husbands were participants and the median age of respondents was older. The differences between the 1979 and 1982 samples were likely to be functions of the stratified selection, since there were characteristic differences between patient/ family units who were enrolled in the Hospice Program and those who were not. Younger persons, persons with greater incomes and more formal education, persons with dependent children still at home, and persons under the medical direction of a Medical Oncologist were more likely to be Hospice Program participants.

Bearing in mind the probability of selection bias when patients were referred to the Patient Care Coordinator, the only valid comparison to be made is between the aggregate responses of the 76 participants in 1982 to the historical "pre-intervention" group of 29 affected family members in the 1979 sample.

RESULTS

Fisher's exact test of association was applied to test associations.

Supportive Service Data

Testing at the .05 level of significance, there were no differences in reported needs for services in general or in reported needs for any specific supportive service. However, statistically significant increases in knowledge of existing services were noted in the areas of personal care assistance, respite care for the family, emotional counseling, transportation and legal assistance. Increases, although not statistically significant, were noted regarding awareness of services for companionship, meals, equipment and bereavement support.

Increased use of community services was noted for every need except recreation and child care. Proportionate in-

creases in use which were statistically significant involved
the use of services for those who expressed the following
needs: personal care, emotional counseling for the patient,
companionship for the patient and legal services.

Seventy-six to 100% of the family members who used a
service reported each community service as effective in addressing the need.

Symptom Management Data

Family members in the 1982 study reported only one
statistically significant improvement in effective management
of patients' physical symptoms, that involving bowel incontinence. A statistically significant decline in effective
management of ambulation difficulties was noted. We believe
that this decline is directly related to the home care emphasis of our interventions. The fact that our interventions
did not proportionately improve symptom management is not surprising since the Hospice Program was not intended to alter
physicians' methods of practice.

General Satisfaction

The 1982 group reported a greater degree of satisfaction
with the medical care system than the 1979 group. For example,
in 1979, 48% of the family members of deceased patients
wished there had been a special terminal care team involved
in the patient's care, but only 19 or 25% of the 1982 group
expressed this wish.

As mentioned earlier, numerous characteristic differences
were noted between the patients enrolled in the Hospice Program and those not enrolled in the Program. The consequent
bias makes it difficult to compare any outcomes between these
groups. However, we noted some encouraging patterns. While
there were no differences in reported awareness of services
between the groups participating and not participating in
the Program, it was noted that Hospice Program participants
used community services more, experienced home death more
frequently, and when hospitalized, experienced shorter lengths
of stay in a hospital prior to death than did persons not
served by the Hospice Program.

CONCLUSIONS

Our future directions for the Program based on this evaluation are: 1) to continue to facilitate the use of existing
community services to enable home care, 2) to enlist the explicit involvement of the physician in providing direction for
care, 3) to eliminate selection bias through professional
education, thus potentially removing barriers to patient and
family access, and 4) when evaluating future changes in the
Program to consider random assignment of patients, since the
limitations in this study design inhibit us from flatly
stating that one approach is superior to another.

REFERENCES

Grobe ME, Ahmann DL, Ilstrup DM (1982). Needs Assessment
for Advanced Cancer Patients and Their Families. Oncology
Nursing Forum Vol 9, 4:26.
Grobe ME, Ahmann DL, Ilstrup DM (1980). Needs Assessment
for Terminally Ill Cancer Patients in a Tri-County Area
Surrounding Rochester, MN. Proceedings of the 1980 Annual
Meeting of the American Society of Clinical Oncology.
Grobe ME, Ilstrup DM, Ahmann DL (1981). Skills Needed by
Family Members to Maintain the Care of an Advanced Cancer
Patient. Cancer Nursing Vol 4, 5:371.

ACKNOWLEDGMENT

This study was supported, in part, by Grants CA 15083
and CA 29354 from the National Cancer Institute, National
Institutes of Health, Bethesda, Maryland.

Progress in Cancer Control IV: Research in the Cancer Center, pages 417–424

CLERGY AS INTERMEDIARY — AN APPROACH TO CANCER CONTROL

Delores G. Askey, M.S.; Dorothy Parker, M.H.S.;
Darralyn Alexander, R.N.; Jack E. White, M.D.
Howard University Cancer Center, College of
Medicine
2041 Georgia Avenue, N.W., Washington, D.C. 20060

The Black Church in America has played a significant
role in influencing standards of conduct and educating and
caring for children. The church has served as a resource
center for the black family and has played a role in its
survival.

The Black Church continues to be the main social institution for blacks. In a study conducted by distinguished
social scientist E. Franklin Frazier, the church is defined
as "an agency of social control," "an economic cooperative,"
and an "educational institution." (Frazier 1964) Like any
important institution of society, the Black Church has a
number of roles and functions, and thus an impact upon its
membership. These functions--political, economic, social,
and security, all attest to the secular scope of the Black
Church. Many schools of thought have been voiced regarding
the secular scope of the Black Church. Joseph Washington,
in "Black Religion: The Negro and Christianity in the U.S.,"
(1964) refers to the work of the late Rev. Martin Luther King,
Jr., as an extension of ther religious role of the church
into the civil rights area. Although Washington viewed
King's philosophy as a perversion of the uses of Christian
theology, his rationale was based on a lack of emphasis on
theology in the Black Church. Other writers have tended to
support the view that, on balance, the function of the Black
Church was not so much to foster the spiritual growth of its
members by it adherence to and development of the normative
Christian theology of the Church, as it was to serve their
spiritually related secular needs.

In a study of the Black Church in Chicago, it was concluded that "The Negro Church is ostensibly a religious organization, but Bronzeville expects it, too, to 'advance the race.'" "Negro Baptists think of their congregation as a 'race church,' and their leaders concern themselves with such matters as fighting the job ceiling and demanding equal economic opportunity as well as 'serving the Lord.'" (Drake, Cayton 1970)

The many functions and interest of the Church underscore the increased necessity for it to be responsive to the social needs of the Black community. The nature of these social needs becomes urgent by the genesis of new problems and concerns. The Black community continues to look to the Black Church for services to meet the ever-changing needs of its community.

In a study conducted by the Institute for Urban Affairs, at Howard University (Walters-Brown 1980), 94% of the 98 respondents felt that Black Churches should take an active role in social service and community action activities. The "Attitudes of Blacks Towards Cancer" study, conducted by the EVAXX corporation for the American Cancer Society in 1981 (ACS 1981), further strengthens this concept by pointing to the need to intervene through community organizations in an effort to reach large numbers of black people. This need has been further documented by discussions on the clergy's responsibilities in the community by Blizzard in 1956 and Reeves in 1971, and studies done on the role of the clergy in the management of the terminally ill by Reeves in 1971 and Weisman in 1975.

Through the leadership of the black preacher, the Black Church in America has provided an effective organization of groups, an approved and tolerated place for social activities, a forum for expression, an outlet for emotional repressions, and a plan for social living. (Hamilton 1972) The black ministry continues to be a concept cushioned in feelings of trust and mutual loyalty not found in other relationships. The phrase "my pastor" frequently enters into discussions held amongst church affiliated blacks; and when the phrase is used, there is a strong sense of mutual, personal attachment. For many black people, the Church is the only institution they belong to which is decidedly and exclusively theirs. Thus, over the years a very personal relationship has developed between the black preacher and his parishioners

Since the black culture is characterized by an oral tradition, knowledge, attitudes, ideas, and notions, are traditionally transmitted orally, not through the written word. It is not unusual then, that the natural leader among religious tradition, the successful black preacher, is an expert orator. By his mere presence and continued leadership, he offers a steady figure with which the people can identify. He represents continuity and, in an important sense, stability--the only stable strand in the lives of many people who have been wracked by instability and abrupt changes. Thus, it becomes increasingly obvious that the Black Church has a physical presence and constituency already organized in the community. It has availed itself as a vehicle by which the Christian community can deal substantively and effectively with the urban crisis and its related illnesses.

The Black Church has enormous potential for having a positive impact upon the lifestyle choices of its church community. Its resources extend beyond the religious fellowship and emphasize the importance of directing the whole person. It is for these reasons, the need arises to utilize the potential of the Black Church in improving education and behavior toward positive lifestyle habits displayed by people within the community. It has been noted that "clergymen counsel more troubled people than any other helping profession," and that "the immense health contributions of organized religion will be released only as increasing numbers of churches become centers of health and growth." (Hamilton 1972)

Washington, D.C. has been identified as having very high cancer mortality rates. Cancer rates of nonwhites in the District of Columbia are among the highest in the nation. (White, Enterline 1980) Blacks make up approximately 70% of the city's population. Cancers of the breast, colon, lung, and esophagus are reported to be extremely high among D.C. residents. With the exception of esophageal cancer, each of these high risk cancers can be controlled, to some degree, by primary and/or secondary prevention activities. Lung, and possibly colon cancers have associated risk factors which are controllable. The prognosis of both breast and colon cancers can be dramatically improved through early detection and treatment. (Axtell 1976)

The need for cancer control services in the District of Columbia, e.g., health education and screening has been documented. (Parker, White 1979) More than 1,500 Washington, D.C.

residents die from cancer each year. Traditional prejudices have contributed to preventing many people from learning more about cancer, and the meaning of cancer control and prevention. In the survey on attitudes of blacks towards cancer, conducted by EVAXX for the American Cancer Society, it was also found that for many black people, myths and misconceptions about cancer have influenced their ability to make informed judgments. Examination of such projects as that in Eastern Maine entitled "Ecumenical Approach to Health Education" (Campbell 1966), the San Fernando Community project entitled "The Pastor as Encourager of Community Development, the "Black Churches Project" at the University of North Carolina at Chapel Hill (Hatch, Eure 1981), and others, all point to the importance of the preacher in influencing attitudes and beliefs of people towards their lifestyle habits. Elaborate evaluative instruments (semantic differentials, death anxiety scales, familiarity and willingness scales) have been designed to document knowledge and attitudes of ministers towards specific cancer topics. Such instruments have been implemented at the University of Alabama in their "Development and Evaluation of a Clinical Cancer Education for the Clergy" program. (Daffin 1979)

The Howard University Cancer Center, in its efforts to reach large numbers of people constituting high risk populations in the District of Columbia, has chosen to increase local awareness of cancer and its preventable aspects through the involvement of the black preacher who, as discussed earlier, has served as an influential factor for our target group.

The ultimate goal of the "Clergy as Intermediary Project" is to integrate the expertise of the black preacher in developing cancer information and education programs which could conceivably promote cancer risk reduction behavior in the religious and non-religious community. The PRECEDE model developed by Green et al., was chosen as the framework used to help plan the most effective program while integrating the most scientific theories and educational technologies. PRECEDE is an acronym for predisposing, reinforcing, and enabling causes in educational diagnosis and evaluation. These terms will be further discussed as we proceed.

Following the format of PRECEDE, the Social Problem of cancer morbidity and mortality was identified, the Health Problem of high cancer rates of lung, breast, esophagus, and

colon in the District of Columbia was identified; thus, lead-
ing us to the identification of specific cancer-related
Preventive Behaviors that appeared to be linked to the Health
Problem.   These Preventive Behaviors were identified as:

(1) stop smoking or don't start
(2) drink responsibly or don't start
(3) conduct regular breast self-examination
(4) conduct regular Pap smear
(5) follow recommended dietary guidelines.

It was felt that these behaviors could be affected by
the recognition of three sets of factors Green refers to as
predisposing, enabling and reinforcing. Predisposing factors
are a person's attitudes, beliefs, values and perceptions
which facilitate or hinder personal motivation for change.
Enabling factors are the skills and resources necessary to
perform health behaviors, e.g., health facilities, training
and education programs, outreach clinics. Enabling factors
also pertain to the accessibility of needed resources.
Reinforcing factors are factors related to the feedback the
learner receives from others, the results of which either
encourage or discourage behavioral changes.

Accordingly, in sorting and categorizing the factors
that seemed to have direct impact on the behaviors, and those
that were important and changeable within the available
resources at the Cancer Center, the factors were identified
as: Predisposing - increase knowledge about cancer and
health enhancing factors, influence positive attitudes about
cancer, influence cancer salience. Enabling - access to
education programs, access to training programs (BSE, Quit
Smoking), influence the lack of specific health skills
related to lowering risk for cancer. Reinforcing - influence
negative and uninformed judgments about cancer made by peers
and adults, help ministers and ministerial staff to become
better informed transferors of cancer education information,
influence family and community. Thus the Education Strategy
for impacting on these factors was developed as follows:

1. Further collect data on cancer problem in the District of Columbia and the need to intervene at the level of
the local clergy.

2. Further review existing health education programs
aimed at clergy.

3. Identify local ministers. Identify the demographic makeup of the local clergy to be involved.

4. Develop some sense of the attitudes and beliefs of local clergy towards cancer, health education in the church, their perceived roles and functions, and what, in fact, is currently taking place in their individuial churches to educate people about lifestyle habits.

5. In conducting a telephone survey of local ministers, we chose the sample size such that if the true proportion in the population was .05, we could be .95 confident that the estimate obtained by our sample would be within .05 of the true population value. This led to a sample size of approximately 250 people. Preliminary results of this survey indicated that 89% of the ministers felt that cancer is a particularly serious problem among blacks, that 63% realized the seriousness of the cancer problem in the District of Columbia, 26% were not sure if there was anything one could do to lower his or her risk of getting cancer, 79% felt that the church should play a role in health education while the remaining 21% did not know, only 39% felt they knew enough about cancer to be able to talk freely about it with their congregation, and 87% were interested in attending a cancer training seminar to gain further education and information about cancer. These findings are more thoroughly discussed in another paper entitled "Attitudes and Knowledge about Cancer Held by Black Clergy." (Askey, White 1982)

6. Contact was made with key ministerial organizations and significant clergy.

7. A planning task force was created. Preliminary findings from the survey were shared and suggestions and plans discussed and developed.

8. An introductory course in cancer education for clergy in the metropolitan area was developed. This course was devloped in an effort to increase their knowledge about cancer. The effectiveness of training courses in educating transferors of information about cancer was documented in 1981. (Parker 1981) The training course provided information on the cancer experience in the District of Columbia, what cancer is, current treatment, sociological and psychological effects of cancer, diet and alcohol and their relationship to cancer, nutrition and its role in cancer

prevention, and pastoral counseling of the cancer patient. The overall impression of the three-day course was strongly positive. Area ministers expressed their appreciation to the Cancer Center, by awarding the Cancer Center a Certificate of Appreciation.

Follow-up to the three-day course has been in the form of constant contact with the minister, sharing information about cancer and its risk factors via newsletter, and most importantly, participating ministers have identified liaisons within their church to work with us in the design of tailored cancer education programs and activities for their respective congregations. Such activities are presently underway in many of our churches.

Conclusion

The need for health education intervention at the Clergy level became evident from the review of the data collected on the role of the clergy in the black community and the data on the cancer experience in the United States and specifically in the District of Columbia. It is commonly felt by many health professionals that education is an essential element to reducing risk associated with cancer and other diseases. It is also understood that there are an infinite number of variables in play in one's environment that might have an effect upon the desired outcomes. Certainly, knowledge of health facts does not always assure desirable health behavior, yet one cannot practice what one does not know.

While the impact of the Clergy as Intermediary Project has yet to be determined, initial reactions from the course participants, the planning team, and several community clergy have been quite favorable. The Cancer Center has been urged to offer the "Introductory Course in Cancer Education for Clergy" on an annual basis, and to offer another level of information for those clergy who have completed the introductory course. A course in the Psychosocial Aspects of cancer is presently being planned for those who have completed the introductory course, and the Cancer Center has decided to offer the introductory course annually.

The Clergy as Intermediary Project, based on the use of the PRECEDE model, represents one method of intervention at the community level. This approach could be useful to other communities interested in reaching large groups of people with information on cancer or disease prevention.

REFERENCES

American Cancer Society (1981) "Black Americans' Attitudes Towards Cancer and Cancer Tests, Final Report and Unpublished Tabulations.

Askey DG, White JE (1982) Unpublished paper "Attitudes and Knowledge about Cancer Held by Clergy."

Axtel LM, Asure AJ, Myers MH (eds) (1976) Cancer Patient Survival: Report Number Five, U.S. Department of Health, Education and Welfare, DHEW No. (NIH) 77-992.

Blizzard S (1956) The Ministers Dilemma, "The Christian Century" 508-510.

Campbell MM (1966) An Ecumenical Approach to Health. IN Health Educators at Work, 17:45-49.

Daffin R, Maisiak R, Durant J (1979) The Development and Evaluation of a Clinical Cancer Program for the Clergy.

Drake SC, Cayton HR (1970) "Black Metropolis: A Study of Negro Life in a Northern City," New York: Harcourt, Brace and World.

Frazier EF (1964) "The Negro Church in America", New York: Schocken Books.

Green LW, Kreuter MW, Deeds SG, Partridge KB (1980) "Health Education Planning: A Diagnostic Approach" Palo Alto: Mayfield Publishing Company, 146.

Hamilton CV (1972) "The Black Preacher in America," New York: Morrow.

Hatch JW, Eure MA (1981) The Community Health Education and Resources Utilization Program. Paper presented at the 109th Annual Meeting of the American Public Health Association.

Parker DF, White JE (1979) "The Distribution of Cancer Mortality in Washington, D.C.: 1971-1976" Washington, D.C. Cancer Coordinating Council for Metropolitan Washington.

Reeves RB (1971) Professionalism and Compassion in the Care of the Dying. "Pastoral Psychology" 22:7-14.

Walters RW, Brown DR (1980) "Exploring the Role of the Black Church in America" Mental Health Research and Development Center, Institute for Urban Affairs, Howard University.

Washington JR (1964) "Black Religion: The Negro and Christianity in the United States." Boston: Beacon Press.

Weisman A, Sachtleben C, Worden JW "Psychosocial Analysis of Cancer Deaths. "Omega" 6:61-75.

White JE, Enterline JP (1980) Cancer in Nonwhite Americans. IN "Current Problems in Cancer," Year Book Medical Publishers, Inc., 4:16-18.

Progress in Cancer Control IV: Research in the Cancer Center, pages 425–432
© **1983 Alan R. Liss, Inc., 150 Fifth Avenue, New York, NY 10011**

DEMONSTRATION OF THE EFFECTIVENESS OF THE PROFESSIONAL
EDUCATION COMPONENT OF A COMPREHENSIVE CANCER CONTROL
PROJECT USING SERIAL "PATTERNS OF CARE" (POC) STUDIES

William P. Vaughan, M.D.
Laura L. Morlock, Ph.D.
Raymond E. Lenhard, M.D.
Gregory P. Rausch, M.D.
Stanley P. Watkins, M.D.
Joyce M. Kane
T. Phillip Waalkes, Ph.D., M.D.

The Johns Hopkins Oncology Center and
School of Hygiene and Public Health
Baltimore, Maryland, 21205

Virtually all patients with cancer are diagnosed and
have their initial therapy decisions made in the primary
care setting, and the majority (78-80%) of patients receive all of their cancer care in community hospitals. The
initial evaluation and treatment decisions are the most
critical in cancer management and significant advances in
the management of a variety of cancers have been made in the
past decade. Many of these advances require increased
sophistication of the cancer care delivery team. These
factors have resulted in increased demand from within and
outside the health care professions for the institution of
programs and procedures to assure that optimum cancer care is
provided at the community hospital level. In response to
this need, "Models of Care" and care systems have been promoted formally and informally by the American College of
Surgeons, the National Cancer Institute, the American Cancer
Society, the Cooperative Groups and the Regional Cancer
Centers. These models generally include multidisciplinary
involvement in management, evaluation through registries and
conferences, professional education activities, and participation in protocol management or the development of management guidelines.

Formal cancer control research and evaluation efforts have been ongoing at The Johns Hopkins Oncology Center (JHOC) since 1973. Early projects included a major survey of all Maryland acute care general hospitals in order to determine: 1) estimates of the incidence and distribution of cancer related hospitalizations throughout the State; and 2) the degree of development of hospital-based program elements in cancer control including the presence/absence, composition and level of activity of a multidisciplinary cancer committee; presence/absence of a hospital tumor registry; and the nature and scope of other hospital-based cancer control activities.

By 1977, we had established a series of major cancer control efforts in the area of management (Table 1) as well as a framework for the evaluation of interventions where feasible.

Table 1
Major Johns Hopkins Oncology Center Maryland Cancer
Control Management Interventions 1977-1982

Comprehensive Demonstration Projects
Cancer Care Network Organization
Promotion of Formalized Community Hospital Cancer
  Programs
Assistance in Cancer Registry Development
Professional Education for Physicians and Nurses
  - Assistance with local program development
  - JHOC based post-graduate program including:
    weekly multidisciplinary conference
    monthly regional physicians meeting
    annual two-day post-graduate course

The underlying assumption of these efforts, in terms of the Donabedian model(Donabedian 1966), is that interventions aimed at improving the structural and process variables in the care of patients will improve outcome. For use as a process measure in this evaluation effort we designed "Patterns of Care" (POC)(Kramer and Herring, 1976) type studies for the initial management of cancers of cervix, lung, large bowel and breast. For use as outcome measures we developed patient questionnaires which included CES scales for depression and disability to assess morbidity, and planned to use tumor registries to assess mortality. Additional morbidity measures also included time to recurrence (from the registry) and total days in hospital for diagnosis and initial treatment, as well as subsequent hospitalizations (from the charts).

The chart and registry based studies were performed for patients whose diagnosis and initial management took place in 1975-6 in four cooperating hospitals within Maryland. These studies have all been repeated in those four hospitals for the original four primary sites in 1982 (1980-81 cases). In addition, two new POC instruments have been developed for evaluation of the management of pleural effusion occurring in patients with malignancy and the management of cerebral metastases. Thus, a "quasi-experimental" design (Cook, Campbell 1977) was established for evaluating interventions during the 1975-1980 time period aimed at improving cancer care.

The results of the 1977 POC studies in these four Maryland Communities have been analyzed and permit several important conclusions (Vaughan et al 1983). First, though there was significant variation in POC within hospitals, there was significantly more consistency to POC for each of the four cancer sites within the hospitals studied than there was between hospitals. This occurred despite the fact that for general and gynecologic surgery there were up to five different groups or solo practitioners in each hospital and in every hospital at least two groups or solo practitioners in each specialty. Such conformity suggests a tendency for different practitioners involved with diseases requiring multidisciplinary management to communicate among themselves regarding quality of care rather than through specialty societies or other regional organizations. This strongly supports the contention that the individual local hospitals and medical staffs are the most promising targets for cancer control interventions in the area of management. Second, there was some suggestion of an underlying logic to the within hospital consistency in POC, perhaps related to that hospital's own experience with the disease. For example, in the case of breast cancer, the one hospital (Hospital 2, Table 2) where the majority of patients had mammography performed, as part of their work-up had the highest percentage of small primaries, the most consistent effort to determine the extent of disease prior to surgery, was still performing the more extensive surgery and was not yet obtaining estrogen receptor data.

Table 2
Frequency of Selected Staging Procedures Performed On
Breast Cancer Patients at Four Community Hospitals,
Stage of Primary, Use of Standard Radical Mastectomy
and Frequency of Estrogen Receptor Determination

	Hospital			
	1	2	3	4
Mammography	.08	.81	.16	.20
Alkaline Phosphatase	.96	1.00	.13	.40
Primary <4cm	.28	.41	.19	.24
Standard Radical Mastectomy	.04	.88	.07	.24
Estrogen Receptors	.57	0	.31	.32

Hospitals 3 and 4 in this survey are very similar
with respect to bed size (just under 300 beds), size and
character of the medical staff (e.g. 5 general surgeons each),
type of community served, and distance from the Baltimore
and Washington metropolitan areas. Both hospitals are the
sole source of hospital services for well defined population
bases and both hospital staffs had substantial ties to
Hopkins in general and the JHOC in particular. As can be
seen from Table 2, these 2 hospitals had very similar POC
for breast cancer patients in 1975.

In 1977, a comprehensive Cancer Control Demonstration
Project was begun in Hospital 3 (Vaughan, Waalkes, Lundahl
1981). In this community all of the process and morbidity
studies were performed and integrated with community health
and civic leadership reconnaissance, population and provider
surveys. This information served to evaluate a number of
efforts in the community including
community organization, public education, screening and detection programs as well as management and rehabilitation programs. In the area of management a JHOC faculty
member established a management education and assistance program based upon an inpatient and outpatient consultation
service at the hospital. Review of discharge diagnosis data
for the first two years of that involvement demonstrated that
virtually all patients admitted for management of metastatic
disease or initial management of high risk of recurrence
disease were seen formally. By not accepting total care of
any patients (although he did supervise the administration
of chemotherapy) the JHOC faculty member was able to maintain the desired position of educator of providers rather

than provider _per_ _se_. While not promoting specific guidelines for the management of individual patients, he did
organize a targeted education program (Table 3) and concen-
trated his own individual effort in order to focus on perceived deficiencies in management and the rapid introduction
of new technology, especially in the management of breast
cancer

Table 3
Hospital 3 Cancer Control Project
Target Education Program

1. Breast Cancer - routine estrogen receptor assay
2. Breast and colon cancer - routine lymph node counting
   and sectioning of grossly negative nodes
3. Unusual tumors and presentations - frequent pre-op
   consultations
4. Ovarian cancer - routine abdominal exploration, omen-
   tectomy and sectioning of grossly negative omenta
5. Breast cancer - separate diagnostic and therapeutic
   surgery
6. Increased vigilance against unnecessary morbidity, e.g.
   skeletal
7. Increased proficiency in general cancer patient care
   and more appropriate referral
8. Routine consideration of adjuvant chemotherapy

Data from the 1982 POC studies for breast cancer are
now available (Table 4), and demonstrate a significant increase between 1975 and 1980 in the number of diagnostic
studies performed as part of the initial diagnosis and
management of patients with breast cancer in Hospital 3 as
compared to the closely matched control hospital (Hospital 4).

Table 4

Change in Rates of Performance of Selected Tests Used in the Evaluation of Patients
With Suspected Breast Cancer at Hospital 3 vs. Hospital 4 1975/1980

	Hospital 3			Hospital 4			Hospital 3 vs. Hospital 4*	
	1975	1980	p*	1975	1980	p*	1975	1980
Mammography	16%	48%	<.01	20%	20%	NS	NS	<.05
Liver Chemistries	19%	60%	<.01	16%	28%	NS	NS	<.05
Alkaline Phosphatase	13%	60%	<.001	40%	32%	NS	<.02	<.05
Bone Scan or Survey	6%	56%	<.001	12%	24%	NS	NS	<.05
Liver Scan	3%	52%	<.001	8%	8%	NS	NS	<.001
CEA	9%	80%	<.001	4%	20%	NS	NS	<.001
Estrogen Receptors	32%	96%	<.001	32%	72%	<.01	NS	<.05

* All p values by χ^2

Further data analysis will determine to what extent the significant increase in these performance rates represents appropriate management for the patients on whom they were performed but at the same time there was improved performance of cancer screening procedures at Hospital 3 relative to Hospital 4 and no substantial rate of performance of clearly unnecessary tests for the work-up of breast cancer at either hospital (Table 5).

Table 5
Rates of Performance of Selected Tests Performed on Suspected Breast Cancer Patients in Two Maryland Hospitals, 1980

	Hospital 3	Hospital 4	$p(\chi^2)$
Brain Scan	4%	0%	NS
Bone Marrow	4%	0%	NS
Intravenous Pyelogram	4%	0%	NS
Upper Gastrointestinal Series	0%	0%	NS
Pap Smear	96%	60%	<.01
Digital Rectal Examination	76%	12%	<.01
Stool for Occult Blood	4%	0%	NS

Of course, it cannot yet be determined whether the significant change which has occurred in the POC for breast cancer in Hospital 3 will be associated with a significantly greater improvement in five year survival than in the control hospital, and if so whether that improvement occurred as a result of the alteration in POC or some other process change which resulted from the intervention such as better management of metastatic disease. However, future data accumulation and analysis will determine whether there was improved survival after the development of metastatic disease as well as address other alternative hypotheses. In the meantime, we have demonstrated that significant changes in POC have taken place in one community where an especially direct and disease specific educational intervention took place, but not in another where only less intense efforts existed.

Cook TD, Campbell DT (1979). "Quasi-Experimentation: Design and Analysis Issues for Field Settings." Chicago: Rand McNally.
Donabedian A (1966). Evaluating the quality of medical care. Milbank Meml Fund Quart 44:166.

Kramer S, Herring DF (1976). The patterns of care study: a nationwide evaluation of the practice of radiation therapy in cancer management. Int J Radiation Oncol Biol Phys 1:1231.

Vaughan WP, Waalkes TP, Lundahl S (1981). A model for community hospital/regional oncology center collaboration in cancer control. In Mettlin C, Murphy GP (eds): "Progress in Cancer Control," New York: Alan R. Liss, p 223.

Vaughan WP, Waalkes TP, Lenhard RE, Watkins SP, Sadler WP, Stout DA, Carney SP, Del Carmen BV, Herring DF (1983). Patterns of care in oncology: an approach to medical and utilization audit. In Engstrom P, Anderson PM, Mortenson LE (eds): "Advances in Cancer Control: Research and Development," New York: Alan R. Liss, (in press).

Partial support: NCI-CA-17448

Progress in Cancer Control IV: Research in the Cancer Center, pages 433-442
© 1983 Alan R. Liss, Inc., 150 Fifth Avenue, New York, NY 10011

COLORECTAL CANCER PATIENT REHABILITATION AND CONTINUING CARE
NEEDS: A PRELIMINARY ASSESSMENT OF SERVICES PROVIDED BY A
VOLUNTARY CANCER AGENCY*

William A. Stengle, M.P.H. and Dorothy Eckert, Ph.D.

Michigan Cancer Foundation
110 East Warren Avenue
Detroit, Michigan 48201

INTRODUCTION

With tremendous advances in cancer diagnosis and treatment cancer patient management has become increasingly complex. Ideally, a cancer care system should encompass: 1)
prompt initiation of treatment, 2) continuity of care during
the course of disease, 3) a structure to facilitate dissemination of new oncological knowledge and technology to the
disciplines involved in patient care, 4) treatment services
available and convenient for the patient and, 5) all the
supportive services necessary for the cancer patient both in
and out of the hospital setting (Greenwald, 1980). Con-
curring with these goals, this study examines the existing
supportive services of the Michigan Cancer Foundation (MCF)
for the colorectal cancer patient.

Like other cancer control organizations, the MCF is
confronting several important issues: changing community
service needs, the need to transfer non-paying service
activities to those capable of receiving reimbursement, and
economic necessity which dictates that we make better use of
limited community financial resources to help achieve the
above model.

The MCF is located in Metropolitan Detroit which consists of three urban counties with a population of 4.3

*Supported by Grant #CA-29023-03; Exploratory Grant
for Cancer Centers awarded by the National Cancer
Institute.

million people residing in 2022 square miles (UCS, 1982).
There are 65 hospitals, 3200+ physicians, 2 medical schools
and 44 home care organizations. The Comprehensive Cancer
Center of Metropolitan Detroit is comprised of the MCF,
Wayne State University School of Medicine, and institutions
in the Detroit Medical Center complex. Other voluntary
organizations such as the American Cancer Society and the
usual social agencies found in an urban area contribute to
the network of cancer care.

The Michigan Cancer Foundation engages in basic and
clinical cancer research, is part of the National Cancer
Institute (NCI), Survey Epidemiology and End Results (SEER)
program and is a pioneer in community-based cancer patient
services. Beginning in the late 1940's all services were
provided by volunteers. Since the late 1960's, it has com-
plemented its volunteer program by supporting and training
professionals in cancer detection and screening, rehabilitation, home nursing, home hospice and social work. During
the late 1970's MCF, as a recipient of an NCI community-based

TABLE 1

MICHIGAN CANCER FOUNDATION REHABILITATION
AND CONTINUING CARE SERVICE PROGRAMS

	Service	Carried Out By
1.	Speech Rehabilitation Laryngectomy Visitors	Speech Therapists Volunteers
2.	Rehabilitation Nursing and Counseling	Rehabilitation Nursing Specialist Enterostomal Therapist Social Workers (MSW) Social Work Technician
3.	Individual, Group and Family Counseling	Social Workers (MSW)
4.	Home Care Services/Home Hospice	Oncology Nurse Specialists Homemakers, Social Workers, Home Health Aide
5.	Patient Supportive Services supplies, equipment, comfort items, dressings, transporta- tion, friendly assistance	Volunteers in 9 regional offices
6.	Program Development and Coordination	Director, Cancer Control (MD) Administrative Staff (MPH, MHA)

cancer control program, (the Metropolitan Detroit Cancer
Control Program - MDCCP), established four regional outreach
centers in densely populated areas. These centers offered
communities cancer screening, information, referrals, and
professional counseling together with the more traditional
volunteer functions (Table 1). The regional centers'
clients are referred by self, hospital or physician.

METHODOLOGY

Traditionally, the greater portion of MCF services has
been for both breast and colorectal cancer patients. Colorectal cancer ranks as one of the major forms of cancer
facing our community with an average of 2100 new cases
diagnosed annually (Table 2). The age-adjusted incidence
rates for this type of cancer are exceeded only by the age
adjusted rates for cancer of the lung, the leading form of
cancer for both sexes (Young, 1981). The relative survival
rates for those diagnosed with colorectal cancer are substantially better than the rates for lung cancer, e.g., the
relative survival rates for colorectal cancer in Metropolitan Detroit are 68.4% at one year, 49.1% at 3 years and
41.6% at five years. In contrast the comparable rates for
lung cancer patients are 30.1%, 11.9% and 8.4% (Metropolitan
Detroit SEER 1973-1980).

TABLE 2

NEWLY DIAGNOSED COLORECTAL CANCER CASES IN
METROPOLITAN DETROIT BY YEAR AND RACE (SEER)

	1973	1974	1975	1976	1977	1978	1979	1980
White	1549	1624	1562	1658	1729	1805	1886	1870
Black	246	257	269	273	327	353	356	402
Total	1795	1881	1831	1931	2056	2158	2242	2272

As in indicator for future planning, this study views retrospectively the type of services requested and provided for colorectal patients by the MCF (1978-1981). The colorectal site is investigated because it includes both sexes. For this site a comparison is made between the served population and the total population of newly diagnosed cases as a measure of the extent of demand from the community. Also reviewed are: 1) age, (Table 7) and hospital of treatment for newly diagnosed cases (Table 3), 2) a profile of patient service needs compiled for all colorectal cancer patients served during the MDCCP (Table 4), and 3) a survey of new, and recently active colorectal cancer cases served by the regional centers is conducted to assess source of referral to MCF, client satisfaction with services rendered and degree of additional unmet needs (Tables 5).

TABLE 3

COLORECTAL CANCER CASES BY NUMBER
OF CASES DIAGNOSED PER HOSPITAL (1980)*

Number of Hospitals	Percent of Hospitals	Colorectal Cancer Cases Per Year	Colorectal Cancer Cases all Institutions	Percent of Total Cases
36	53.8	1-24	367	15.2
15	22.4	25-49	546	22.6
11	16.4	50-99	760	31.5
5	7.4	100 +	743	30.7
67	100.0		2,416	100.0

*Metropolitan Detroit Cancer Surveillance, Epidemiology and End Results Program (SEER)

TABLE 4

MICHIGAN CANCER FOUNDATION PROFESSIONAL SERVICES TO COLORECTAL CANCER PATIENTS
METROPOLITAN DETROIT CANCER CONTROL PROGRAM (JULY 1977 – APRIL 1981)

	N=708	
	n	Percent
Home Care Nursing	158	22.3
Social Work Counseling	173	24.4
Social Work – service assistance	121	17.1
Rehabilitation Nursing	347	48.9
Case Aid Assistance	161	22.7

MICHIGAN CANCER FOUNDATION VOLUNTEER SUPPORTIVE SERVICES TO ALL PATIENTS
METROPOLITAN DETROIT CANCER CONTROL PROGRAM (JULY 1977 – APRIL 1981)

	Patients all Diagnoses				Colorectal Patient Survey January 1982 – September 1982 N=206
	Year 2 N–1986	Year 3 N=2191	Year 4 N=2075	Year 5 N=1710	
	%	%	%	%	%
Dressings	32	34	35	40	44
Equipment	43	44	44	44	29
Supplies	22	22	22.5	19	41
Transportation	17	19	18	16	7

TABLE 5

COLORECTAL PATIENT SERVICE SURVEY

Referral Sources for Colorectal Cancer Patients to MCF
for Patient Supportive Services (January 1982 – September 1982)

N=206

1.	Health professional external to MCF	35%
2.	Self, family, friend	30%
3.	MCF professional staff	18%
4.	Other community agencies	9%
5.	Unknown	8%

Service Information Provided by Hospital and or Doctor at Discharge and use of
Services by Colorectal Cancer Patients (January 1982 – September 1982)

Service	Information Provided N=70		Services Used
	n	%*	n
Michigan Cancer Foundation	40	57	42
American Cancer Society	8	11	8
Home Care Agency	32	45	31
Family Services Agency	2	3	1
Ostomy Association	2	3	–
Other Agencies	3	4	2
Information on Home Care Only	10	14	–
No information provided	18	26	31

*does not total 100 because information on several sources provided to patients

DISCUSSION

In reviewing the data it is found that colorectal cancer cases are treated in 67 hospitals. A small number of
hospitals (5) account for one-third of all treatment given.
The remaining two-thirds of the patients are seen in 62
geographically widely dispersed hospitals. Seventy-six percent of the hospitals treat fewer than 50 patients per year

(Table 3); 53% of the hospitals are treating fewer than 24 cases per year. It is hypothesized that, in the main, hospitals with fewer cases may be less likely to have colorectal support services. In order for the regional centers to effectively reach those patients, the establishment and maintenance of a permanent referral mechanism with the hospitals in a given region is required.

The services rendered by the regional centers fall into two categories, professional and volunteer. Rehabilitation nursing, including counseling in ostomy management and adjustment to surgical procedures, accounted for half the services rendered. Equal numbers of patients (22%, 24%) received home care nursing assistance and individual, social work, psychological and counseling services. Approximately 40% of the patients required assistance with physical needs, supplies, finances and/or other short term needs which could be handled by a triage social worker or case aid .

Patients of all diagnoses receiving volunteer supportive services through the MCF regional network averaged 2077 patients per year, of which 17% were colorectal cancer patients. Volunteer services provided during the first 10 months of 1982 are compared to those provided to all patients (Table 4). During years 2-5 of the MDCCP, the level of services provided by MCF to all cancer patients varied only 28% while the mix of the services rendered did not vary greatly from year to year. While data is not available for previous years, patients recently entering the MCF service structure required assistance with dressings (44%) and medical supplies (41%).

Data as to the origins of referrals was collected in a telephone survey of 107 patients/family members who had received services from January to September 1982 (Tables 5-6). In addition to this information, those interviewed were asked if there were present needs unmet. Few responses to the latter were obtained. The source of referral, reported by regional centers, roughly correlated with the responses given in the survey. In the survey, 35% came from health professionals and hospitals and 38% came from the MCF community network (self, family, friend, volunteers, and MCF professionals). A small percentage (9%) were referred by other community service organizations. Survey participants were asked if they were provided information at the time of discharge by hospital or medical personnel about the types of services available in the community to help them in their post-surgical treatment. Fifty-seven percent were informed of MCF services at the time of discharge, 45% were given information about home health nursing services, 26% received no information about any available community services (Table 5). Over 80% of participants surveyed judged the MCF provided services to be very satisfactory and useful.

Because we are interested in the proportion of colorectal cancer patients in the community who turn to MCF for assistance, we have compared the number of patients requesting services with incident cases (Table 6).

TABLE 6

MICHIGAN CANCER FOUNDATION-METROPOLITAN DETROIT CANCER CONTROL PROGRAM
SERVICES TO COLORECTAL CANCER PATIENTS COMPARED TO NUMBER OF NEWLY
DIAGNOSED COLORECTAL CANCER CASES IN METROPOLITAN DETROIT (1978-1980)

Year	Professional Services Patients	Volunteer Assistance Patients	MCF Colorectal Patients/all MCF Patients	Professional Services/all Colorectal Patients*	Volunteer Services Patients/all Colorectal Patients*
	N	N	%	%	%
program year 3	212	359	16.4	9.8	16.6
program year 4	274	366	17.6	12.2	16.3
program year 5	156	369	18.1	6.9	16.2

*Metropolitan Detroit Surveillance Epidemiology End Results Program (SEER)
1978:2158, 79:2242, 80:2272

A constant 16% of all newly diagnosed colorectal cancer cases are requesting volunteer-assisted supportive services. The percentage of new cases requesting professional service assistance varies from 6.9% to 12.2% over the three reported years. The fraction of colorectal patients serviced in comparison to all other cancer patient diagnoses varies from 16.4% to 18.1% during the same period.

The age distribution of MCF colorectal patients compared to all colorectal cancer cases are similar. Seventy-seven percent of the service center patients were 61+ versus 73% of the SEER cases and 83% of the survey respondents. Thus, the population presently served is a bit older and possibly subject to more social and economic needs than those of the general population of colorectal patients (Table 7).

TABLE 7

PROFILE OF COLORECTAL CANCER PATIENTS RECEIVING SERVICES IN
MICHIGAN CANCER FOUNDATION OFFICE BY AGE AS COMPARED TO ALL NEWLY
DIAGNOSED COLORECTAL CANCER CASES IN METROPOLITAN DETROIT (SEER 1973-80)

Age	All Cases (SEER) %	Service Center Patients January 82 - September 82 N=206		Survey Colorectal Patient/Family N=70*	
		n	%	n	%
<30	.01	1	.5	-	-
31-40	1.4	4	1.9	-	-
41-50	6.0	5	2.4	2	2.9
51-60	18.0	36	17.5	9	12.9
61-70	27.4	68	33.0	21	30.0
71-80	28.4	54	26.2	23	32.9
81+	17.4	38	18.4	14	20.

*1 age unknown.

SUMMARY

The data of the MDCCP and the Patient/Family Survey reveal a relatively constant level of colorectal cancer patients/families requesting services from MCF, both professional and volunteer. There is a sizable group of individuals for whom these services fulfill a specific need. That some colorectal patients report not being informed of community services indicates a departure from the ideal model. Needs assessments reported elsewhere cite this as a basic barrier to access community supportive services for cancer patients especially for the elderly (Greenleigh 1979, Lehman 1978, Snider 1982).

These preliminary data on MCF services serve as the basis for development of a more comprehensive study as to how social, psychological and other support services are provided to colorectal patients throughout the community. Such a study will be useful in indicating the direction our cancer agency should take and whether or not a change of role is indicated for the Michigan Cancer Foundation.

REFERENCES

Greenleigh Associates (1979). Report on the Social Economic, and Psychological Needs of Cancer Patients in California. American Cancer Society, California Division.

Greenwald HP (1980). Social Problems in Cancer Control. Cambridge: Ballinger, p 37.

Harven R, Hollis M, Jellinek M, Habeck R (1982). Cancer Rehabilitation An Analysis of 36 Program Approaches. JAMA 247:2127-2131.

Lehman J, Delisa J, Warren CG (1978). Cancer Rehabilitation: Assessment of Need, Development and Evaluation of a Model of Care. Arch Phys Med Rehab 59:419-419.

Snider EL (1982). Health Policy and the Elderly. Social Indicators Research 4:405-419.

United Community Services of Metropolitan Detroit (1982). What Lies Ahead for Human Services in the Detroit Area?

Young JL, Percy AJ, Asire AJ (1981). Surveillance, Epidemiology and End Results. National Institute of Health, Bethesda.

Progress in Cancer Control IV: Research in the Cancer Center, pages 443–453
© 1983 Alan R. Liss, Inc., 150 Fifth Avenue, New York, NY 10011

CANCER REHABILITATION ISSUES
FOR OCCUPATIONAL AND PHYSICAL THERAPISTS:
A CONFERENCE REPORT

Patricia D. Lynch, M.S.,Sarajane Schaefer, A.C.S.W.
and Dorothy Eckert, Ph.D.
Comprehensive Cancer Center of Metropolitan
   Detroit
110 East Warren Ave., Detroit, MI 48201

INTRODUCTION

In spite of improved survival for patients diagnosed
with cancer, they have often not been considered eligible
for rehabilitation. Until recently, rehabilitation from
cancer or its treatment has not been widely practiced. This
was true regardless of whether the patient was judged to be
cured, controlled or in an advanced stage of disease. "The
initial goals of rehabilitation are the elimination, reduction, or alleviation of disability, while the ultimate goal
is the reestablishment of the patient as a functional individual in his or her own environment." (Dietz, 1981) To
avoid unrealistic expectations in cancer and other chronic
diseases, perhaps readaptation should be used as a synonym
for rehabilitation. It would be defined as "accommodation
or adjustment to personal needs for physical, psychological,
financial and vocational survival." (Dietz, 1981)

Cancer patients have unique rehabilitation needs
throughout the course of their disease (Cobb, 1973; Cobb,
1974). It is important to remember that these needs can
range from post-surgical rehabilitation to the care required
during the palliative and terminal phases of the disease
(Dietz, 1981). Therefore, it is essential that rehabilitation professionals be part of the multidisciplinary cancer
team, and that they are prepared both technically and psychologically to offer their skills to the cancer patients.

This paper will report on the development, implementation, and implications of an Oncology Rehabilitation

Conference that was organized through the Comprehensive Cancer Center of Metropolitan Detroit. The First Michigan Regional Oncology Rehabilitation Conference, entitled, "The Role of Occupational and Physical Therapists in Assuring Quality Living," was held in suburban Detroit, June 11 and 12, 1982. Conferences similar to this one have been held in other parts of the country, but this is the first one of its kind to be held in the midwestern part of the United States.

The conference focused on two primary goals: to teach and discuss rehabilitation skills for professionals treating cancer patients, and to promote the attitude that all cancer patients, regardless of stage, have rehabilitation potential (Dietz, 1981). The conference offered the opportunity for a wider sharing of the Center's experience with rehabilitation of cancer patients. In addition to reflecting our own experience in Detroit, we were fortunate to have J. Herbert Dietz, Jr., M.D., Emeritus Chief of Rehabilitation Services at the Memorial Sloan-Kettering Cancer Center, to share his extensive experience in practice and program development. As a result of this conference, we hope to see an increase in the acceptance of the Occupational and Physical Therapist's place on the cancer team, and the development and expansion of oncology rehabilitation programs in existing settings and institutions.

Since April, 1980, the Patient and Family Services Department of the Michigan Cancer Foundation has sponsored half-day oncology rehabilitation seminars for health professionals in the Detroit area. There was strong interest in these programs, and we began to suspect that there were similar needs and interests outside of Metropolitan Detroit. As we interacted with health professionals and cancer patients, it became clear that rehabilitation services routinely available to cancer patients were less than optimal.

In order to accurately assess the current state of rehabilitation programs in Detroit, we conducted a survey of the Metropolitan Detroit hospitals. The survey examined the type of personnel who provide rehabilitation services in the hospitals, whether services are provided on an inpatient or outpatient basis, what the referral patterns are, and any specific types of programs which are available. Although somewhat informal, the results of the survey indicated that rehabilitation services are organized in many different ways, and that there is an extreme variety in the type of program a cancer patient can expect, depending on the hospital where he or she is admitted. Certainly at the time of diagnosis, most cancer patients are interested in treatment and are not prepared to shop around to find the hospital with the type of rehabilitation program they might need. In fact, many patients are unaware that such support services exist (Sorkin, 1975). In general, the larger hospitals offered more services, as would be expected, but we were occasionally surprised at the number of services which some of the smaller hospitals indicated they provided. A number of hospitals have a full complement of rehabilitation personnel, but provide very few services for cancer patients. For some hospitals, their cancer patient population is small, so they refer them to other agencies for services. Some reported they are planning to initiate more services for cancer patients in the future.

In January, 1982, the Comprehensive Cancer Center of Metropolitan Detroit received funding from the National Cancer Institute for a Cancer Communications Network Office. This contract allowed us to develop and implement as a special project the Oncology Rehabilitation Conference. The project was jointly sponsored by the Cancer Communications Network Office and the Patient and Family Services Department.

METHODS

To plan the actual conference, we recruited a multidisciplinary planning committee. The group represented the major rehabilitation disciplines, including Occupational Therapy, Physical Therapy, Rehabilitation Social Work, and Vocational Rehabilitation. The committee also included the Chief of Rehabilitation at MCF, and both the Health Educator and Evaluator from the Cancer Communications Office. Problems of time, distance and availability prevented us from including members from outside the Detroit area. Participants on the committee were selected from some of the more active Occupational Therapy and Physical Therapy departments around the Detroit area. We selected representatives from the large and small hospitals, as well as home care agencies.

The planning committee had major responsibility for selecting the topic areas, the format of the conference, learning objectives, and speakers. In addition, they provided expertise about the organization of Occupational and Physical Therapy groups, insight into special problems and needs of the therapists.

Program Description

One of the major difficulties in planning a conference such as this one is in determining the level of knowledge and expertise of the target audience. Our planning committee felt that most Occupational Therapists and Physical Therapists did not have a great deal of background information about cancer, did not have the opportunity or did not take the opportunity to see cancer patients in their practices, and were somewhat unsure of how to deal with some of the psychological issues involved -- both for themselves and for their patients. Many recent Occupational Therapy and Physical Therapy graduates have not been exposed to oncology during their training.

The program format was designed to deal with some of the issues that the planning committee felt are most important for Occupational Therapists and Physical Therapists. Our keynote speaker addressed current issues and perspectives on rehabilitation; a practicing oncologist did an extensive presentation on cancer diagnosis and treatment. In the afternoon, the Chief of Clinical Social Work at the Michigan Cancer Foundation discussed the psychosocial aspects of cancer and cancer care, as well as coping with patients' reactions to the disease. During the last part of the first day, participants met in small groups with a cancer patient. These sessions each lasted 45 minutes. These patients were chosen from among those who have received services through the Michigan Cancer Foundation; some were also suggested by members of the planning committee. Patients varied according to diagnosis, and whether they had received appropriate rehabilitation services. Some had participated in good programs, while others had experienced major difficulties before they had received any services. Conference participants were assigned to two groups so that the patients they met with were not too similar. Discussion in the small groups was facilitated by staff social workers, experienced in group processes, who were assigned to each group.

The second morning began with four workshops. The workshops lasted 90 minutes each and were run twice. Each

conference participant had the opportunity to attend two
workshops. Each program dealt with a different phase of rehabilitation and different cancer topics: Preventive Rehabi-
litation--Mastectomy, Restorative--Head and Neck Cancer,
Supportive--Central Nervous System Tumors, Palliative--the
Terminally Ill. Participants chose two workshops when they
pre-registered, and the participants were fairly evenly distributed over the workshops.

In the afternoon, Dr. Dietz discussed some of the ways
to sell rehabilitation programs to physicians and hospital
administrations. He was able to share a number of experiences about setting up an Oncology Rehabilitation Program
in New York, as well as to offer concrete suggestions and
strategies for participants to utilize. Another area which
the planning committee felt was particularly important was
the area of therapist burn-out, and we had a registered Physical Therapist discuss strategies for staff support. The
afternoon was concluded with a panel discussion of post-
hospital care options. These presentations included discussions of a large home care program, a description of vocational rehabilitation resources, the concept of hospice and
its role in the terminal phases of disease, and a description
of potential community resources and strategies to access
them.

Program Audience

The target audience for the Oncology Rehabilitation
Conference was primarily practicing Occupational and Physical Therapists. In order to attract the appropriate audience, we adopted a number of different strategies. Our
primary approach was direct mail. We purchased two mailing
lists; one from the National Occupational Therapy Association,
and the other from a large mailing list house. Obviously,
the quality of the mailing list can have a huge impact on the
type of audience that can be reached. We learned that Occupational Therapists must belong to the national organization,
but are not required to belong to their state one. Physical
Therapists, on the other hand, are required to belong to the
state organization, and national membership is optional. In
this case, it is not entirely clear how much this affected
registrations for the conference. More Occupational Therapists attended the conference, and a number of Physical
Therapists from different areas reported that they had never

received a brochure at all. They had heard about the conference through friends, or their institution had received a brochure from a separate mailing list. Unfortunately, experience is often the best predictor of a mailing list's value.

In addition to the direct mail to therapists, we distributed brochures to the Metropolitan Detroit hospitals, all members of the National Association of Rehabilitation Agencies, and all Comprehensive Cancer Centers in the United States. We also submitted notices about the meeting to both the national Occupational and Physical Therapy journals, the monthly newspaper, Oncology Times, and a local health oriented weekly newspaper, The Health Care News.

Attendance at the conference was limited to 150 persons because of the type of presentations and format that the planning committee felt would be most effective. In spite of the large direct mail campaign of about 17,000 pieces, we were only able to attract 79 participants. We suspect that a number of different factors influenced the small turn out. We are aware that in our area, travel budgets have been severely reduced, and most health professionals are attending fewer meetings. Many Occupational Therapists and Physical Therapists are paid on fee-for-service basis, and their institutions are reluctant to give them time off. Another possible factor is the problem of other conflicting meetings. There also appeared to be some reluctance to fund travel for a "single disease" conference. A number of people reported that their institutions prefer more generic conferences which might have more widely applied benefits.

RESULTS

The conference attracted the desired target audience. About 56% of the participants were practicing Occupational Therapists; 29% were Physical Therapists. Most participants were from the state of Michigan (Table 1), but with reasonable representation from neighboring states. The majority of participants have received their licenses since 1970, and only 22% received them prior to 1968. Three students expect to receive licenses in 1983. Participants represented a number of different settings, but hospitals predominated with nearly 70% working in a hospital setting. A large proportion of those working in hospitals are affiliated with teaching hospitals. Participants were also drawn from home care

Table 1

FIRST MICHIGAN REGIONAL ONCOLOGY REHABILITATION CONFERENCE
June 11-12, 1982

States Represented by Conference Registrants

N=79

Michigan	35
Ohio	11
Illinois	11
Indiana	6
Wisconsin	5
Kentucky	3
Pennsylvania	2
New York	2
Minnesota	1
Virginia	1
Unknown	2
Total	79

programs, extended care facilities, including nursing homes, hospices, private practice and a health department (Table 2). Nearly 90% of those attending the conference were involved in providing direct patient care, and patient care accounts for more than 50% of their time.

The planning committee suggested that the Occupational Therapists and Physical Therapists should be exposed to professionals who are active participants on the cancer treatment team. There was a fairly even distribution of conference participants at the four workshops. Nearly ninety percent of the participants attended two workshops. Many people indicated on their evaluation forms that they would have been very interested in attending all four workshops. In general, the workshops were well-received. Most participants rated the content highly, and stated that the subject was pertinent to their needs and interests. The most variability in the responses occurred in the evaluation of the workshop dealing with the terminally ill. It suggests that this was a much more sensitive issue for many participants, and perhaps confirms that the planning committee correctly identified this as a problem area for many Occupational Therapists and Physical Therapists.

We evaluated the conference using a pre-test/post-test design. Pre-test scores (Table 3) indicated a wide range of knowledge about cancer prior to the conference. Out of a possible 98 correct responses, 39% of the participants fell between 66-76 correct responses. Scores ranged from a low 17 to a high of 87 on the pre-test. Post-test scores showed a marked improvement in knowledge. These scores ranged from 17 to 91, with more than 70% of the participants scoring 77 or more correct responses.

Conference attendees were also asked to evaluate how well the conference met its learning objectives. Basic cancer information and issues and concepts in oncology rehabilitation were the most successfully met. Both received 96.6% "yes" responses respectively. The lowest rated objectives were those which related to the therapists' skills in coping with patient reactions and dealing with dying patients, but it is interesting to note that the objective to increase knowledge about the psychosocial impact of cancer was one of the highest rated.

Table 2

FIRST MICHIGAN REGIONAL ONCOLOGY REHABILITATION CONFERENCE
June 11-12, 1982

Work Settings Represented
by Conference Registrants

	N	%
Hospitals	55	69.6
Home Care	6	7.5
Extended Care Facility	5	6.3
Hospice	3	3.7
Consultant/Private Practice	3	3.7
Health Department	1	1.2
Unknown	6	7.5
Total	79	99.5

Table 3

FIRST MICHIGAN REGIONAL ONCOLOGY REHABILITATION CONFERENCE
June 11-12, 1982

Scores of Pre- and Post-Test
Correct Answers
Possible Score=98

Pre-Test = N=78			Post-Test = N=63		
Test Scores	N	%	Test Scores	N	%
17-50	15	19.2	17-50	1	1.6
51-65	20	25.6	51-65	7	11.1
66-76	30	38.5	66-76	10	15.9
77-87	13	19.7	77-87	37	58.7
			88-91	8	12.7
Total	78	100.0	Total	63	100.0

DISCUSSION AND IMPLICATIONS

Our first goal was to provide an opportunity for professionals to learn rehabilitation skills which could be applied
to cancer patients. Post-test scores and participants'
evaluation of the learning objectives both strongly indicate
that we were successful in meeting this primary goal. Promoting the attitude that all cancer patients have rehabilitation potential is obviously a more complicated process, and
is one that can be difficult to assess. Lecture presentations, especially the one by Dr. Dietz, dealt with the ideal
of rehabilitation potential on a cognitive level, and we hope
that the small group discussions with cancer patients made
this information a bit more concrete and personal for the
therapists. Individual comments on the evaluation forms indicated that for many people the small group discussion was
the high point of the conference.

At the conference, we were able to present examples of
team-oriented programs which effectively include Occupational
and Physical Therapists. As a result, participants were exposed to programs, as well as role models, and we hope that
this will lead these professionals to actively explore their
own role in oncology rehabilitation.

During the conference, one of the Occupational Therapists met with other Occupational Therapists in the group who
were interested in starting an oncology section in the National
Occupational Therapy Association. We hope this indicates
growing interest in oncology and promotes cooperation among
peers to establish programs in their own areas.

Efforts to influence the amount and quality of rehabilitation which cancer patients receive are determined by many
different variables. This conference focused on Occupational
Therapists and Physical Therapists, and attempted to increase
their knowledge about cancer and cancer rehabilitation, and
also sought to reinforce the importance of rehabilitation
for the cancer patient. Clearly, this is only a beginning.
Members of the planning committee suggested that fear of the
unknown and fears about their own coping skills are two factors which influence the Occupational Therapist's and Physical Therapist's willingness to be actively involved in cancer
patient care. Obviously, these are areas which are difficult
to influence or change because they require not only knowledge, but readiness on the part of the therapist.

Medical professionals must be aware of the rehabilitation potential of cancer patients, and be willing to include rehabilitation professionals on the cancer team. Another significant factor in the availability of rehabilitation services is reimbursement by third-party payers. A conference of this type cannot be expected to single-handedly alter the practice of medicine, but it can convene appropriate professional groups, and provide needed information that will be utilized to influence the number and quality of rehabilitation programs available to cancer patients.

REFERENCES

Cobb, Beatrix A. Medical and Psychological Aspects of Disability. Springfield, Illinois, 1973.

Cobb, Beatrix A. Special Problems in Rehabilitation. Springfield, Illinois, 1974.

Dietz, J. Herbert, Jr. Rehabilitation Oncology. New York, 1981.

Office of Cancer Communications. Pretesting in Health Communications. DHHS, NIH No. 81-1493. Revised November, 1980.

Sorkin, Alan L. Health Economics. Lexington, Massachusetts, 1975.

Progress in Cancer Control IV: Research in the Cancer Center, pages 455–463
© 1983 Alan R. Liss, Inc., 150 Fifth Avenue, New York, NY 10011

QUALITY OF CANCER CARE EVALUATION IN ITALY

A.LIBERATI, G.MASERA[+], G.TOGNONI, M.G.ZURLO[+]

Istituto di Ricerche Farmacologiche Mario Negri,

Via Eritrea 62, 20157 Milano,Italy

[+]Cattedra di Puericultura, Università di Milano,

Milano, Italy

How to make best available to the largest possible number of cancer patients the few clinically encouraging results
obtained in controlled trials has been recently indicated as
a priority goal, since no major breakthroughs are expected
for the reasonably near future (Carter, 1982). Development
of systematic programs to promote higher standards of care
is particularly important where resources are being reallo-
cated as part of the overall reorganization of the NHS.
The Italian situation can be considered a model case, as
some excellence centers have long held leading roles in
selected areas; however no attempt had been made to aggregate general hospitals in collaborative programs.

Summarized here are the results of two retrospective
surveys based on medical records, planned by our groups with
the aim of assessing the feasibility of auditing procedures
as part of routine hospital activity. Data to be collected
was selected so as to provide information on some outcome
variables and to check whether the standard of care was in
any way related to the degree of curability of the disease.
Pediatric and adult cancers were chosen, as they represent
different levels of health care organization.

The reliability of the information provided has been
discussed elsewhere (Liberati et al. 1982b) together with the

general methodology, which is summarized here. Medical
records of all patients in the study were screened with the
agreement of medical staff in charge by medically qualified
investigators trained and tested for comparative reliability
in transferring data from medical records to specific forms
including pre-coded items and free-text reporting. For
adult cancers a set of diagnostic and therapeutic procedures
was established, through a peer review analysis, as reference standard for evaluating the actual performance of different hospitals.
Sample of relevant findings are reported separately for the
pediatrics and adult populations.

Pediatric cases : In childhood acute lymphoblastic leukaemia (ALL) survival of all new cases (267) diagnosed in the
period 1974-1978 and treated in 94 pediatric wards of the
Lombardy Region (8.9 million inhabitants) has been found to
differ significantly in specialized teaching centers compar-
pared to general and community hospitals (95% vs 76% at 12
mos; 64% vs 42% at 36 mos) (Figure 1)

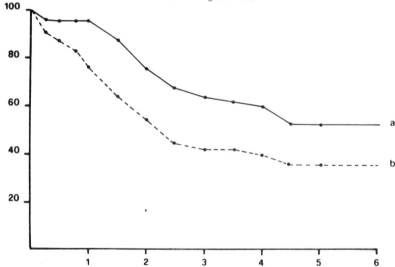

Figure 1. Life-Table analysis by type of treating hospital
of children aged 0-9 years, resident in Lombardy region,
affected with acute lymphoblastic leukemia and treated in
hospitals of the region (1974-1978).
a=hospitals treating 15-20 new cases/year (124 pts)
b=hospitals treating 1-4 new cases/year (143 pts)

Deaths during the first 3 months after diagnosis are respectively 4.5% and 2.8% in the two teaching centers and 9.7% in general and community hospitals(Zurlo et al.1983).Global survival is similar to that observed in the Manchester region for the period 1972-1977 (Birch et al.1981) it remains however consistently lower than ALL prognosis.

No immediate explanation has been found for these differences. A bias due to selection of higher risk cases in smaller hospitals does not seem evident from the data, which indicate a casual distribution of patients at the two levels of care, possibly more as a consequence of different patterns and criteria of referral of the caring physician than because of geographical distances. The phenomenon is sizeable as more than half of the total ALL population (143 vs 124 cases) is admitted to non-specialized centers, which include small and large general hospitals. The fact that the difference in fatal cases is already fully evident in the first three months and the survival trend is not different after one year suggests unsatisfactory accuracy of staging and of antitumor treatment and failure of intensive supportive care as causal factors in the different outcomes.

Adult cancers : The patterns of care versus standards set in accepted protocols were evaluated in 4913 patients (2406 breast cancer, 1692 lung cancer, 303 non-Hodgkin lymphoma, 277 ovarian cancer, 235 Hodgkin lymphoma) in 31 hospitals representing five Italian regions.

The overall results are summarized in Table 1,centering general indicators of care, which broadly agree with the few comparable data available in similar studies (Kramer, 1977; Kramer, Herring 1976).

Lag-time between first symptom and diagnosis seems to be the single most clinically relevant feature for breast cancer(Liberati et al.1982a).Comparison with similar findings for delayed diagnosis of endometrial cancer in Italy (Franceschi,et al.1983) suggests an inherent local problem.

The majority of patients with ovarian and lung cancers (67% and 73% respectively) are treated with chemotherapy, but a very small proportion follow recommended protocols. Because of the lack of evidence of any real benefit even with accepted regimens for these two types of cancer, such treatments are very likely to be more of a source of risk

TABLE 1 – Quality of cancer care according to four indicators of the quality of the diagnostic/therapeutic process

	Hodgkin lymphoma (%)	Breast cancer (%)	Non-Hodgkin lymphomas (%)	Ovarian cancer (%)	Lung cancer (%)
Lag-time between first symptom and diagnosis ⩾ 6 months	22	25	23	19	17
Standard stage classifications	64	44	42	28	14
Recommended chemotherapy[#] protocols	92	78	79	55	48
Patients in follow-up	60	50	54	47	24

Value are expressed as percentages of the relative sample; Tumours are presented ir scending order of curability (from left to right).

[#]Percentage of total patients treated

and suffering than of benefit.

In agreement with the findings of MacLean(1981), there seems to be no clear relationship between hospital qualification and quality of care delivery. The generally better profile of more qualified centers as regards lung cancer (Liberati et al. 1983) cannot mask the poor performance of some of them (Table 2), suggesting that concentration of cases in larger centers cannot be equated with better expectations (the same holds true as regards the ALL data). To check whether the poor performance that was a general feature of the care of less-curable tumours had any bearing on the outcome of the patients treated, long-term evaluation of the survival of ovarian cancer patients has been planned. Tracing up cases three-five years after diagnosis has been successful and data are now being processed. There is however already a suggestion that a monitoring program of the "natural" evolution of this population cared for outside standard protocol regimens is feasible and could provide an interesting reference series against which to assess the real benefit of clinical trials (La Vecchia et al. 1983)

Comments and Conclusions

The following points appear to merit specific attention in future studies :
1) Philosophy of cancer care organization. Our data confirm the importance of investigating the unsettled question of whether concentrating patients in specialized centers is a requisite for good care delivery. While this does seem to emerge from the ALL series of pediatric patients and from the overall favorable trend observed for adult cancers, it is worth emphasizing that an acceptable degree of performance is noted more in places where highly motivated, re-search-active teams are at work than in purely formally "qualified" groups. This possibly reproduces the apparently contradictory findings of two major studies (Sylvester,1981; Begg et al.1982)wherethe discriminant factor is better seen in the intensive problem-oriented training made available also to small hospitals of the U.S.A. series, which perform very well, in contrast with the EORTC experience where hospitals are recruited with no ad hoc auditing or intervention strategy.

2) Results of clinical trials and community care. Scant data has been collected from which to assess to what extent the population recruited for selective controlled trials

TABLE 2 - Differences between hospitals in performance in lung cancer care according to quality of care indicators

	Hospitals with oncological services		Hospitals without oncological services		x^2
	Proportion of patients	(%)	Proportion of patients	(%)	(D.F. = 1)
Diagnostic [No information	249/901	(28)	420/791	(51)	49.29 (p<0.001)
Clinical Stage only	46/901	(5)	11/791	(1)	16.72 (p<0.001)
Profile [Stage and histology	153/901	(17)	7/791	(1)	106.97 (p<0.001)
No.patients treated for neoplasm	719/901	(80)	512/791	(65)	7.66 (p<0.01)
Recommended chemotherapy protocols	339/566	(60)	110/343	(32)	27.49 (p<0.001)
Follow-up	231/901	(26)	90/791	(11)	38.38 (p<0.001)

really reflects the care available and actually delivered to
the majority of the same population seen in community or
general centers. The poor staging and, more important, the
delay in diagnosis observed in our series of patients suggest there is no direct inference from any benefit shown in
clinical trials, where rigid criteria are observed at every
step of the care process, to the attributable benefit measured in the health care system at large. Ad hoc series of
patients should perhaps be monitored appropriately to enable
investigators and planners to make documented decisions on
priorities and resources.

3) Impact of education-intervention studies on the quality
of care. In a recent survey on the impact of clinical
trials in the practice of community hospitals affiliated to
a research group (E.C.O.G.Boston) the authors concluded that
apart from the 16% of patients who enter research protocols,
a further 35% have their treatment plan influenced by a
protocol(Begg et al.1983).The search for the best way of
involving participating centers in educational, self-evalu-
ating programs needs to be combined with an effort to
devise simple methods for obtaining reliable and interpretable results from routine care. In this respect our
results seems promising as they suggest that something less
than the accumulation of data required by formal clinical
trials could be sufficient for routine collection and peri-
odical auditing. Larger networks could provide complementary and compatible data for quick assessment of the interaction, if any, between reference and general hospitals.

The above considerations led to the formulation of two
long-term research projects now in progress :
a) the follow-up of all childhood ALL cases treated in our
region in order to re assess the difference, if any, in
survival weighted by prognostic factors and to identify
causes of death and their distribution, to pinpoint the
critical steps in medical care organization;
b) prospective evaluation of diagnostic/therapeutic
approaches applicable to breast cancer to assess the
consistency of our previous findings and to define the role
of in- and out-patients assistance in producing the overall
quality of care. To start assessing the impact of educational programs, a group of centers which have officially
adopted the procedures recommended by the Italian National
Breast Cancer Task Force has been included in the study. A
complementary line of investigation through questionnaires

will provide information on the general practitioner's role in the overall process of care and the quality of life of patients (quality of survival, reaction to therapies, determinants of positive and negative compliance).

References

Begg CB, Carbone P.P., Elson PJ, Zelen M (1982). Participation of community hospitals in clinical trials. Analysis of five years of experience in the Eastern Cooperative Oncology Group. N Engl J Med 306: 1076.

Begg C, Zelen M, Carbone P, McFadden E, Bradawsky H, Engstrom P (1983). Cooperative groups and community hospitals: Measurement of impact in the community hospitals. To be published.

Birch JM, Swindell R, Marsden HB, Morris Jones PH (1981). Childhood leukaemia in North-West England 1954-1977: Epidemiology, incidence and survival. Br J Cancer 43: 324.

Carter SK (1982). Clinical trials in patients with cancer. N Engl J Med 306: 1105.

Franceschi S, La Vecchia C, Gallus G, Decarli A, Colombo E, Mangioni C, Tognoni G (1983). Delayed diagnosis of endometrial cancer in Italy. Cancer in press.

Kramer S (1977). The study of the patterns of cancer care in radiation therapy. Cancer 39 suppl.: 780.

Kramer S, Herring DF (1976). The patterns of care study: A nationwide evaluation of the practice of radiation therapy in cancer management. Int J Radiat Oncol Biol Phys 1: 1231.

La Vecchia C, Franceschi S, Liberati A, Gallus G, Tognoni G (1983). The clinical relevance of the epidemiology of ovarian cancer. To be published.

Liberati A, Andreani A, Colombo F, Confalonieri C, Franceschi S, La Vecchia C, Tognoni G (1982b). Quality of breast cancer care in Italian general hospitals. Lancet 2: 258.

Liberati A, Andreani A, Colombo F, Confalonieri C, Tognoni G (1982a). Care of cancer patients in thirty-one Italian general hospitals. Methodological aspects and general findings. Eur J Cancer Clin Oncol in press.

Liberati A, Confalonieri C, Andreani A, Colombo F, Franceschi S, La Vecchia C, Talamini R, Tognoni G (1983). Lung cancer patient care in general hospitals. To be published.

MacLean CJ, Davis LW, Herring DF, Powers WE, Kramer S (1981). Variation in work-up and treatment procedures among types of radiation therapy facilities. Cancer 48: 1346.

Sylvester RJ, Pinedo HM, De Pauw M, Staquet MJ, Buyse ME, Renard J, Bonadonna G (1981). Quality of institutional participation in multicenter clinical trials. N Engl J Med 305: 852.

Zurlo MG, Rossi MR, Marchi A, Pastore G, Ugazio GA, Masera G (1983). Epidemiologia descrittiva delle leucemie dei bambini in età 0-9 anni residenti in regione Lombardia 1974-1978. Hematologica, in press.

Progress in Cancer Control IV: Research in the Cancer Center, pages 465-476

DATA BASES FOR PATTERNS OF CARE STUDIES IN DEFINED POPULATIONS*

Lorenz J. Finison, Ph.D.,[1] Paul Jacques, M.S.,[2] Sharon J. Spaight, B.A.,[1] William Fine, M.S.,[1] W. Bradford Patterson, M.D.,[1] Richard Clapp, M.P.H.,[3] Cynthia Burghard, B.A.,[4] Vincent O'Sullivan, M.A.[5]

[1]Division of Cancer Control, Dana-Farber Cancer Institute, Boston, MA. 02115, [2]U.S.D.A. Nutrition Research Center on Aging at Tufts University, Boston, MA. 02111, [3]Department of Public Health, Commmonwealth of Massachusetts, Boston, MA. 02116, [4]Massachusetts Health Data Consortium, Waltham, MA. 02154, [5]Cancer Registry Program, Brockton Hospital, Brockton, MA. 02402

INTRODUCTION

Patterns of care studies typically suffer from a defect in terms of making inferences about the cancer care received by population groups. They are ordinarily carried out with samples of patients from volunteering hospitals, which may be non-representative of hospitals in a given region. This problem can be avoided by utilizing data from regional or state registries. Many such registries, however, collect information only on incidence and not on treatment. Nevertheless, all registries collect cancer stage information which would be useful for patterns of care studies, if augmented by treatment data.

Other sources of treatment data might be utilized at low cost to study cancer management patterns. One

*This investigation was supported by PHS grant number 16408, awarded by the National Cancer Institute, DHHS.

obvious source of such information is hospital discharge
data files, but hospital discharge data are episodic,
rather than case-based. Furthermore, they do not
include stage of cancer, which is critical for any
patterns of cancer care study.

A solution, described in this paper, is to merge
registry and hospital discharge data to provide staged
treatment data on a case by case basis. The method is
based on the assumption that it is of vital importance
to assure the confidentiality of patient records. Thus,
the method studied does not utilize patient-specific
identifiers in establishing the linkages of registry and
hospital discharge data.

The resulting case reports, which include both
cancer stage and treatment information, can be
aggregated in a number of ways, for example, by
hospital, by region of treatment, or region of
residence. Such aggregated case reports may be utilized
in making comparisons of treatment practices or
establishing baselines for evaluating the long-term
effects of cancer control interventions.

METHOD

Incident female breast cancer cases were identified
through a cancer registry and linked to hospital
discharge reports to develop composite case reports.
The two data bases may be linked by elements which are
common to both. For hospital discharge data, these
elements will be found in the Uniform Hospital Discharge
Data Set (U.S. National Committee on Vital and Health
Statistics, 1978), UHDDS. While there is not any such
formally established minimum data set for cancer
registries, a recent survey conducted by the Minnesota
Department of Public Health indicates which elements are
commonly collected. The elements collected in the UHDDS
and by cancer registries are listed in Table 1.
Examination of this table indicates that the demographic
variables which are common to both data sets include
patient code number, date of birth, zip code of
residence, hospital code number, sex, and race. Patient
code number, sex, and race were not used to link the two
data sets. The variable patient code number was

	Element	UHDDS	Cancer Registries
1.	Patient Name		X
2.	Patient Address		X
3.	Patient Code Number	X	X
4.	Date of Birth*	X	X
5.	Sex	X	X
6.	Zip Code of Address	X	X
7.	Hospital Code Number	X	X
8.	Admission Date	X	
9.	Discharge Date	X	
10.	Diagnosis	X	X
11.	Procedures	X	
12.	Expected Principal Source of Payment	X	
13.	Service at Discharge	X	
14.	Race	X	X
15.	Date of Procedure	X	
16.	Disposition of Patient	X	
17.	Admission Status	X	
18.	Special Care Units	X	
19.	Special Care Days	X	
20.	Attending Physician Code Number	X	
21.	Operating Physician Code Number	X	
22.	Primary Site of Cancer		X
23.	Stage of Cancer		X
24.	Histology		X
25.	Confirmation Method		X
26.	Vital Status		X
27.	Place of Diagnosis		X

* Although date of birth is reported in UHDDS, some abstracting services may report age rather than date of birth to health data consortia.

Sources: Massachusetts Cancer Incidence Registry, Massachusetts Department of Public Health; Massachusetts Health Data Consortium

Table 1. Data elements in hospital discharge data systems and cancer registries.

excluded for several reasons, including incomparable coding systems across hospitals, concerns about patient confidentiality, and multiple code numbers for patients receiving treatment at several hospitals. Race was not used as a variable by which to link the two because of suspected problems in coding. The variable sex, also common to both, was not employed because female breast cancer was the cancer under study.

All incident cases of female breast cancer (n=419) diagnosed during the period October 1, 1979 through September 30, 1980 were identified for the 13 hospitals from HSA V which are included in the Southeastern Massachusetts Cancer Registry (SEMCARE), a regional hospital-based cancer registry. This registry was chosen for the test of the matching and linking procedures instead of the statewide cancer incidence registry because the latter has been in operation for only a year and thus could not be used to match the available hospital discharge records. Registry information included stage of disease at diagnosis, date of birth, hospital of diagnosis, and zip code of residence at the time of diagnosis. Treatment information was available from a computer file of hospital discharge data held by the Massachusetts Health Data Consortium (MHDC). All discharge records (n=1539) for the period October 10, 1979 through December 31, 1980 for hospitals in HSA V were identified for which there was a diagnosis of breast cancer, a diagnostic or treatment procedure related to breast cancer, or a history of breast cancer. Each discharge summary record also included either date of birth or age, hospital of treatment, and zip code of residence at time of discharge. Patient names or code numbers were not available from MHDC.

For this test, 52 cases were excluded from the analysis because of an indication of a prior primary cancer. Cases from six hospitals, representing 248 registry cases, were excluded because of the manner in which they reported discharge data to MHDC. Five of these hospitals reported age at discharge rather than date of birth. Since the matching procedure currently being tested uses date of birth as the primary matching variable, cases from these hospitals were not included. The remaining hospital was excluded because of irregularities in the reporting of discharge data to MHDC.

In future analyses, the cases from the excluded hospitals may be linked to discharge data. After verifying the matches for the current procedure, they will be used to determine whether age can replace date of birth as the primary matching variable. If so, records from the five hospitals reporting age will be linked to registry data. It will be possible to perform the linkage using date of birth for the sixth hospital, but since it defined the reporting year differently from the other 12 hospitals, it will be handled separately.

Figure 1 summarizes the breakdown of incident breast cancer cases available for the study. Of the 1539 MHDC records, which represented both incident and prevalent cases, 151 were suitable to test the matching and linking procedures in that they matched at least one registry identified case on the basis of date of birth. Having just the same date of birth was not sufficient for the two to be considered matched. When a match was

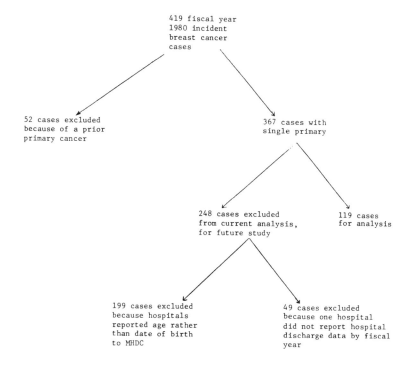

Figure 1. Breakdown of incident breast cancer cases from cancer registry.

made, the appropriate registry and MHDC records were linked. Each registry case was allowed to be linked with up to five records.

Verification of Matching

A sample of matched records was checked to determine whether registry cases were correctly matched to their hospital discharge records. Those matches for which date of birth, zip code, and hospital were the same were verified at MHDC as were those matches for which only date of birth and hospital were the same. For those matches where date of birth and zip code were the same, but hospitals of diagnosis and discharge were not, verification was performed using SEMCARE files. One of registry records without any matching MHDC records was also verified as not being treated in the region through SEMCARE files.

RESULTS

The procedures under study were highly successful in matching registry and hospital discharge records which contained patient date of birth. One hundred forty-one of the 151 discharge records matched an incident registry case on the basis of date of birth and zip code of residence and/or hospital code number. The remaining 10 MHDC records shared only the same date of birth of a registry case and therefore were not considered valid matches. Considering incident cases only, 115 of 119 were found to have corresponding treatment information. These results are summarized in Figures 2 and 3.

Verification of the matching procedure using samples of matched cases and records as presented in Figure 4 indicates that matching on the basis of date of birth and either zip code of residence or hospital code number will likely yield a true match. Matching solely on the basis of date of birth, where neither zip code of residence nor hospital match, will likely yield a false match. In addition, one of the four cases without any matched treatment records was verified as receiving treatment outside of the region. Thus, our initial

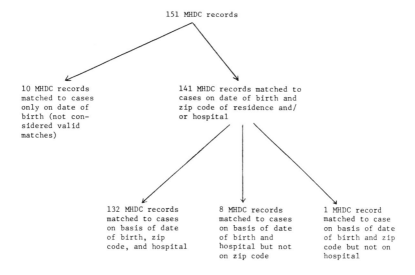

Figure 2. Results of matching hospital discharge records
        to incident breast cancer cases.

goal, to develop a procedure which will match registry
and hospital discharge records without utilizing
patient-specific identifiers, must be termed a success.
The next step in the process will involve studying those
records for which age rather than date of birth is
available.

    There are a number of possible uses of the
resulting matched hospital discharge records. Any of
the UHDDS variables listed in Table 1 might form the
basis of a patterns of care study, in which cancer care
could be analyzed by cancer stage, hospital of
treatment, or place of residence. To illustrate
possible uses of these data, treatment information for
the 119 cases has been analyzed.

A preponderance of registry identified cases had a unilateral simple mastectomy or a unilateral extended

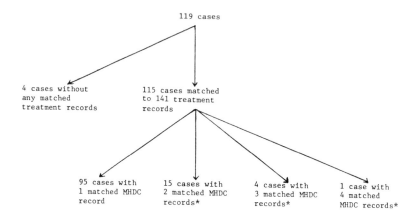

* A case with more than one matching MHDC record indicates multiple hospital admissions (and discharges) for a single individual.

Figure 3. Results of matching incident breast cancer cases to hospital discharge records.

simple mastectomy (UE), which includes extended simple mastectomy, modified radical mastectomy, and simple mastectomy with excision of regional lymph nodes. Ninety-four of 119 cases (79 percent) included such a procedure. Only one case included a more radical procedure, a unilateral radical mastectomy. Three percent of the cases involved procedures which removed less than the total breast. Thirteen cases (10 percent) reported local excision, breast biopsy, or other diagnostic procedures without any treatment procedures to the breast. Eight cases, or seven percent, did not report any diagnostic or treatment procedures. These data are presented by stage in Figure 5.

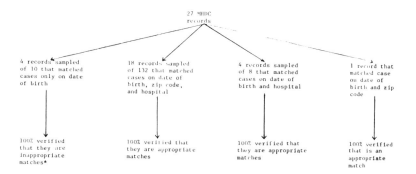

Figure 4. Results of verification of sample of matches between hospital discharge records and incident cases.

An examination of these data discloses several interesting points. One might note the extreme preponderance of procedures which remove the entire breast. Few diagnosed cases received less invasive procedures at community hospitals in southeastern Massachusetts in 1980. At the same time, the Halsted radical mastectomy virtually disappeared in this area. There is little or no surgical treatment variation by stage of cancer for stages 0-3. It appears, however, that few stage 4 breast cancer patients receive mastectomies at community hospitals in southeastern Massachusetts.

The scope of this study did not allow an examination of all treatment of breast cancer patients who were diagnosed at Massachusetts hospitals. First, hospital discharge data for other regions were not available at the time of the study. Therefore, any information regarding referral and treatment of these Boston teaching hospitals was not available. Second, the hospital discharge data available from MHDC do not

include adjuvant therapy given in a physician's office
or in a radiation therapy facility.

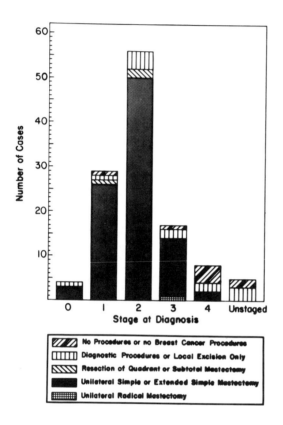

Figure 5. Breast cancer procedures by stage of disease.

Potential for Data Base Linkage in Other States

There are approximately 40 population-based cancer
registries in the United States and its territories. Of
these, about half are statewide registries with five
operating in states that also have statewide hospital

discharge data consortia. These five states include Connecticut, Massachusetts, New York, North Carolina and Rhode Island. The patterns of care study described in this paper, therefore, has potential application in at least five statewide data bases.

Problems involved in such data linkage studies include data accessibility and data quality. Statewide hospital discharge data and cancer registry data are collected by both private non-profit organizations and state agencies. Although protocols for access to the data vary, a request for the data required in a record linkage study as described in this paper universally would be reviewed by a technical or research review committee prior to release of data. In some cases, Rhode Island and Connecticut, hospital discharge data cannot be released without the consent of individual hospitals. In addition, the approval of the request by a Technical Review Committee or similar body and/or other protocols is required in Connecticut, Massachusetts, New York, North Carolina, and Rhode Island. In Connecticut, non-government researchers must obtain approval from a Human Investigating Committee to get access to cancer registry data. A Research Subcommittee must approve release of individually identified cancer registry data in Massachusetts and similar mechanisms for access exist in New York and North Carolina.

The overriding concern in any patient care study, however, is data quality. Both hospital discharge data held in health data consortia and staging information held in centralized cancer registries may be of widely varying quality. Staging is of importance because meaningful analysis of cancer care is dependent upon an accurate description of extent of disease. Since hospital discharge data originate from medical record rooms, they are therefore potentially subject to the problems identified by the Institute of Medicine in its study of the quality of discharge data (Institute of Medicine, 1977). Problems in interpretation of the data will result unless some quality assurance checks are performed on a sample of staged treatment reports. Other studies could be considered in states without statewide cancer registries or discharge data consortia. For example, small states that have a single hospital record abstracting service for all hospitals or cancer registries covering counties or other subdivisions might provide data for record linkage. In these situations, data accessibility and completeness must be evaluated before proposing studies of patterns of care for defined populations.

REFERENCES

Institute of Medicine (1977). "Reliability of hospital discharge data." Washington, D.C.: National Academy of Sciences.

U.S. National Committee on Vital and Health Statistics (1978). "Final summary report of activities: U.S. National Committee on Vital and Health Statistics, 1975-1978." Washington, D.C.: Government Printing Office.

Progress in Cancer Control IV: Research in the Cancer Center, pages 477–481
© **1983 Alan R. Liss, Inc., 150 Fifth Avenue, New York, NY 10011**

THE UNIVERSITY OF TEXAS M. D. ANDERSON HOSPITAL PATIENT
SURVEILLANCE SYSTEM

Vincent F. Guinee, M.D., M.P.H.
Luceli Cuasay, M.P.H.
Department of Patient Studies, University of
   Texas M. D. Anderson Hospital
Houston, Texas 77030

Because so many research activities involve the
ascertainment of the vital status of the patient who has
cancer, optimal patient surveillance is essential to a
cancer center. This article presents the approach used at
the University of Texas M. D. Anderson Hospital in the
Department of Patient Studies. This system has evolved over
6-7 years. We should note at the outset that we keep in
touch with the patient directly, not through the referring
physician. Actual data from recent surveillance activity
are presented.

U.T. MDAH Patient Surveillance

Computer Selection

Epi Master file	171,134
Deceased	83,990
Benign not traced	36,595
Cancer, not known dead	50,549

Basic data on all patients registered at M. D. Anderson
Hospital since it opened in 1944 are stored on computer
disk. Activities of the surveillance system are scheduled
on a quarterly cycle. First, patients known to have died
are substracted from the file. Next, patients who have
come to the hospital for diagnosis and were found not to
have cancer are removed from the file. The resulting cohort
of 50,549 patients had a diagnosis of cancer and are not
known to have died.

U.T. MDAH Patient Surveillance

Computer Match

	(July '82)
Texas deaths	9,392
Patients with cancer	50,549
Status - death	220

This cohort of 50,549 patients is next matched against death certificate information sent to use, on tape, on a monthly basis from the Texas State Health Department. In a typical month's match, 50,549 MDAH patients with cancer were matched against 9,392 reported deaths. There were 220 new deaths found.

U.T. MDAH Patient Surveillance

Computer Match

Accounts receivable	34,477
Physician charges	29,868
Patients with cancer	50,549
Status - alive	24,654

The cohort of 50,549 is also matched against billing information. There are two separate patient billing systems, one for tests, etc. (accounts receivable) and the other for physician services. When a patient has charges on both systems, their status is considered alive as of the data they were seen by the physician. This date is then stored on the computer as "last date of contact." We see that nearly half (24,654) of the cohort can be updated in this fashion.

U.T. MDAH Patient Surveillance

Computer Subtraction

	(July '82)
Contact within 12 months	9,745
Pediatric	8,790
Scheduled appt/new infor	2,032
Registered before 1961	2,399

The remainder of the cohort, approximately 25,000

patients, undergoes a subtraction process to eliminate:
1) patients who have "contact" information within the past
12 months, 2) pediatric patients (who are followed
independently by that department), 3) patients with appointments scheduled in the next six months, and finally 4) a
small group of patients registered before 1961. Depending o
on the particular surveillance cycle, this leaves approximately
3 to 4 thousand patients who enter the mailing cycle.

U.T. MDAH Patient Surveillance

3 Letter Cycle

	Mailed	Reply
Sept. 81	4,498	85%
Feb. 82	3,807	79%
Apr. 82	2,837	70%
July 82	2,854	64%
Oct. 82	3,090	81%*

* 2 letters

Letters are produced by the computer, addressed to the
patient. Each is personally signed by a staff member. We
ask the patient to write a short note at the bottom of the
page and return it to us in a business reply envelope.

As is seen here, we are moving into a quarterly mailing
schedule. The percent reply, which is based on up to 3
letters to each patient, does show considerable variation.
The mailings sent in September 1981 and October 1982 had an
excellent response of approximately 85%. This could be
related to the time of year or to the composition of that
particular group of patients.

Post office returns also influence these results. The
highest post office return for a single mailing was 9.7% for
the first letter of July 1982. Reasons for this variation
will be the subject of future analyses.

U.T. MDAH Patient Surveillance

Response to July '82 Mailing

Letter	Mailed	Reply	%
1st	2,854	1,196	42
2nd	1,427	276	19
3rd	1,105	342	31
		1,814	64

Each letter has slightly different wording. The second and third refer to the fact that previous correspondence has not been answered.

The variation in response to the individual mailings is seen here. Interestingly, the percent reply does not always decrease with each successive mailing. The third mailing of the July 1982 cycle had a markedly better response than the second. What is important is that the third letter does engender response and does "pay for itself."

U.T. MDAH Patient Surveillance

Exclusions form Phone Cycle

Phone Cycle	Sept. 81	Feb. 82	Apr. 82
Non-USA	685	805	822
Chart Info	117	143	158
New Death	6	3	6

After the responses from the three letters have been received, the remainder of the groups is turned over to our phone follow-up staff. At this point, patients are removed from the system if: 1) they are residents of other countries, 2) information is found in the chart indicating contact at this time is not necessary, or 3) if they have died recently.

It should be noted that this point is the first time that the patient's chart is used for initiating a step in the surveillance process. All previous actions have been performed by the staff utilizing computer output only.

U.T. MDAH Patient Surveillance

Phone Cycle

	Call	Completed	%
Sept. 81	430	416	97%
Feb. 82	537	495	92%
Apr. 82	548	510	93%

In phone surveillance, attempts are made to call the patient first. If that is unsuccessful, relatives, friends, local physicians, hospitals, and tumor registries are contacted. Response to phone calls has been uniformly high, i.e., over 90%. The variation of the three cycles shown can be accounted for by calls not completed in recent time periods. The percent completed in the February 1982 and April 1982 groups should approximate 97% when the cycle activities are finished.

U.T. MDAH Patient Surveillance

Response Mail/Phone Cycles

Sept. 81	96%
Feb. 82	95%
Apr. 82	92%

The overall results of the mail/phone cycles are the ascertainment of vital status in well over 90% of our patient population that is "not known dead" at the time the first letter is printed.

Another estimation of the success of this program would be to calculate its efficiency in relation to the original cohort of approximately 50,000 patients minus the pediatric patients and those patients admitted prior to 1961. Using this criterion, this surveillance system is capable of maintaining current vital status information on 98% of approximately 40,000 patients annually.

Progress in Cancer Control IV: Research in the Cancer Center, pages 483–491
© **1983 Alan R. Liss, Inc., 150 Fifth Avenue, New York, NY 10011**

STATEWIDE CANCER MANAGEMENT OUTLINES: AN AID IN PATIENT-
ORIENTED CANCER CONTROL

T. C. Hall, M.D., G. Batten, M.D., G. D. Murfin,
Ph.D., R. N. Denney, AICP and P. H. King, Ph.D.
Cancer Center of Hawaii, Univ. of Hawaii - Manoa
1236 Lauhala Street, Honolulu, HI 96813

I   INTRODUCTION

The cancer management outlines development project grew
out of a concern that the medical community in Hawaii be
provided up-to-date information in the latest and best
methods for the diagnosis and treatment of cancer, and
enhance the quality of cancer care on the Neighbor Islands
away from the concentration of specialists on Oahu. A long-
term goal was to improve neighbor island cancer care such
that patients would not have to travel to and remain in
Honolulu for treatment, with costs in money, emotional
distress and family disruption. Another purpose was to provide information useful to nurses and other medical personnel in care of cancer patients.

II   PHASE I - CCPH

A. The project comprised two periods. First, the five
sites chosen in the statewide Community Based Cancer Control
Program (CCPH) operative in Hawaii from 1977 to 1982.
Thereafter, the rest of the sites under Hawaii Medical
Association (HMA) sponsorship, initially under a one-year
subcontract from the CCPH, and thereafter with local support
for a second year.

B. The CBCCP Implementation Plan for Year 03,
Objective 3.2.1 called for the preparation of outlines
covering the continuum of cancer control for each target
site: Breast, Lung, Colon and Gynecologic; during Year 03,

skin cancer-melanoma was added.

C. Working committees of physicians were established for each site. Articles pertinent to the outlines development were collected and questions regarding their content and usefulness developed by the CCPH staff and mailed to the committee members for review and comment. Comments were returned by mail, recorded and collated by staff. This process was repeated with outlines developed in Grand Rapids, Rochester, Virginia, Boston, and Detroit. From the feedback, drafts were developed by staff and reviewed by committee members in an iterative fashion. Figure 1 shows the sources consulted.

Chapters were also created on unproved methods, clinical trials and nutrition.

Participation of the medical community is evidenced by the number of physicians and other medical professionals involved. A list of committee members from all sites is included in Figure 2.

CANCER MANAGEMENT OUTLINES

Prior Guidelines Used

1. University of Rochester Syllabus

2. Boston ACS Handbook

3. Grand Rapids Guidelines

4. American College of Surgeons' Followup Guidelines

5. Fred Hutchinson Guidelines

6. Detroit-Michigan Cancer Foundation Guidelines

7. Tidewater Virginia Guidelines

8. Vanderbilt Guidelines

9. Kapiolani Gyn Guidelines

Figure I

CANCER MANAGEMENT OUTLINES

Physician Involvement on Site Committees

1.	GI	27
2.	Breast	35
3.	Skin Cancer/ Melanoma	56
4.	Lung	24
5.	Gyn	18
6.	Bone	5
7.	Central Nervous System	6
8.	Eye and Orbit	3
9.	GU	6
10.	Leukemia	9
11.	Lymphoma	6
		195

Figure 2

Through March 31, 1982, about 7,000 hours of volunteer time had been devoted to the outlines. The total dollar value of physician plus other medical professional time contributed was $763,713.

D. Management Outline Development--Committee Membership and Participation.

Other cancer sites, bone, central nervous system, eye and orbit, genitourinary tract, gynecologic, head and neck, leukemias, lymphomas, sarcomas of soft tissue, and pediatric solid tumors were subcontract to the HMA. The project expressed a primary goal of CCPH: exchange of information and coordination among all health professionals which are also central to HMA purposes. The HMA agreed to assume responsibility for future regular periodic updating. The compendium of Outlines will be in looseleaf form. The subcontract covered August 1, 1980 to January 31, 1982. It was the first time in the United States that a three-way collaboration took place among the NCI, a State Medical Society, and a community-oriented agency such as CCPH in the development of management outlines. The HMA obtained local funding for the completion of all their site outlines.

III PHASE II - HMA SPONSORSHIP

A. The unfamiliarity of the local medical community with standardized management criteria led to initial resistance to developing the outlines. This included a concern that the product would be "cook book" medicine, insensitive to the particular idiosyncracies of individual cases and the role of clinical judgement. This concern was dispelled in two ways. First, the word "outlines" was substituted for "guidelines", which eliminated connotations of compulsion. Second, concern was dispelled by Dr. Edward Moorhead in his talk to the local medical community in November of 1979. He described the process by which committees of physicians from five Grand Rapids hospitals successfully put together guidelines. The Grand Rapids model and Dr. Moorhead's enthusiastic presentation were important factors in generating local motivation and interest in the creation of management outlines for Hawaii.

B. Method of HMA Implementation

The process for the HMA sites differed somewhat from the mail-response system used for the CCPH sites.

Committees were formed and met as a group with the project's Staff Coordinators to determine outline structure and content. The coordinators were an MD with extensive experience in surgical oncology and tumor registries, and a health planner with a long-standing interest in cancer programs.

Each Committee was chaired by one or two physician experts in the field. He or she chose 6-12 or more physician members.

In the preparation of each Outline, the following steps were taken: the Coordinator assembled journal articles and other relevant materials relating to specific cancers. Outlines from Grand Rapids, Rochester, Boston, Virginia, Seattle, Detroit, and elsewhere were studied. Materials were collated and compared, and questions raised as to how they might be updated and adapted to the unique, insular, ethnic and occupational realities of Hawaii.

Current practices were also described by examination of Tumor Registry data, analysis of anonymous hospital cases and through consultations among colleagues. All cases studies were anonymous as to patient, physician and hospital.

Epidemiological and etiological information was also gathered, and a section on these topics written by members of the Epidemiology Program of the Cancer Center. This material is specific to the cancer problem of Hawaii.

Approval of final outlines will be given by the HMA Council after review and recommendations from the HMA Cancer Committee.

Final draft outlines are to be distributed to relevant professional societies, hospital cancer committees and specialists not otherwise involved in the program for input and recommendations.

Copies of the Outlines will be provided to the approximately 2,500 practicing physicians in the State. Medical students, nurses and other health professionals will have easy access to the Outlines through copies made available to all libraries and hospital wards.

IV   RESULTS

The CCPH site outlines and the Sections on nutrition
were completed by the end of the CCPH contract. The HMA
site outlines were started later and designed to extend to
July 31, 1982, by which time the HMA and CCPH components
were to be integrated into one document, printed and distributed. Budgetary cutbacks at NCI resulted in the elimination of funds for the final six months of the HMA
subcontract. When CCPH was prohibited from funding the project beyond January 31, 1982, other sources for completion
of the project were found, to enable support through January
15, 1983, by which time all sections will be complete and
ready for reproduction.

V   EVALUATION

Evaluation of the Outlines project includes assessment
of 1) the process of outline development, 2) the results of
outline implementation, and 3) the accuracy, pertinence and
currency of outline content as time passes.

1) Process: The process of outline development was
successful. The active, prolonged volunteer participation
of the medical community was elicited and sustained and the
outlines were produced, in spite of the elimination of funds
for the last six months of the HMA subcontract. Both the
CCPH and HMA methods of development were successful. Members of the CCPH Site Committees actively participated by
mail, and members of the smaller HMA Committees actively
participated through face-to-face meetings. The large membership of the committees served the crucial function of
helping to legitimize the project in the medical community.
CCPH target site cancers. The mail response format utilized
for CCPH outlines was not compromised by the larger committee sizes, as the committee members did their work individually. The smaller sizes of the HMA committees were
similarly appropriate to their group process of outline
development. While more face-to-face meetings were used
(particularly luncheon meetings supported by HMA), mailings
were used for distribution of drafts for input and critique.
Most meetings had at least 50% attendance. There was a high
proportion of active participants, with most members providing original copy for the sites for which they were
experts.

The development process was more lengthy than might have otherwise been the case because of 1) the overlapping sequential (rather than contemporaneous) work periods of the CCPH and HMA segments. Four site coordinators, the CCPH staff medical consultant, CCPH Assistant Director for Programs and for Planning, and two graduate students had substantial roles. A concentration of staff responsibility in, for example, one Coordinator with a graduate student assistant, may be a more efficient and more focused structure for outlines development.

2) Implementation: Implementation of the Management Outlines in the community was not accomplished in the work period covered by the CCPH conract for reasons previously discussed. However, a procedure for evaluating their usage and impact was devised, and will be implemented as a Phase IV research project under a proposed Cancer Control Research Unit contract.

Evaluation for the management outlines was process rather than impact oriented. Actual implementation of the outlines in any form was not proposed as a CCPH function. For evaluation purposes, two instruments were developed and tested. The first was the Management Outline Checklist. These were developed by physicians and corresponded to various procedures identified in the outline for the major target cancer sites.

In order to ascertain which of the various procedures were most important, the checklist was sent to local physicians who were asked to rank the items on the list relative to their importance to the assessment of care for a patient. These rankings were developed on each target site by stage. Figure 3 illustrates the form used to rank order items on Breast Cancer and a summary of the ranking for Breast cancer on admission. These values change for different procedures desired at different stages.

The usage and impact evaluation procedure includes the assessment of the management of cases from medical records according to criteria drawn from the outlines themselves. For the CCPH target sites, diagnostic, treatment, follow-up and rehabilitation procedures were abstracted from the outlines, formed into a checklist, and each item rated by the committees on a three-point scale of importance: 3 =

very important to proper management, 2 = somewhat important, and 1 = not important. Individual committee member ratings were averaged to determine overall importance weights to be utilized in case management evaluation For example, in a clinical case where a very important procedure on the checklist was in fact performed, the score would be 1 (performed) x 3 (very important) = 3. The sum of each performance (1 = performed, 0 = not performed) times its associated importance weight, over all checklist items, constituted the score for the management of the individual case. In this manner, relative correspondence of actual case management by site and stage to outline recommendations was accomplished for a group of pilot cases, and can be used to evaluate future changes resulting from the Outlines.

COMMUNITY HOSPITAL ONCOLOGY PROGRAM

MANAGEMENT CHECKLIST

Assessment Codes: CRITICAL to know or do = 3
HELPFUL to know or to do = 2
SOMETIMES HELPFUL, but can be
omitted without affecting
management of this cancer = 1

BREAST CANCER

		1X̄	2X̄	3X̄	4X̄
I. Pre-Rx Work-Up					
A. Patient History					
1.	Weight Loss	1.4	1.7	2.1	2.8
2.	Mass in Breast	2.4	2.8	2.8	2.6
3.	Anorexia	1.1	1.4	1.7	2.3
4.	Heaviness of Breast	1.2	1.1	1.4	1.3
5.	Nipple Discharge	2.1	2.0	2.3	1.8
6.	Nipple Thickening, Cracking	2.0	2.1	2.3	1.8
7.	Pain	1.4	1.6	1.6	2.2
8.	Nodes - Neck	2.4	2.8	3.0	2.9
9.	P.E. - Breast Exam	3.0	3.0	3.0	2.9
	- Nodes: Axilla & Neck	3.0	3.0	3.0	3.0
	- Hepatomegaly	2.1	2.2	2.3	2.8
	- Ascites	1.8	2.1	2.2	2.6
	- Mass	1.8	2.2	2.3	2.7
	- Jaundice	1.8	2.0	2.1	2.4
B. Lab Data					
1.	CBC	2.8	2.9	2.5	3.0
2.	Liver Function				
	- Alk. P'tase	2.1	2.4	2.7	2.9
	- Bilirubin	1.6	1.8	2.0	2.2
	- LDH	1.6	1.8	2.0	2.2
	- CEA	1.2	1.7	1.9	2.3
3.	X-Ray				
	- Mammogram	3.0	3.0	2.8	2.4
	- Chest Film	2.9	3.0	2.9	3.0
	- Bone Scan	1.9	2.0	2.9	3.0
	- Metastatic Spine Series	1.0	1.2	1.9	2.1
C. Diagnostic Procedures					
1.	Needle Biopsy	1.5	1.5	1.8	1.8
2.	Open Biopsy	3.0	3.0	2.8	2.6
3.	Ultrasound	1.0	1.0	1.4	1.3
4.	Estrogen Receptors	2.5	2.9	2.9	3.0

Figure 4

Users' surveys of target audiences (physicians, nurses, medical students and other medical professionals) can also be done to determine outline usage level, purpose and the extent to which medical case management decisions are explicitly based on outline recommendations.

Hawaii Tumor Registry records will also be used to corroborate treatment pattern results, by assessments of the extent to which treatment patterns correspond to Outlines criteria.

Grand Rapids, which is the only other community that we are aware of having done this, has found a significant increase in cases being treated according to its Management Guidelines over the period in which they have been available in that community. We hope to study the impact of the Outlines on this community in a similar manner. In addition, survival and quality of life will be monitored over the long term through the Tumor Registry and compared between Outline complier and non-complier treatment patterns. We have requested support for such an undertaking as part of a proposed Cancer Control Research Unit for the State of Hawaii.

3) Outlines Content: Evaluation of outlines content will be a continuous process. Relevant outlines will be discussed at Tumor Board Meetings and suggested revisions noted. An updating of the Outlines will take place every other year by members of the HMA Cancer Site Sub-Committees who will review the materials and comment on changes to be recommended to the HMA Cancer Committee. This Committee will review, comment, and recommend to the HMA Council. Revised papers will then be distributed for insertion into each volume of the Management Outlines.

VI   OVERALL LESSONS LEARNED

Whether, by whom and to what extent the management outlines are utilized will be determined only after their upcoming implementation. The impact on morbidity and mortality of changes in management practices prompted by the outlines will take place and can be measured after that time. Lessons learned to date from the management outlines project, therefore, are limited to the processes of project development and outlines production in the local community.

The most important of these lessons are:

1) The sanctioning of the outlines project by the appropriate State-wide medical organizations is important, if not essential, to the cooperation of local physicians in the production process.

2) The involvement of central organization (i.e., CCPH, HMA) with specifically assigned personnel in the outlines development process is very helpful in sustaining the production process to completion.

3) Staff coordination and administration of the outline development process is very important, given physicians' limited time availability.

4) Wide-spread involvement of the medical community in the production process enhances acceptance of the outlines, but lengthens and complicates the process.

5) Since acceptance of the outlines by the local community is necessary to project success, community input and evaluation are necessary for a project to be optimally accepted.

6) Outlines should be conceived of and presented as authoritative, informational but non-directive, rather than as rigid rules for case management decision-making.

7) Outlines development can serve as an integrating activity to strengthen and extend communication patterns among individual physicians and other health professionals and among local medical organizations.

8) The Outlines can be evaluted in a quantitative fashion based upon mostly physician management practice, and a long-term impact on survivorship as revealed by a regional Tumor Registry.

Supported in part by NCI Contract Number NO1-CN-75399

Progress in Cancer Control IV: Research in the Cancer Center, pages 493–502
© **1983 Alan R. Liss, Inc., 150 Fifth Avenue, New York, NY 10011**

A PROGRAM TO ENCOURAGE EARLY DETECTION AND TREATMENT OF
BREAST CANCER BY GIVING INFORMATION AND EMOTIONAL SUPPORT

Rose Kushner, Executive Director
Breast Cancer Advisory Center
Rockville, Maryland 20850

INTRODUCTION

Ask any woman what disease she dreads most, and she
will say " breast cancer." Mammary carcinoma is now almost
epidemic in the United States: it is estimated that about
112,000 new cases were discovered in 1982, and one of 11
American women can expect to develop breast cancer at some
time in her life. It accounts for 28 per cent of all female
cancers; about 40,000 women, diagnosed in previous years,
died of the disease. (American Cancer Society [ACS] 1982).
Since nine of ten breast problems are harmless, this means
that the vast majority of symptomatic women in this country
underwent one or more evaluation procedures of some kind to
find the expected 112,000 patients who had positive diagnoses; almost one million women endured the stress and anxiety
of facing breast cancer to find the one-tenth who were actually found to have the disease (Schain 1976).

Of course the physical traumata resulting from a radical mastectomy must be addressed. But this statistic suggests that health professionals in all disciplines should
also pay attention to the emotional problems of symptomatic
women before breast cancer is diagnosed, in addition to
helping them cope with the problems encountered afterward.

The best known breast-cancer program, "Reach to Recovery," was begun in the early 1950s by Terese Lasser, a
mastectomee, and her organization was incorporated into
the ACS in 1969. However, the pre-diagnostic emotional
problems of women were not, and still are not, considered

to be within Reach to Recovery's scope (Lasser 1972). Indeed, although women facing a possible diagnosis of and
treatment for breast cancer urgently need attention, almost
all existing cancer-control programs are designed to help
them find a symptom of disease or to deal with psychological
and physical rehabilitation. There is a gap in the middle.

In addition, asymptomatic women -- continually exposed
to mass media threats of breast cancer -- need help. Anecdotal evidence shows that thousands of symptom-free women
(especially those over 35) find that constant reminders of
breast cancer are most traumatic and stressful. Some become
obsessive paranoics; others develop a denial so intense that
they cannot feel a symptom, should one be found (Breast
Cancer Advisory Center 1975-83).

There has been some work done in this crucial "before"
period, but the research has primarily been retrospective to
study women who had already been diagnosed and treated. For
example, psychologists analyzed the "avoidance," "delay,"
"lagtime," etc. (patients' and physicians) between women's
discovery of a symptom and its eventual diagnosis (Magarey
1976; Cameron, Hinton 1968; Worden, Weisman 1975; Buls
1976). Other work compared anxiety levels before and after
a biopsy to see if women who were found to have cancer had
higher anxiety levels than those who did not (Greer, Morris
1976). There have also been studies of the avoidance behaviors (denial) of asymptomatic women, behaviors that inhibits them from dealing with breast cancer in any way.

The most studied behavior is the denial that prevents
women from practicing Breast Self-Examination (BSE). But
even this was not recognized to be the serious problem it is
until 1973 when a Gallup poll, "How Women Think about Breast
Cancer", was commissioned by the ACS. For this poll, 1,007
women older than 18 were surveyed via personal, in-depth interviews. Although 56 per cent of the sample said that this
disease was their most serious medical problem, fewer than
one-third of them had ever examined their breasts (Gallup Organization 1973). This ACS poll seems to be the first time
attention was given to women's anxieties about breast cancer
before the disease struck.

Except for the studies of delay cited above, pre-treatment emotional problems were not even recognized until the
late 1960s when a clinical trial showed that breast self-

examination (BSE) could detect tumors at early, curable stages (Strax 1969). Health professionals were surprised to learn that women's refusal to think about breast cancer was an obstacle to their looking for symptoms: society's obsession with two firm and beautiful mammary glands out-weighed women's fears of dying of cancer (Strax 1974).

In late 1974, the mastectomies of Betty Ford and Happy Rockefeller caused an world-wide breast-cancer panic, and women packed doctors' offices and screening centers for examinations. Six years later, to see if the "panic" had bequeathed a lasting change of attitude, the National Can-cer Institute (NCI) ordered a second poll -- Breast Cancer: A Measure of Progress in Public Understanding. Asked what their most serious health problem was, the majority (58 per cent) of 1,580 healthy, adult women again said, "breast cancer." (Paradoxically, about 60 per cent of them had never examined their breasts.*) (NCI 1980).

Thus, both surveys showed that a woman's anxiety -- her "coping with breast cancer" -- begins long before a scalpel touches her breast. Both the ACS and the NCI res-ponded by launching large public-education programs about the importance of early detection and campaigns to teach BSE. And, since few women in the surveys had accurate knowledge of the disease, information bombarded the public via television, films and printed publications (ACS, NCI 1974-83). No programs, however, were launched to help anxious women afraid of finding a symptom or those facing the ordeal of biopsy and, possibly, mastectomy.

According to the 1980 census, about 50 million women in the United States are in the "at risk" age group older than 35, so the sheer magnitude of numbers makes it impos-

---

*Most non-practicing women said they "didn't think of it," but many health professionals felt the reason was ac-tually lack of confidence. Thus, programs for publicity, improved teaching materials, training classes, etc. were instituted. A growing number of health professionals, how-ever, believe women do not practice BSE because they do not want to find what they are looking for: Why spend time and effort to find something the size of an apple seed if it will be treated with the same operation used to treat a lump as large as an apple? (Ingall 1980).

sible to help all of them. A great deal, however, can be
done to aid the hundreds of thousands of women who endure
weeks or months of "pre-clinical anxiety," even though the
vast majority will not have the disease. This can involve
giving information, explanations, referrals and a "shoulder
to cry on" during the endless waiting periods they must endure. Some examples follow (Breast Cancer Advisory Center
Data Bank 1975-83).

FINDING A SYMPTOM

Women who practice BSE usually feel apprehensive before every self-examination, and many do not ask their
doctors questions, because they are too timid. Moreover,
most women do not examine themselves or have professional
examinations. They may find a mass accidentally or partners
find lumps during lovemaking. Some have no personal physicians. All women need an agency to refer them to a breast
specialist; all should have a prepared list of questions
to ask as well as data about their histories give the physician for a personal risk-assessment.

CHOOSING A DOCTOR

The best way to judge a doctor for expertise in breast
diseases is by his/her breast examination. Yet few women
know a thorough exam should also include palpation of both
axillas. Nor do many know they should be asked to lift and
stretch their arms to be sure sure both breasts respond
identically without "dimpling" or "puckering." Women should
also know their nipples must be squeezed gently to check
for any discharge. Most need to be assured that they may
request a referral to an expert.

THE CLINICAL EXAMINATION

Women usually go to a doctor alone the first time. On
the table, they must be nude from the waist up while he/she
examines them. Often, a specialist can determine whether
or not a mass is harmless simply by manual palpation, but
the mass may require needle aspiration by a surgeon. This
means waiting once more, and support is urgently needed.

NEEDLE BIOPSIES

A surgeon (who is usually a total stranger) may use a

fine needle to try to withdraw fluid from the mass, and
once more the woman must wait -- now for the cytologist's
report. If a mass is solid, nothing flows into the syringe,
and most surgeons immediately recommend a surgical biopsy.
However, women should be informed that a Trocar or Tru-cut
wide-bore needle can often be used to avoid surgery, saving
money as well as an operating-room visit.

DIAGNOSIS

If nothing is removed by either type of needle biopsy,
women should know that if they are younger than 30 and have
no family history, they may be advised to wait and return
after one or two menstrual cycles. Symptomatic women older
than 40, regardless of family history, are usually sent directly for mammography. Because of past adverse publicity
about breast X-rays, most women need assurance that the benefit of the small amount of radiation outweighs its risk.
They may also want to know about xerography and other well
advertised tests like ultrasonography, diaphanography and
thermography. In addition to information, they again need
support while waiting for the radiologist's diagnosis.

SURGICAL BIOPSY

Regardless of age, history or a negative mammogram,
every woman with a persistent breast symptom will end her
odyssey in a surgeon's office and will have a surgical biopsy, usually as an in-patient under general anesthesia.

As stated earlier, nine of ten breast symptoms are benign, and to find the estimated 112,000 new cases of cancer
in 1982, almost a million women waited anxiously for space
on operating-room schedules. Most were asked to sign a
form giving the surgeon permission to perform an immediate
mastectomy if cancer was found. While this practice has
been gradually changing since 1979, the diagnostic biopsy
is still usually followed by immediate definitive treatment
in a one-stage procedure. The rage of awakening to learn
that a breast was amputated while they are unconscious cannot be measured. Of course, many women prefer to be asleep,
but all women expecting biopsy should know there is a choice.

ESTROGEN- AND PROGESTERONE-RECEPTOR ASSAYS

Every patient anticipating a biopsy should know that

her surgeon must order estrogen- and progesterone-receptor
assays (ERAs and PRAs), if the tumor is malignant (Jensen
1976). Large medical centers prepare specimens for the
tests routinely, but this is not always the case in smaller
hospitals, and it is often wise for the patient to make
advance arrangements in the event that carcinoma is found.

WAITING FOR THE "PERMANENT SECTION"

Women who have biopsies done separately must endure an
additional waiting period of two or three days for results
of the "permanent section," and health professionals can
provide much-needed support during this painful time.

STAGING

For patients whose diagnoses showed cancer, staging
is, perhaps, the most stressful part of pre-clinical anxiety. Most women believe breast cancer metastasizes from one
breast to the other and do not know the disease can spread
first to distant organs. Thus, the reason for the examinations must be explained and frightening tests must be described, e.g., that nuclear scans do not burn and are not
dangerous. (Women who have a onestage procedure should be
staged before the biopsy.)

CHOOSING "DEFINITIVE TREATMENT"

While most surgeons in the United States believe ampu-
tation is the only safe treatment for breast cancer, there
are different kinds of mastectomies. For example, the modified radical mastectomy is now called a "total mastectomy
with axillary dissection" (NCI 1979). Women may fear they
will have more extensive surgery since the term sounds more
terrifying. Some may wonder about the simple (or total)
mastectomy and should be told that at least some of the
axillary nodes must be excised to see if adjuvant therapy
will be necessary. By the same token, elderly or infirm women are usually not given cytotoxic drugs, even if malignant
nodes are found. These patients should, therefore, be told
why axillary dissection or sampling may not be performed.

A growing number of specialists, however, now treat
the disease with breast-conserving procedures in which
only the tumor and axillary lymph nodes are removed. Radiotherapy, instead of surgery, is used to eradicate other

foci of cancer that may be elsewhere in the breast. Women
anticipating a one-stage procedure must discuss alternatives
with their surgeons in advance of the biopsy; those who
chose a waiting period after the biopsy can use the time to
investigate other treatment options.

Less-than-mastectomy procedures may be grouped under
the general term, "segmental resection," and these are
usually accompanied by removal of some axillary nodes and
are followed by radiotherapy to the preserved breast. Some
experts, however, omit the radiation in certain cases. Indeed, the multiple combinations and permutions of current
breast-cancer treatments are confusing even to health professionals. To the average women, the array of choice is
overwhelming, frightening and must be carefully explained.

Radiotherapy

Women who will be treated by radiotherapy instead of
surgery face unique problems that must be detailed in advance. For example, they must know they will be irradiated
daily (usually in a hospital) for at least five weeks and
that afterward, they may be isolated for several days while
"boosters" in the tumor site make them "radioactive."

WAITING FOR A DIAGNOSIS OF THE AXILLARY LYMPH NODES

If axillary nodes are malignant, some kind of adjuvant
therapy involving combinations of drugs, hormones and anti-
estrogens may be given as soon after surgery as possible.
Patients should know that such therapy depends on their
nodal and receptor status and not on the primary treatment
done. All patients must wait for several days until the
pathology report is completed before knowing their fates.
Plans reconstruction must be delayed if nodes are malignant.

ADJUVANT THERAPY

Because of wide publicity in mass media about the
success of anti-cancer agents, patients today are usually
aware of the controversies surrounding various therapies.
Since all substances, dosages, schedules and durations are
still experimental, most patients are partipants in some
clinical trial. They must understand that no one yet knows
what regimen is "best" (Fisher 1982).

Waiting for the results of pre-surgical staging examinations is stressful and traumatic, but there are no toxicities, the wait is short and the answers come quickly. On the other hand, adjuvant therapy continues for at least six months and usually longer. Breast cancer does not make women bald or ill: these toxic side-effects are caused by the medications. Unlike patients treated for measurable metastatic disease, these women have nothing that can be seen on scans, X-rays or other tests. In their doctors' or clinics' waiting rooms, they meet and talk with other patients whose ages, nodal and receptor status are identical to theirs. Yet these other patients are receiving different drugs for different lengths of time.

And, of course, there is still no way to know if the prophylactic anti-cancer agents will prevent or delay a recurrence. The only way a woman knows whether or not the substances are effective is that the cancer does not return. So they must cope with its toxicities and uncertainties on faith, without knowing if their treatment is "right" or "wrong." Breast-cancer patients receiving cytotoxic adjuvant therapy have the greatest burden of all and urgently need a support program to help them bear it.

LIVING WITH RECURRENT DISEASE

Patients whose cancers have metastasized are faced with the same painful dilemma, except that the progression or regression of their disease can be measured. Women must often be encouraged to continue treatment in spite of toxic side-effects; switching to quackery must be fought.

LIVING WITH FEAR OF RECURRENCE

About 25 per cent of node-negative patients will develop metastastic disease in spite of the absence of cancer in their axillas; those who had positive nodes have, of course, a higher risk of recurrence (NCI, SEER Report 1981). So all women treated for breast cancer face added years of watching, waiting and worrying about unusual bone pain, hoarseness, coughing and digestive problems. Moreover, women who have had cancer in one breast have a higher risk of developing another in the remaining breast. Periodic follow-up examinations, with all their stress and anxiety, become new patterns of their lives.

The hundreds of thousands of women whose biopsied lumps were benign also face years of anguish and anxiety, because they are now in the high-risk category. Some will opt for prophylactic mastectomies. All women -- after suffering through weeks or months of waiting, multiple examinations and, finally, diagnostic surgery -- know they may endure the ordeals many times for the rest of their lives.

SUMMARY

There is a great need for an organized program to give all women information, referrals and emotional support for breast diseases before detection, diagnosis and treatment. This provides an excellent opportunity for public and private agencies concerned with cancer-control to fill the wide gap. At this time, there are no organized programs between those that teach women how to do BSE and -- much later -- to help them "cope with cancer." With the 2-stage procedure becoming more common and available to women, the time should be used for education before primary treatment.

Breast cancer is more than a disease; it is a "process" having many phases. BSE and worrying about finding a symptom is the first and may last a lifetime. Primary treatment is second; the need for support continues throughout. The purpose of this presentation is to urge health professionals to recognize the great need and fill the wide gap.

#

American Cancer Society (1974). Basic facts about Breast Cancer. American Cancer Society. "1982 Cancer Facts & Figures."

Breast Cancer Advisory Center Data Bank (1975-83). Kensington, Maryland, USA 20895.

Buls JG, et al (1976). Women's attitudes to mastectomy for breast cancer. Med J of Australia 2:336-338.

Cameron A, Hinton J (1968). Delay in seeking treatment for mammary tumors. Cancer 21: 121-1126.

Fisher B (1982). Personal Communication.

Gallup Organization, Inc. (1973). Women's attitudes regarding breast cancer. American Cancer Society.

Greer S, Morris T ( ). Psychological attributes of women who develop breast cancer. J Psychosomatic Research 19: 147-53.

Ingall J MD (July 1980). Personal communication. London.

Lasser T (1972). "Reach to Recovery." Amer Cancer Society.

Magarey J, Todd, PB (1976). Breast loss and delay in breast cancer: Behavioral science in surgical research. Australia-New Zealand J Surg. 46: 391-393.

National Cancer Institute (1979). Consensus Development Conference: Treatment of Primary Breast Cancer.

National Cancer Institute (Dec. 10, 1980). New cancer survey shows progress in understanding of breast cancer: Report of survey done by Opinion Research Corp.

National Cancer Institute (1982). SEER (Surveillance, Epidemiology and End Results).

Schain W (1976). Psychological impact of the diagnosis of breast cancer on the patient. In Vaeth (ed): "Breast Cancer."

Shapiro, S (1966). Evaluation of Periodic Breast Cancer Screening with Mammography. J Amer Med Assn. 195 :731-738.

Strax P (1974). "Early Detection." New York: Harper & Row.

Worden JW, Weisman AD (1975). Psychosocial components of lagtime in cancer diagnosis. J Psychosomatic Research. 19: 69-79.

Index

Acquired immune deficiency syndrome
(AIDS), 217–226
  Azimexon, 226
  Burkitt's lymphoma, 220–221
  CMV, 218, 220–221
  EBV, 220
  Flagyl treatment, history of, 219
  in haemophilia A, 220
  hepatitis, history of, 219
  homosexuals, male, 217, 219, 221–223
  interferon, 225–226
  Kaposi's sarcoma, 217–218; *see also*
    Kaposi's sarcoma
  lymphoma, 217
  lysozymes, 218, 219
  mononucleosis, 220–221
  nitrites, 219
  Pneumocystis carinii pneumonia, 217, 218
  prevention, 221–223
  radiosensitive suppressor cells, 218
  recreational drug use, 219
  semen, 220, 224
  squamous cell cancer, 217
  syphilis, history of, 219
  T cells, 222
  therapy, 221, 225–226
  thymosin, 218, 223
  transmissible agent, 220
Adenocarcinoma
  nasal, in furniture workers, 47–48, 53
  tumor regrowth prevention by β-carotene and vitamin A, 237–245
    combined therapy 242–244
  X-ray induced tumor regression, 238–245
    radiation dosage, 244–245
Adolescence
  cancer in, 85–89
  smoking, 273, 275
Adria Laboratories and adolescent
  cancer, 85
Africa, West, Kaposi's sarcoma in, 218
Age
  and breast cancer, 351, 354–356, 358
  and Breast Examination Training
    centers, 287
  and breast self-examination, 296, 297, 299, 300
  and cancer, 59, 113–114, 123–124
  and Cancer Information Service use, 146–148, 150, 153, 164–166
  correlation with low cancer
    knowledge, 140
  at first coitus, and cervical
    intraepithelial
    dysplasia, 204, 206, 213–214
  and Kaposi's sarcoma, 218
  at marriage and cancer, 60
  see also Elderly
AIDS. *See* Acquired immune deficiency
  syndrome
Air pollution, 61
Alcohol
  and cancer, 60
  and cervical intrapethelial dysplasia, 208, 213
Alkaline phosphatase, 428, 430
Alternative therapies, 193–194; *see also*
  Laetrile clinical trials

American Cancer Society
and American College of Surgeons,
37
cancer prevention and control, 29–35
Cancer Prevention Study I and II,
33, 34
and cigarette smoking, 34
Crusade, 143
early detection, 32
environmental etiologies, 33
Great American Smokeout, 34
monoclonal antibodies, 32
National Conference on Smoking and
Health, 34
network approach, 35
organizational activity, 29–30
Pap test, 30–31
recommendations, changes in, 31
survey of black attitudes toward
cancer, 418
American College of Surgeons
and American Cancer Society, 37
Annual Hospital Activity Reports,
41–42
-approved cancer control research,
37–43
breast, 38–40
audits of management, 38
Commission on Cancer, 37–43
provision of comparative statistical
data, 43
American Pharmaceutical Association,
Helping Smokers Quit program,
99–102
Amygdalin. *See* Laetrile
Anderson, M.D. *See* University of
Texas M.D. Anderson
Hospital Patient Surveillance
System
Antigen, carcinoembryonic (CEA), 430
Arsenic, 61
Asbestos, 51–54, 61
Association of American Cancer
Institutes, 3
Attitudes
black, towards cancer, 418

elderly, towards physicians, 128,
130, 131
negative, as deterrent, 115–116
Azimexon and AIDS, 226

Behavior
ascertaining, and cancer prevention,
146, 147
Cancer: The Behavioral Dimension,
58
change
elderly as target population, 124
after public education program,
138–140
and knowledge, 93, 141, 372
public, surveys. *See under* Cancer
prevention/detection
sexual and reproductive. *See* Sexual
behavior
see also Cancer prevention/detection,
lifestyle changes
Benzene, 75, 77
Benzo(a)pyrene, 61
Birth control pills. *See* Contraceptives,
oral
Blacks
attitudes towards cancer, American
Cancer
Society study, 418
church, 417–423
clergy as cancer control
intermediary, 417–423
and Howard University Cancer
Information Service, 171–181
cancer sites, 173
male cf. female, 172–174
percentage of callers, 172
and printed media, 174–175, 180
TV and radio, 173, 174, 180
types of questions, 173
urban cf. suburban, 172–173
prevention of cancer, 249, 257–259
relative risks of cancer vs. whites,
252
see also Communications strategies,
cancer; Race

Bladder stones, 59
Booklets, adolescent cancer, 88–89
  comic books, 135–139, 141–144
  see also Media
Breast cancer
  and American College of Surgeons,
    38–40
  care/therapy in Italy, 457–459
  control, approaches, 283
  detection demonstration projects,
    110, 111, 341–342
  frequency of inquiries to Cancer
    Information Service, 162, 165–
    169
  high rates in Washington, D.C.,
    420–421
  incidence, 283, 313, 372
  intervention, primary cf. secondary,
    313
  management checklist (HMA), 489
  mortality, 313, 331, 372
  Network Registry, 295
  patterns of care, 427–428, 466–470
  physician beliefs about value of early
    detection, 366–367
  physician delay and risk factors,
    351–360
    delay components, 357
    family history, 354–359
    lump cf. other symptoms, 351
    patient age, 351, 354–356, 358
    race, 351
    risk factor index, 356, 358, 369
  procedures by disease stage, 474
  professional education in community
    hospitals, 429–431
  screening, 345–348
  suspected, tests, 427–431
Breast examination, family physicians'
  feelings about, 361, 363, 366–367
Breast feeding, 60
Breast self-examination, 107–110
  and breast cancer control, 283
  and community-based cancer control
    programs (NCI), 273–280
  competency, 313–321
    predictors, 336–337

    scoring, 333–337
  education and age, 296, 297, 299,
    300
  effectiveness analysis, 293–295
  and the elderly, 124–125
  evaluation, 332–333
  frequency, 314, 316, 318, 324–326,
    328
    correlated with lump detection,
      323–328
    predictors, 336–337
  lump detection
    correlated with frequency and
      technique, 323–328
    size threshold, 306, 309
    statistics regarding, 331–332
  cf. mammography, 309; *see also*
    Mammography
  mass media, 299, 301
  method (technoque), 305–309, 315–
    316, 318, 324–328
  in minority women, 276–277
  pamphlet and videotape, 324, 327
  performance before and after
    training, 307–308
  post-mastectomy, 293–303
    cf. pre-mastectomy practice, 296,
      299–302
  silicone breast model, 306–307, 323–
    328
  size threshold for lump detection,
    306, 309
  socio-demographic factors, 296, 297,
    333
  and stage of disease at diagnosis, 332
  students and their mothers, 314, 317,
    319
  teaching, 285, 305–306
  telephone survey, 333
  training, 324–326, 328, 335
  training centers, 284–285
    effect of age, 287
    effect of race, 288
    follow-up evaluation, 285–291
    hospital community, 289–290
Burkitt's lymphoma and AIDS, 220–221
Burns, 59

Cancer
and age, 113–114, 123–124
in aging population, 123, 132
beliefs of elderly, 128, 129
and blacks. *See* Blacks
care/therapy. *See* Management,
cancer
center and health department
linkages, New York State, 67–
80
DES and vaginal cancer in
offspring, 68–70
Love Canal, 75–79
New York State Cancer Registry,
70, 75
prevention, 80
trends in female cancer, 70–75
detection. *See* Cancer prevention/
detection
and diet, 61, 114
changing habits, 62, 64
education. *See* Education
and elderly. *See* Elderly
etiology, terminology standardization,
(UICC), 16
high-risk population, 251–258
and immune system, 114; *see also*
Acquired immune deficiency
syndrome (AIDS)
incidence, 250, 251, 256; *see also*
under specific sites and types
intervention. *See* Intervention, cancer
knowledge
ascertaining level of, 146, 147
and behavior change, 91, 96
correlation with age, 140
transfer problems, 372
see also Education
management. *See* Management,
cancer
mortality. *See* Mortality
occupational. *See* Occupational
cancer
patterns of care. *See* Pattern of care
studies
phobia, modified by consumer
education, 186–190
public interest, 193
registry. *See* Registry, cancer

screening. *See* Screening
survival
five-year, 254-255
and stage at diagnosis, 343
see also specific sites and types
Cancer control
clergy of black church as
intermediary, 417–423
community-based programs. *See*
under Community
community hospitals. *See* Hospital(s)
Consortium of Ohio (CCCO), 264-
265
mortality report, 266–267
definition, 19, 261
Donabedian model, 426
in the elderly, 123–132; *see also*
Elderly
epidemiology, 264
and etiologic factors, 3–5
history, 29
international resources, 3–17; *see*
also specific agencies
model for estimating effects of
preventive activities, 249–252
application, 252–258
cf. other diseases, 5–6
phases I-V, 19–20, 68
PRECEDE model, 420–421
priorities, 21
see also specific cancers and
organizations
Cancer Information Line, 110, 142–143
Cancer Information Services (CIS)
audience targeting, 157–158
fatalists cf. diligent, 157
categories of information requested,
168, 169
and elderly, 158, 168
Howard University, 171–181; *see*
also Blacks
methodology for cancer control
(Michigan), 161–169
Michigan, 167–169
NCI Task Force, 154–159
potential user population assessment,
145–152
by age, race, sex, and income,
146–148, 150, 153, 164–166

cancer-related knowledge levels, 147
concern about health, 147, 149, 150
perceived adequacy of community resources, 150, 151
visibility, 152
promotion, 153–160
PSAs, 154
social marketing techniques, 154–160
Public Response Program, 161, 161
sites, telephone call analysis, 162, 164–169
social support, 167–169
telephone inquiry service, 145, 146, 153
user characteristics (sex, age, race, income), 146–148, 150, 153
use statistics, 153
who calls for whom, 166–169
Cancer prevention/detection, 80
behaviors, ascertaining, 146, 147
among blacks, 249, 257–259; *see also* Blacks
conditions associated with cancer, 59–61
and drugs, 93; *see also* Alcohol, Drugs
environmental factors, 93
host factors, 93
lifestyle changes, 55–65
dietary habits, 61, 62, 64, 114
role of physician, 63–65
smoking, 62, 64
steps, 55–56
model for estimating effectiveness, 249–252
application, 252–258
model, statistical, for planning, 258–259
occupational hazards, 93
preventive oncology as new field, 57
primary vs. secondary, 67
public behavior, three surveys, 103–112
questionnaires, 104
results, 108–110
sampling, 104–106
site-specific questions, 107–108, 110
women cf. men, 108
school-age risk reduction curriculum, 91–97
sexual and reproductive behavior, 93
stress, 93
sun exposure, 60, 61, 93
see also Breast self-examination, Screening
Cancer: The Behavioral Dimensions, 58
CANSAT, 16
Carcinoembryonic antigen (CEA), 430
β-Carotene, prevention of regrowth of adenocarcinoma C3HBA, 237–245
CCOP, 23, 25, 26
Cells, T, and AIDS, 218, 222
Cerebral metastases, 427
Cervical cancer
continuum from cervical dysplasia, 203
criteria for management among community physicians, 371–373
incidence and mortality in North Carolina, 372
invasive, declining rates, 203
mildly contagious, 203
physician's belief about value of early detection, 366–367
screening, 348
sexual transmission, 203
Cervical intraepthelial dysplaisa
age at first coitus, 204, 206, 213–214
alcohol/drugs, 208, 213
and carcinoma in situ, 203, 213
case-control study, 204–211
cigarette smoking, 204, 205, 208, 213
contraceptives, 204–208, 211, 213
and invasive cervical cancer, 203
marital status, 206–207, 211–212
medical history, 208–212, 214
number of sexual partners, 204, 206–207, 213
race, 205, 206
risk factors, multivariate analysis, 211, 212

Chemotherapy compliance. *See*
Compliance, chemotherapy,
CHOP, 23
Chronic disease control, community-
based programs in Los
Angeles, 271–280
Cigarette smoking. *See* Smoking
Circumcision, 60
Cirrhosis, 59
Clark, R. Lee, 37
Clergy as Intermediary Project
(Washington, D.C.), 417–423
CMF and chemotherapy compliance,
380
Coffee, 60
Colorants, 61
Colorectal cancer
chemotherapy compliance, 393
frequency of inquiries to cancer
information service, 162, 165–
169
high rates in Washington, D.C.,
420–421
incidence, 435, 436
physician's belief about value of
early detection, 366–367
rehabilitation and continuing care
age distribution and patient
profile, 441
economic considerations, 433
referral services, 438–440
requests, 440–441
types of services, 437
voluntary agencies, service
assessment, 433–442
screening, 343–345
stage at diagnosis and survival, 343
Comic books, 135–139, 141–144
Committees, county cancer, 265–266
Communicable diseases, 59, 203
Communications strategies, cancer
and blacks, 171
health professionals in community
outreach, 179–180
mass media, 171, 177–178
social marketing approach, 175–178

goals, 175–176
media objectives, 177
primary audience and target
group, 176–177
sociological factors, 171, 178–179,
181
see also Blacks, Media
Community
-based cancer control programs,
NCI, 271–280
cumulative effects, 275–276
eligibility criteria, 276
empirical limitations, 277–278
financing, 279, 280
future planning, 272–278
lead time for establishment and
effectiveness, 274–275
media use, 272–273
planning and monitoring at
national levels, 278–280
smoking cessation, 273, 275
staffing and skills, 278–279
-based cancer education for elderly,
113–122
hospice approaches, 411–415
hospitals. *See* Hospitals
involvement, role of WHO, 10
Compliance, chemotherapy
and assessment of treatment
effectiveness, 379
blood levels, 380
CMF, 380
for colorectal cancer, 393
complexity of regimen, 381
education, patient, 383–384, 399
hematologic malignancies, 379–380
home structuring and visits, 386–387
ignorance, patient, 391–392, 396–
399
informed consent, 391–399
federal regulations, 391
patient decision-making process,
393
patient understanding of forms,
391–392
physician–patient interview, 396

sociodemographic characteristics, 393–395
intervention design, 379–387
for lung cancer, 393
MOPP, 380
noncompliance
consequences, 379–380
extent, 380–381
factors affecting, 381–382
fear, 382
management, 383–387
and side effects, 381–382
patient program, shaping, 385
support, 386–387
Congenital abnormalities, 59
Contagiousness, cervical cancer, 203
Contraceptives, oral, 190
and cervical intrapethelial dysplasia, 204–208, 211, 213
and smoking, 99
see also Endometrial cancer, Estrogen
Country cancer committees, 265–266
Cytomegalovirus and AIDS, 218, 220–221

Data
bases
merging registry and discharge data, 466, 470, 471
interstate linkage, 474–476
for pattern of care studies in defined populations, 465–476
collection
adolescent cancer, 86–87
cancer management criteria, 374–375
occupational cancer, 48–59
limitations in cancer mortality, 261–262
Demographics
breast self-examination, 296, 297, 333
and chemotherapy compliance, informed consent, 393–395

Depression, 59
Detection. *See* Cancer prevention/detection, Screening
Diagnostic errors, 61
Diet, 60, 61, 62, 64, 114
Diethylstilbestrol (DES), 68–70
Dietz, J. Herbert Jr., 444, 452
Doll, Sir Richard, 53, 56
Donabedian model, 426
Drugs, 61, 93
and AIDS, 219, 224–225
and cervical intrapethelial dysplasia, 208, 213
Dysplasia, cervical intraepithelial. *See* Cervical intraepithelial dysplasia

Education
breast self-examination, 296, 297, 299, 300
knowledge and behavior, 141, 372
knowledge transfer, 141, 372
knowledge transfer, 372
needs and adolescent cancer, 85–89
patient, and chemotherapy compliance, 383–384, 399
professional, community hospitals, on breast cancer, 429–431
public
behavior changes following, 137–140
community-based, for elderly, 113–122
concerning estrogen use and endometrial carcinoma, 186–190
cultural factors and, 116
and mass media coverage of medical events, 193, 200
modification of cancer phobia, 186–190
school-age cancer risk reduction curriculum, 91–97
see also Cancer Information Service (CIS)
Effusion, pleural, 427

Elderly
  attitudes towards physicians, 128,
    130, 131
  breast self-examination, 124–125
  cancer beliefs, 128, 129
  cancer control, 123–132
  cancer education, 113–122, 125
  and Cancer Information Service,
    158, 168
  data from Title XX nutrition centers,
    126
  in screening program, 125
  value of communication, 131
Endometrial carcinoma
  criteria for management among
    community physicians, 371–
    378
  and estrogen use, 183, 185–186
  incidence in women with normal
    menstrual cycles, 185
  modification of cancer phobia and
    public education, 186–190
  see also Cervical cancer, Cervical
    intraepithelial
    dysplasia, Estrogen
Environment and environmental
    pollution, 33, 61, 93
Esophagus cancer, 50
  high rates in Washington, D.C.,
    420–421
Estrogen
  and endometrial carcinoma, 183,
    185–186; see also
    Endometrial carcinoma
  osteoporosis prevention, 183–185
  with progestogens, 183, 186, 190
  receptors in breast cancer, 427, 428,
    430
  "Should I or Shouldn't I" program,
    186–190
  "unopposed," 186
Ethnicity, 60
Eye color, 59

Family
  history, 59
    breast cancer, 354–359
  size, 60

Fat, 61
Fear and chemotherapy compliance, 382
Financing/funding
  cancer intervention programs, 263,
    269
  community-based cancer control
    programs, 279, 280
  screening, 349
Flagyl and AIDS, 219
Foods, processed, 61
Ford, Betty, 299
Fox Chase Cancer Center, 295, 393
  Program for Older Citizens, 125–
    126, 132
Furniture workers and nasal
    adenocarcinoma, 47–48, 53

Geographic
  identification of high risk patients,
    262
  location and cancer, 60
Gliomas, 401
Guidelines for Development of a
    Comprehensive Cancer Center
    (UICC), 15
Gynecologic cancer, 70–75; see also
    specific sites and types

Haemophilia A and AIDS, 220
Hair color, 59
Haitians and Kaposi's sarcoma, 218
Hawaii
  Breast Cancer Demonstration
    Program, 110, 111
  Health Awareness Surveys, 103–112,
    135
  Medical Association, 483, 485–490
  skin cancer/melanoma control
    program, 135–144
  risk factor identification, 136
  statewide cancer management
    guidelines, 483–491
Health Awareness Surveys (Hawaii),
    103–112, 135
Health Belief Model, 301
Health departments. See Cancer center
    and health department linkages
Health Insurance Plan (HIP) of Greater

New York, 283
Health professionals in community
    outreach, 179–180; *see also*
    Physicians, Pharmacists
Health Promotion Center, 268
Helping Smokers Quit program
    (American Pharmaceutical
    Association and NCI), 99–102
Hematologic malignancies and
    chemotherapy compliance, 379–
    380
Hemoccult, 343–345
    family physicians' feelings about,
        361, 363, 365, 366–367
    see also Colorectal cancer, Screening
Hemophilia A and AIDS, 220
Hepatitis and AIDS, 219
Herbicides, 61
Heyman, James, 4
HLA DR5 and BW35 in Kaposi's
    sarcoma, 219
Hodgkin's disease
    care/therapy in Italy, 457–459
    chemotherapy compliance, 380
Homosexuals, male, and AIDS, 217,
    219, 221–223
Hospice, coordinated community
    approach, 411–415
Hospital(s)
    American College of Surgeons
        Annual Hospital Activity
        Reports, 41–42
    Breast Examination Training centers,
        289–290
    community
        cancer control, 425–431
        professional education on breast
            cancer, 429–431
    different cancer management criteria,
        376
    rehabilitation, small vs. large
        hospitals, 445
Host factors and cancer risk, 93
Howard University Cancer
    Communications Network, 171;
    see also Blacks
Hydrocephalus and medulloblastoma,
    407

Hygiene, 60

Iatrogenic effects, 61
ICRETT, 14
ICREW, 14
Immune system, 114
Immunosuppression, 61
Incidence of cancer, 250, 251, 256
Income and Cancer Information Service
    use, 146–148, 150, 153
Industry. *See* Occupational cancer and
    cancer institutes
Informed consent, 391–399
Intercourse, 60
Interferon and AIDS, 225–226
International Academy of Oncology
    (UICC), 17
International Agency for Research in
    Cancer (IARC), 5, 8, 10
International Cancer Patient Data
    Exchange System (ICPDES,
    UICC), 14–15
International Cancer Research Data
    Bank (NCI), 12–14
International Directory of Specialized
    Cancer
        Research and Treatment
            Establishments, 14
International Union Against Cancer
    (UICC)
    Committee on International
        Collaborative Activities
        (CICA), 7–17
    cancer etiology terminology
        standardization, 16
    CANSAT, 16
    Guidelines for Development of a
        Comprehensive Cancer
        Center, 15
    ICRETT, 14
    ICREW, 14
    Organization, 12
    regional associations of world
        cancer centers, 15–16
    10th International Congress (1970),
        11–12
    13th International Congress (1982),
        6–7

Intervention, cancer
  breast cancer, primary vs. secondary,
    313
  chemotherapy compliance, 379–387;
    see also Compliance,
    chemotherapy
  design (CIPD), 263
  financial resources, 269
  local (county) cancer committees,
    265–266
  Ohio's mortality-based system for
    site identification, 261–270
  site choice, 264
Ionizing radiation, 61
Irritation, tissue, 59, 61
Italian National Breast Cancer Task
    Force, 461
Italy, cancer care/therapy
  acute lymphoblastic leukemia, 456–
    457
  impact of education-intervention
    studies, 461–462
  medical records study, 455–456
  organizational philosophy, 459
  quality evaluation, 455–462
  results of clinical trials, 459, 461
  various cancers, 457–460

Jews and Kaposi's sarcoma, 217
Johns Hopkins Oncology Center, 426

Kaposi's sarcoma
  age distribution by race, 218
  in AIDS, 217–218
    epidemiology, 221–223
  in Haitians, 218
  HLA DR5 and BW35, 219
  in Jews, 217
  and lupus, 219
  after transplantation, 219–220
  treatment, 221, 225–226
  usual victim, 217
  in West Africa, 218
  see also Acquired immune deficiency
    syndrome (AIDS)
Keratoses, skin, 59

Kidney stones, 59
King, Martin Luther, 417
Knowledge
  ascertaining, and cancer prevention,
    146, 147
  and Cancer Information Service use,
    147
  change after public education
    program, 137–138
  relationship with behavior, 141, 372
  transfer, cancer, 372; see also
    Education
Kottmeir, H.L., 4

Laetrile (Amygdalin) clinical trials,
    193–200
  background, 194
  newsclip analysis, 195–199
  participating cancer centers, 194
Leukemia
  care/therapy in Italy, 456–457
  chemotherapy, 380
  and Love Canal, 76–78
Lifestyle. See Cancer prevention/
    detection, lifestyle changes
Liver cancer and Love Canal, 76–78
Los Angeles, community-based chronic
    disease control programs, 271–
    280
Love Canal, 75–79
Lung cancer
  care/therapy in Italy, 457–459, 460
  chemotherapy compliance, 393
  frequency of inquiries to cancer
    information service, 162, 165–
    169
  high rates in Washington, D.C.,
    420–421
  respiratory cancer and Love Canal,
    77–79
Lupus and Kaposi's sarcoma, 219
Lymphoma
  and AIDS, 217
  Burkitt's and AIDS, 220–221
  care/therapy in Italy, 457–459
  and Love Canal, 76–78

Lysozymes and AIDS, 219, 223

Mammography, 294, 342, 346–348,
    427, 428
  cf. breast self-examination, 309
  family physicians' feelings about,
    361, 363–368
  see also Screening
Management, cancer
  audits of management, American
    College of Surgeons, 38
  breast cancer
    checklist (HMA), 489
    professional education in
      community hospitals, 429–
      431
  endometrial carcinoma, criteria
    among community physicians,
    371–373
    adherence, 376–377
    data collection, 374–375
    differences, hospital-to-hospital,
      376
    establishment, 373–374
    feedback, 375
  statewide guidelines (Hawaii), 483–
    491
  symptom, 414
Marijuana, 60
Marital status/marriage, 60
  and cervical intrapethelial dysplasia,
    206–207, 211–212
Marketing, Cancer Information Service,
    155–160;
        see also Communications
            strategies, cancer
Media
  and blacks, 173–175, 180
  and breast self-examination, 299, 301
    pamphlets, 324, 327
  and community-based cancer control
    programs (NCI), 272–273
  coverage of
    Laetrile, clinical trials, 195–199
    medical events, 193, 200
  and Helping Smokers Quit program,

101
  and public education program, 135–
    137
  public service announcements
    (PSAs), 135–136, 144, 154
  videotapes, 88–89, 324, 327
  see also Communications strategies,
    cancer
Medical history, and cervical
    intrapethelial dysplasia, 208–212,
    214
Medulloblastoma
  clinical hydrocephalus, 407
  five-year cure rates, 401–408
    historical trends, 403
  cf. other gliomas, 401
  radiotherapy, 401–408
  recurrence, 402
  stage at presentation, 406, 408
Melanoma. *See* Skin cancer/melanoma
Menarche and menopause, 59
Menstrual cycle and endometrial
    carcinoma, 185
Mental illness, 59
Mesothelioma, 54
Metastases, cerebral, 427
Michigan
  Cancer Foundation, in colorectal
    cancer support services, 433–
    442
  Cancer Information Service, 161–169
Minority. *See* Race
Missouri, Women's Cancer Control
    Program, 342–349
Model
  Donabedian, 426
  Health Belief, 301
  PRECEDE, cancer control, 420–421
  silicone breast, 306–307, 323–328
  statistical, of preventive activities,
    249–252, 258–259
    application, 252–258
Monoclonal antibodies, 32
Mononucleosis and AIDS, 220–221
MOPP and chemotherapy compliance,
    380

Mortality, cancer
-based system for site identification
in intervention, 261–270
black-white differences, 249, 252–258
breast cancer, 313, 331
data limitations, 261–262
effects of incidence and survival on,
250–251
high rates in Washington, D.C., 419–420
in North Carolina, 373
and screening, 361
site-specific, 252
Mouth cleanliness, 60
Narcotics, 60
Nasal adenocarcinoma in furniture
workers, 47–48, 53
National Cancer Institute
and adolescent cancer, 85
Cancer Control Applications
Program, 22–23, 25
cancer control research programs,
19–27
and Cancer Information Services,
154–159; see also Cancer
Information Services
CCOP, 23, 25, 26
CHOP, 23
community-based cancer control
programs. See under
Community
Cooperative Group Outreach
Program, 25
Division of Cancer Prevention and
Control, 21–23
FY 83 budget, 24, 25
establishment, 6
Helping Smokers Quit Program (with
American
Pharmaceutical Association),
99–102
International Cancer Research Data
Bank, 12–14
national distribution of clinical NCI-
funded research activities, 26
prevention, 23, 25
SEER, 38, 252, 434

cancer statistics, 1973–1977, 163
Detroit, 162
and WHO, 9–11
National Cancer Program, 1
National Institute for Aging, 158
Neurologic symptoms, 59
New York State
cancer center and health department
linkages. See under Cancer
Cancer Registry, 70, 75
Health Insurance Plan (HIP), 283
Newspapers. See Media
Nitrites and AIDS, 219, 224–225
North Carolina, cancer mortality, 373

Obesity, 59
Occupational cancer, 61, 93
asbestos, 51–54
data collection and interpretation,
48–49
esophagus cancer, 50
follow-up of effects, 53–54
industry role, 51–52
nonoccupational influences, 51
primary prevention, 47–54
risk
elimination, 51–53
identification, 47–51
secondary prevention and treatment,
54
Swedish National Cancer Registry,
48
vinyl chloride, 51, 52
Occupational therapy, 445–453; see also
Rehabilitation
Ohio, mortality-based system for cancer
intervention
site identification, 261–270
Oncology, preventive, 57
Oncology Rehabilitation Conference
(Detroit, 1982), 443–453
Oral contraceptives. See Contraceptives,
oral
Organization of European Cancer
Institutes, 8–9
Osteoporosis, estrogen for, 183–185; see
also Estrogen
Ovarian cancer, care/therapy in Italy,
457–459

Pamphlets. *See* Media
Pan American Health Organization, 5
Papanicolaou, George Nicholas, 4
Pap test, 30–31, 71–72, 348
    family physicians' feelings about,
      361, 363, 366–367
    see also Screening
Patient(s)
    Care Coordinator, 412
    education. *See* Education
    high-risk, identification, 262
    Surveillance System, M.D.
      Anderson Hospital, 477–481
Pattern of care studies, 425–426
    breast cancer, 427–428, 466–470
    data bases for defined populations,
      465–476; *see also* Data bases
Pepper, Claude, 113
Personality, 59
Pesticides, 61
Pets, 60
Pharmacist, role in smoking prevention
    and cessation, 99–102;
Physical therapy, 445–453; *see also*
    Rehabilitation
Physician(s)
    breast cancer treatment delay. *See*
      under Breast cancer
    community, feedback about cancer
      management criteria, 375
    family, feelings about cancer
      screening tests, 361–368;
      see also specific tests
    role in lifestyle changes and cancer
      prevention, 63–65
    see also Health Professionals,
      Pharmacists
Pill. *See* Contraceptives, oral
Pleural effusion, 427
Pneumocystis carinii penumonia and
    AIDS, 217, 218
Polyvinyl chloride, 61
Populations
    defined, pattern of care studies, 465–
      476
    high cancer risk, 251–258
    see also Blacks, Demographics,
      Elderly

PRECEDE model, cancer control, 420–
    421
Preservatives, food, 61
Press. *See* Media
Preventive oncology, 57; *see also*
    Cancer prevention/detection
Print media. *See* Media
Processed foods, 61
Proctosigmoidoscopy, family
    physicians' feelings about, 361,
    363, 365, 366–367
Professional education. *See* Education
Progesterone, 186
Progestogens and estrogen, 183, 186,
    190; *see also* Estrogens
Project CHOICE, 91–97
Prostate cancer, physician's belief about
    value of early detection, 365,
    366–367
Prosthetics, irritation by, 61
Protein, dietary, 61
Public service snnouncements (PSAs),
    135–136, 144, 154

Questionnaires, public behavior, 104

Race, 60
    and Breast Examination Training
      centers, 288
    and Cancer Information Service use,
      146–148, 150, 153
    and cervical intrapethelial dysplasia,
      205, 206
    and Kaposi's sarcoma, 218
    minority women breast self-
      examination, 276–277
    and physician delay in breast cancer,
      351
    see also Blacks
Radiation
    ionizing, 61
    therapy
      adenocarcinoma C3HBA, 238–
        245
      medulloblastoma, 401–408
Radio. *See* Communications strategies,
    cancer; Media

Radiosensitive suppressor cells and
AIDS, 218
Receptors, estrogen, 427, 428, 430
Rectal examination, digital, family
physicians'feelings about, 361,
363, 364, 366-367
Registry, cancer
breast cancer, 295
interstate linkage, 474-476
merging data with discharge data,
466, 470, 471
New York State, 70, 75
Swedish National, 48
Regulations, chemotherapy compliance,
informed consent, 391
Rehabilitation (and support services)
awareness and utilization, 411-415
colorectal cancer. *See under*
Colorectal cancer
goals, 443, 450
occupational therapy, 445-453
Oncology Rehabilitation Conference
(Detroit, 1982), 443-453
physical therapy, 445-453
program and workshops, 446-447
small cf. large hospitals, 445
symptom management 414
work settings, 451
Reproductive behavior. *See* Sexual
behavior
Respiratory cancer and Love Canal, 77-
79; *see also* Lung cancer
Risk(s) (cancer)
and age, 123-124
black/white, relative, 252
breast cancer
factors, index, 356, 358, 359
physician delay, 351-360
high-risk cancer populations, 251-
258
identification by geographic site,
262
and host factors, 93
identification in skin cancer, 136

multivariate analysis, 211, 212
occupational cancer
elimination, 51-53
identification, 47-51
school-age risk reduction curriculum,
91-97
skin cancer, 136
Rockefeller, Happy, 299

Sarcoma, Kaposi's *See* Kaposi's
sarcoma
Satellite communications, 16
Scars, 59
Schizophrenia, 59
School health curriculum for cancer
prevention, 91-97
classroom observation, 96
data analysis, 95
effectiveness evaluation, 91-92
goal identification, 92-93
test design, experimental vs. control,
94
test instruments, 94-95
see also Education
Screening
breast cancer, 345-348
detection demonstration projects
(BCDDP), 341-342
cervical cancer, 348
colorectal cancer, 343-345
effectiveness, opinions of family
physicians, 365-367
for the elderly, 125
family physicians' feelings about
various tests, 361-368
funding, 349
Hemoccult II, 343-345
mammography. *See* Mammography
and mortality, 361
Pap test. *See* Pap test
recommended frequency, 363-365
uterine cervix cancer, 348
Women's Cancer Control Program
(Missouri), 342-349

see also Breast self-examination, specific procedures
SEER. *See under* National Cancer Institute
Semen and AIDS, 220, 224
Sex, 59
and calls to cancer information service, 164–166
and cancer Information Service, 153
and chemotherapy compliance, 396
Sexual behavior
and cancer prevention, 93
and cervical intrapethelial dysplasia, 204, 206–207, 213–214
intercourse, 60
see also Acquired immune deficiency syndrome (AIDS)
Silicone breast models, 306–307, 323–328; *see also* Breast self-examination
Site-specific cancer mortality, 252
Skin Cancer Foundation, 143
Skin cancer/melanoma
community-based cancer control program in Hawaii, 135–144
risk factor identification, 136
Smoking, 60, 62, 64, 422
and American Cancer Society, 34
adolescence, 273, 275
and cervical intrapethelial dysplasia, 204, 205, 208, 213
cessation
and community-based cancer control programs, 273, 275
Helping Smokers Quit program, 99–102
pharmacist's role, 99–102
and oral contraceptives, 99
Snuff, 60
Social marketing and Cancer Information Service, 154–160; *see also under* Communications strategies, cancer

Sociodemographics. *See* Demographics
Socioeconomic level, 59
Sqaumous cell cancer and AIDS, 217
Statistical model. *See* Hemoccult
Stress, 59, 93
Sun exposure, 60, 61, 93
Supportive service. *See* Rehabilitation (and support services)
Suppressor cells, radiosensitive, and AIDS, 218
Surveys, public behavior. *See under* Cancer prevention and detection
Survival
five-year cancer, 254–255
influence of radiotherapy in medulloblastoma, 402–408
and stage at diagnosis, 343
Swedish National Cancer Registry, 48
Syndrome, acquired immune deficiency. *See* Acquired immune deficiency syndrome (AIDS)
Syphilis and AIDS, 219

T cells and AIDS, 222
Telephone
cycle, M.D. Anderson Hospital Patient Surveillance System, 480, 481
frequency of calls to CIS by site, 162, 164–169
survey, breast-self examination, 333
see also Cancer Information Services (CIS)
Television. *See* Communications strategies, cancer; Media
Terminology, cancer etiology, UICC standardization, 16
Test(s)
design and instruments, school health curriculum
for cancer prevention, 94–95
in suspected breast cancer, 427–431
see also Screening, specific procedures

Therapy, cancer, in Italy. *See* Italy, cancer care/therapy
Thymosin and AIDS, 218, 223
Tobacco. *See* Smoking
Transmission, sexual, of cervical cancer, 203
Transplantation and Kaposi's sarcoma, 219–220
Traumata, 59
Trichlorethylene, 75
Trichomonas infection, 60

UICC. *See* International Union Against Cancer
University of Texas M.D. Anderson Hospital Patient Surveillance System, 477–481
responses, 480
telephone cycle, 480, 481
three-letter cycle, 479, 481
Uranium, 61
Uterine cervix cancer. *See* Cervical cancer

Videotapes
adolescent cancer, 88–89
breast self-examination, 324, 327

see also Media
Vinyl chloride, 51, 52
Vitamin
A in prevention of regrowth of adenocarcinoma C3HBA, 237–245
deficiencies, 61
Voluntary agencies, colorectal cancer rehabilitation.
See under Colorectal cancer

Washington, D.C.
Clergy as Intermediary Project, 417–423
high cancer rates, 420–421
Water pollution, 61
West Africa, Kaposi's sarcoma in, 218
Whites, relative risks of cancer vs. blacks, 252; *see also* Race
Women's Cancer Control Program (Missouri), 342–349
World Health Organization, 5, 8
and NCI, 9–11
promoting community involvement, 10

X rays. *See* Radiation

PROGRESS IN CLINICAL AND BIOLOGICAL RESEARCH

Series Editors

Nathan Back
George J. Brewer
Vincent P. Eijsvoogel
Robert Grover

Kurt Hirschhorn
Seymour S. Kety
Sidney Udenfriend
Jonathan W. Uhr

Vol 1: **Erythrocyte Structure and Function,** George J. Brewer, *Editor*

Vol 2: **Preventability of Perinatal Injury,** Karlis Adamsons, Howard A. Fox, *Editors*

Vol 3: **Infections of the Fetus and the Newborn Infant,** Saul Krugman, Anne A. Gershon, *Editors*

Vol 4: **Conflicts in Childhood Cancer: An Evaluation of Current Management,** Lucius F. Sinks, John O. Godden, *Editors*

Vol 5: **Trace Components of Plasma: Isolation and Clinical Significance,** G.A. Jamieson, T.J. Greenwalt, *Editors*

Vol 6: **Prostatic Disease,** H. Marberger, H. Haschek, H.K.A. Schirmer, J.A.C. Colston, E. Witkin, *Editors*

Vol 7: **Blood Pressure, Edema and Proteinuria in Pregnancy,** Emanuel A. Friedman, *Editor*

Vol 8: **Cell Surface Receptors,** Garth L. Nicolson, Michael A. Raftery, Martin Rodbell, C. Fred Fox, *Editors*

Vol 9: **Membranes and Neoplasia: New Approaches and Strategies,** Vincent T. Marchesi, *Editor*

Vol 10: **Diabetes and Other Endocrine Disorders During Pregnancy and in the Newborn,** Maria I. New, Robert H. Fiser, *Editors*

Vol 11: **Clinical Uses of Frozen-Thawed Red Blood Cells,** John A. Griep, *Editor*

Vol 12: **Breast Cancer,** Albert C.W. Montague, Geary L. Stonesifer, Jr., Edward F. Lewison, *Editors*

Vol 13: **The Granulocyte: Function and Clinical Utilization,** Tibor J. Greenwalt, G.A. Jamieson, *Editors*

Vol 14: **Zinc Metabolism: Current Aspects in Health and Disease,** George J. Brewer, Ananda S. Prasad, *Editors*

Vol 15: **Cellular Neurobiology,** Zach Hall, Regis Kelly, C. Fred Fox, *Editors*

Vol 16: **HLA and Malignancy,** Gerald P. Murphy, *Editor*

Vol 17: **Cell Shape and Surface Architecture,** Jean Paul Revel, Ulf Henning, C. Fred Fox, *Editors*

Vol 18: **Tay-Sachs Disease: Screening and Prevention,** Michael M. Kaback, *Editor*

Vol 19: **Blood Substitutes and Plasma Expanders,** G.A. Jamieson, T.J. Greenwalt, *Editors*

Vol 20: **Erythrocyte Membranes: Recent Clinical and Experimental Advances,** Walter C. Kruckeberg, John W. Eaton, George J. Brewer, *Editors*

Vol 21: **The Red Cell,** George J. Brewer, *Editor*

Vol 22: **Molecular Aspects of Membrane Transport,** Dale Oxender, C. Fred Fox, *Editors*

Vol 23: **Cell Surface Carbohydrates and Biological Recognition,** Vincent T. Marchesi, Victor Ginsburg, Phillips W. Robbins, C. Fred Fox, *Editors*

Vol 24: **Twin Research, Proceedings of the Second International Congress on Twin Studies,** Walter E. Nance, *Editor* Published in 3 volumes: Part A: **Psychology and Methodology** Part B: **Biology and Epidemiology** Part C: **Clinical Studies**

Vol 25: **Recent Advances in Clinical Oncology,** Tapan A. Hazra, Michael C. Beachley, *Editors*

Vol 26: **Origin and Natural History of Cell Lines,** Claudio Barigozzi, *Editor*

Vol 27: **Membrane Mechanisms of Drugs of Abuse,** Charles W. Sharp, Leo G. Abood, *Editors*

Vol 28: **The Blood Platelet in Transfusion Therapy,** G.A. Jamieson, Tibor J. Greenwalt, *Editors*

Vol 29: **Biomedical Applications of the Horseshoe Crab (Limulidae),** Elias Cohen, *Editor-in-Chief*

Vol 30: **Normal and Abnormal Red Cell Membranes,** Samuel E. Lux, Vincent T. Marchesi, C. Fred Fox, *Editors*

Vol 31: **Transmembrane Signaling,** Mark Bitensky, R. John Collier, Donald F. Steiner, C. Fred Fox, *Editors*

Vol 32: **Genetic Analysis of Common Diseases: Applications to Predictive Factors in Coronary Disease,** Charles F. Sing, Mark Skolnick, *Editors*

Vol 33: **Prostate Cancer and Hormone Receptors,** Gerald P. Murphy, Avery A. Sandberg, *Editors*

Vol 34: **The Management of Genetic Disorders,** Constantine J. Papadatos, Christos S. Bartsocas, *Editors*

Vol 35: **Antibiotics and Hospitals,** Carlo Grassi, Giuseppe Ostino, *Editors*

Vol 36: **Drug and Chemical Risks to the Fetus, Newborn,** Richard H. Schwarz, Sumner J. Yaffe, *Editors*

Vol 37: **Models for Prostate Cancer,** Gerald P. Murphy, *Editor*

Vol 38: **Ethics, Humanism, and Medicine,** Marc D. Basson, *Editor*

Vol 39: **Neurochemistry and Clinical Neurology,** Leontino Battistin, George Hashim, Abel Lajtha, *Editors*

Vol 40: **Biological Recognition and Assembly,** David S. Eisenberg, James A. Lake, C. Fred Fox, *Editors*

Vol 41: **Tumor Cell Surfaces and Malignancy,** Richard O. Hynes, C. Fred Fox, *Editors*

Vol 42: **Membranes, Receptors, and the Immune Response: 80 Years After Ehrlich's Side Chain Theory,** Edward P. Cohen, Heinz Köhler, *Editors*

Vol 43: **Immunobiology of the Erythrocyte,** S. Gerald Sandler, Jacob Nusbacher, Moses S. Schanfield, *Editors*

Vol 44: **Perinatal Medicine Today,** Bruce K. Young, *Editor*

Vol 45: **Mammalian Genetics and Cancer: The Jackson Laboratory Fiftieth Anniversary Symposium,** Elizabeth S. Russell, *Editor*

Vol 46: **Etiology of Cleft Lip and Cleft Palate,** Michael Melnick, David Bixler, Edward D. Shields, *Editors*

Vol 47: **New Developments With Human and Veterinary Vaccines,** A. Mizrahi, I. Hertman, M.A. Klingberg, A. Kohn, *Editors*

Vol 48: **Cloning of Human Tumor Stem Cells,** Sidney E. Salmon, *Editor*

Vol 49: **Myelin: Chemistry and Biology,** George A. Hashim, *Editor*

Vol 50: **Rights and Responsibilities in Modern Medicine: The Second Volume in a Series on Ethics, Humanism, and Medicine,** Marc D. Basson, *Editor*

Vol 51: **The Function of Red Blood Cells: Erythrocyte Pathobiology,** Donald F. H. Wallach, *Editor*

Vol 52: **Conduction Velocity Distributions: A Population Approach to Electrophysiology of Nerve,** Leslie J. Dorfman, Kenneth L. Cummins, Lary J. Leifer, *Editors*

Vol 53: **Cancer Among Black Populations,** Curtis Mettlin, Gerald P. Murphy, *Editors*

Vol 54: **Connective Tissue Research: Chemistry, Biology, and Physiology,** Zdenek Deyl, Milan Adam, *Editors*

Vol 55: **The Red Cell: Fifth Ann Arbor Conference,** George J. Brewer, *Editor*

Vol 56: **Erythrocyte Membranes 2: Recent Clinical and Experimental Advances,** Walter C. Kruckeberg, John W. Eaton, George J. Brewer, *Editors*

Vol 57: **Progress in Cancer Control,** Curtis Mettlin, Gerald P. Murphy, *Editors*

Vol 58: **The Lymphocyte,** Kenneth W. Sell, William V. Miller, *Editors*

Vol 59: **Eleventh International Congress of Anatomy,** Enrique Acosta Vidrio, *Editor-in-Chief.* Published in 3 volumes: Part A: **Glial and Neuronal Cell Biology,** Sergey Fedoroff. *Editor* Part B: **Advances in the Morphology of Cells and Tissues,** Miguel A. Galina, *Editor* Part C: **Biological Rhythms in Structure and Function,** Heinz von Mayersbach, Lawrence E. Scheving, John E. Pauly, *Editors*

Vol 60: **Advances in Hemoglobin Analysis,** Samir M. Hanash, George J. Brewer, *Editors*

Vol 61: **Nutrition and Child Health: Perspectives for the 1980s,** Reginald C. Tsang, Buford Lee Nichols, Jr., *Editors*

Vol 62: **Pathophysiological Effects of Endotoxins at the Cellular Level,** Jeannine A. Majde, Robert J. Person, *Editors*

Vol 63: **Membrane Transport and Neuroreceptors,** Dale Oxender, Arthur Blume, Ivan Diamond, C. Fred Fox, *Editors*

Vol 64: **Bacteriophage Assembly,** Michael S. DuBow, *Editor*

Vol 65: **Apheresis: Development, Applications, and Collection Procedures,** C. Harold Mielke, Jr., *Editor*

Vol 66: **Control of Cellular Division and Development,** Dennis Cunningham, Eugene Goldwasser, James Watson, C. Fred Fox, *Editors.* Published in 2 volumes.

Vol 67: **Nutrition in the 1980s: Contraints on Our Knowledge,** Nancy Selvey, Philip L. White, *Editors*

Vol 68: **The Role of Peptides and Amino Acids as Neurotransmitters,** J. Barry Lombardini, Alexander D. Kenny, *Editors*

Vol 69: **Twin Research 3, Proceedings of the Third International Congress on Twin Studies,** Ligi Gedda, Paolo Parisi, Walter E. Nance, *Editors.* Published in 3 volumes: Part A: **Twin Biology and Multiple Pregnancy** Part B: **Intelligence, Personality, and Development** Part C: **Epidemiological and Clinical Studies**

Vol 70: **Reproductive Immunology,** Norbert Gleicher, *Editor*

Vol 71: **Psychopharmacology of Clonidine,** Harbans Lal, Stuart Fielding, *Editors*

Vol 72: **Hemophilia and Hemostasis,** Doris Ménaché, D. MacN. Surgenor, Harlan D. Anderson, *Editors*

Vol 73: **Membrane Biophysics: Structure and Function in Epithelia,** Mumtaz A. Dinno, Arthur B. Callahan, *Editors*

Vol 74: **Physiopathology of Endocrine Diseases and Mechanisms of Hormone Action,** Roberto J. Soto, Alejandro De Nicola, Jorge Blaquier, *Editors*

Vol 75: **The Prostatic Cell: Structure and Function,** Gerald P. Murphy, Avery A. Sandberg, James P. Karr, *Editors.* Published in 2 volumes: Part A: **Morphologic, Secretory, and Biochemical Aspects** Part B: **Prolactin, Carcinogenesis, and Clinical Aspects**

Vol 76: **Troubling Problems in Medical Ethics: The Third Volume in a Series on Ethics, Humanism, and Medicine,** Marc D. Basson, Rachel E. Lipson, Doreen L. Ganos, *Editors*

Vol 77: **Nutrition in Health and Disease and International Development: Symposia From the XII International Congress of Nutrition,** Alfred E. Harper, George K. Davis *Editors*

Vol 78: **Female Incontinence,** Norman R. Zinner, Arthur M. Sterling, *Editors*

Vol 79: **Proteins in the Nervous System: Structure and Function,** Bernard Haber, Jose Regino Perez-Polo, Joe Dan Coulter, *Editors*

Vol 80: **Mechanism and Control of Ciliary Movement,** Charles J. Brokaw, Pedro Verdugo, *Editors*

Vol 81: **Physiology and Biology of Horseshoe Crabs: Studies on Normal and Environmentally Stressed Animals,** Joseph Bonaventura, Celia Bonaventura, Shirley Tesh, *Editors*

Vol 82: **Clinical, Structural, and Biochemical Advances in Hereditary Eye Disorders,** Donna L. Daentl, *Editor*

Vol 83: **Issues in Cancer Screening and Communications,** Curtis Mettlin, Gerald P. Murphy, *Editors*

Vol 84: **Progress in Dermatoglyphic Research,** Christos S. Bartsocas, *Editor*

Vol 85: **Embryonic Development,** Max M. Burger, Rudolf Weber, *Editors.* Published in 2 volumes: Part A: **Genetic Aspects** Part B: **Cellular Aspects**

Vol 86: **The Interaction of Acoustical and Electromagnetic Fields With Biological Systems,** Shiro Takashima, Elliot Postow, *Editors*

Vol 87: **Physiopathology of Hypophysial Disturbances and Diseases of Reproduction,** Alejandro De Nicola, Jorge Blaquier, Roberto J. Soto, *Editors*

Vol 88: **Cytapheresis and Plasma Exchange: Clinical Indications,** W.R. Vogler, *Editor*

Vol 89: **Interaction of Platelets and Tumor Cells,** G.A. Jamieson, *Editor*

Vol 90: **Beta-Carbolines and Tetrahydroisoquinolines,** Floyd Bloom, Jack Barchas, Merton Sandler, Earl Usdin, *Organizers*

Vol 91: **Membranes in Growth and Development,** Joseph F. Hoffman, Gerhard H. Giebisch, Liana Bolis, *Editors*

Vol 92: **The Pineal and Its Hormones,** Russel J. Reiter, *Editor*

Vol 93: **Endotoxins and Their Detection With the Limulus Amebocyte Lysate Test,** Stanley W. Watson, Jack Levin, Thomas J. Novitsky, *Editors*

Vol 94: **Animal Models of Inherited Metabolic Diseases,** Robert J. Desnick, Donald F. Patterson, Dante G. Scarpelli, *Editors*

Vol 95: **Gaucher Disease: A Century of Delineation and Research,** Robert J. Desnick, Shimon Gatt, Gregory A. Grabowski, *Editors*

Vol 96: **Mechanisms of Speciation,** Claudio Barigozzi, *Editor*

Vol 97: **Membranes and Genetic Disease,** John R. Sheppard, V. Elving Anderson, John W. Eaton, *Editors*

Vol 98: **Advances in the Pathophysiology, Diagnosis, and Treatment of Sickle Cell Disease,** Roland B. Scott, *Editor*

Vol 99: **Osteosarcoma: New Trends in Diagnosis and Treatment,** Alexander Katznelson, Jacobo Nerubay, *Editors*

Vol 100: **Renal Tumors: Proceedings of the First International Symposium on Kidney Tumors,** René Küss, Gerald P. Murphy, Saad Khoury, James P. Karr, *Editors*

Vol 101: **Factors and Mechanisms Influencing Bone Growth,** Andrew D. Dixon, Bernard G. Sarnat, *Editors*

Vol 102: **Cell Function and Differentiation,** G. Akoyunoglou, A.E. Evangelopoulos, J. Georgatsos, G. Palaiologos, A. Trakatellis, C.P. Tsiganos, *Editors.* Published in 3 volumes. Part A: **Erythroid Differentiation, Hormone-Gene Interaction, Glycoconjugates, Liposomes, Cell Growth, and Cell-Cell Interaction.** Part B: **Biogenesis of Energy Transducing Membranes and Membrane and Protein Energetics.** Part C: **Enzyme Structure—Mechanism, Metabolic Regulations, and Phosphorylation-Dephosphorylation Processes**

Vol 103: **Human Genetics,** Batsheva Bonné-Tamir, *Editor,* Tirza Cohen, Richard M. Goodman, *Associate Editors.* Published in 2 volumes. Part A: **The Unfolding Genome.** Part B: **Medical Aspects**

Vol 104: **Skeletal Dysplasias,** C.J. Papadatos, C.S. Bartsocas, *Editors*

Vol 105: **Polyomaviruses and Human Neurological Diseases,** John L. Sever, David L. Madden, *Editors*

Vol 106: **Therapeutic Apheresis and Plasma Perfusion,** Richard S.A. Tindall, *Editor*

Vol 107: **Biomedical Thermology,** Michel Gautherie, Ernest Albert, *Editors*

Vol 108: **Massive Transfusion in Surgery and Trauma,** John A. Collins, Kris Murawski, A. William Shafer, *Editors*

Vol 109: **Mutagens in Our Environment,** Marja Sorsa, Harri Vainio, *Editors*

Vol 110: **Limb Development and Regeneration.** Published in 2 volumes. **Part A,** John F. Fallon, Arnold I. Caplan, *Editors.* **Part B,** Robert O. Kelley, Paul F. Goetinck, Jeffrey A. MacCabe, *Editors*

Vol 111: **Molecular and Cellular Aspects of Shock and Trauma,** Allan M. Lefer, William Schumer, *Editors*

Vol 112: **Recent Advances in Fertility Research,** Thomas G. Muldoon, Virendra B. Mahesh, Bautista Pérez-Ballester, *Editors.* Published in two volumes. Part A: **Developments in Reproductive Endocrinology.** Part B: **Developments in the Management of Reproductive Disorders**

Vol 113: **The S-Potential,** Boris D. Drujan, Miguel Laufer, *Editors*

Vol 114: **Enzymology of Carbonyl Metabolism: Aldehyde Dehydrogenase and Aldo/Keto Reductase,** Henry Weiner, Bendicht Wermuth, *Editors*